500 best Healthy recipes

Lynn Roblin, MSc, RD

NUTRITION EDITOR

Robert
ROSE

500 Best Healthy Recipes
Text and photographs copyright © 2004 Robert Rose Inc.

For complete cataloguing information, see page 402.

Disclaimer
The recipes in this book have been carefully tested by our kitchen and our tasters. To the best of our knowledge, they are safe and nutritious for ordinary use and users. For those people with food or other allergies, or who have special food requirements or health issues, please read the suggested contents of each recipe carefully and determine whether or not they may create a problem for you. All recipes are used at the risk of the consumer.

We cannot be responsible for any hazards, loss or damage that may occur as a result of any recipe use.

For those with special needs, allergies, requirements or health problems, in the event of any doubt, please contact your medical advisor prior to the use of any recipe.

Cover image: Chicken Kebabs with Ginger Lemon Marinade (see recipe, page 290)

We acknowledge the financial support of the Government of Canada through the Book Publishing Industry Development Program (BPIDP) for our publishing activities.

Published by Robert Rose Inc.
120 Eglinton Avenue East, Suite 800, Toronto, Ontario, Canada M4P 1E2
Tel: (416) 322-6552; Fax: (416) 322-6936

Printed in Canada

3 4 5 6 7 8 9 FP 12 11 10 09 08

contents

about this book

Most people realize that what they eat makes a difference to being healthy and looking and feeling well. But there is so much conflicting information about nutrition in the media that is it difficult to make informed choices. What is the best diet to follow? Are some foods better than others? Can certain foods help fight against disease? This book not only provides you with more than 500 delicious and healthy recipes, but also helps to answer these and other "top of mind" questions about nutrition, and offers tips and strategies to set you on the road to healthy eating.

While a good diet is a vital component of health, a physically active lifestyle is equally important, as it helps to protect against many health conditions. Eating well and keeping active helps you to feel your best at any age.

eating for health

vary your food choices

Your body needs more than 50 different nutrients to function properly, and no one food offers everything you need. Food provides essential nutrients and other health-promoting components. Eating a variety of wholesome foods, in appropriate quantities, and having fewer less-nutritious foods is the best way to ensure you are eating well. In addition, many foods, especially vegetables and fruits, provide other substances, such as antioxidants, that are important to health.

pay attention to food groups

Foods are categorized into certain groups mostly because they provide similar nutrients. Choosing foods from each group on a daily basis helps you get the nutrient mix you need. Avoiding an entire food group or limiting your food choices, either because you eat the same foods all the time or because you're following a strict diet, limits the variety of nutrients you consume. To get the nutrients your body needs in the right amounts, refer to the chart on page 5, which is based on Canada's Food Guide to Healthy Eating and the United States Food Guide Pyramid.

tips for adding variety to your diet

◆ Choose a food from each group for every meal.

◆ Add one new or different food to your diet every week.

◆ Try exotic or unusual fruits or vegetables such as guava, mangoes, parsnips, fennel, bok choy, kale or kohlrabi.

◆ Experiment with recipes that use less common ingredients such as eggplant, spaghetti squash, sweet potatoes, white beans, water chestnuts, mandarin oranges, sesame seeds, pecans or almonds.

◆ Enjoy foods from different cultures more often.

Guide to food choices and amounts

Food group	Key nutrients	How much do you need each day?	What counts as a serving?
Grain products (bread, cereal, rice and pasta)	Carbohydrates, fiber, protein, thiamin, riboflavin, niacin, folacin, iron, zinc, magnesium	5 to 12 servings	◆ 1 slice of bread ◆ $\frac{1}{2}$ bagel, pita or bun ◆ $\frac{1}{2}$ cup to $1\frac{1}{4}$ cup (30 g) of ready-to-eat cereal ◆ $\frac{3}{4}$ cup (175 mL) hot cereal ◆ $\frac{1}{2}$ cup (125 mL) cooked pasta or rice
Vegetables and fruit	Carbohydrates, fiber, thiamin, folacin, vitamin A, vitamin C, iron, magnesium	5 to 10 servings	◆ 1 medium size vegetable or fruit ◆ $\frac{1}{2}$ cup (125 mL) fresh, frozen or canned vegetables or fruit ◆ 1 cup (250 mL) raw leafy vegetables or salad ◆ $\frac{1}{2}$ cup (125 mL) juice
Milk products and alternatives (milk, yogurt, cheese, fortified soy beverages and calcium alternatives)	Protein, fat, riboflavin, vitamin B_{12}, vitamin A, vitamin D, calcium, zinc, magnesium	2 to 4 servings milk products OR 6 to 8 servings fortified soy beverages and calcium alternatives	◆ 1 cup (250 mL) milk ◆ 2 oz (50 g) cheese ◆ $\frac{3}{4}$ cup (175 g) yogurt ◆ $\frac{1}{2}$ cup (125 mL) calcium-fortified soy beverage or orange juice ◆ $\frac{1}{4}$ cup (50 mL) firm calcium-set tofu ◆ $\frac{1}{4}$ cup (50 mL) almonds ◆ 3 tbsp (45 mL) almond butter ◆ 1 cup (250 mL) cooked or 2 cups (500 mL) raw greens — kale, collards, broccoli or okra ◆ 1 cup (250 mL) beans (soy, white, navy, Great Northern, black turtle beans)
Meat and alternatives (meat, poultry, fish, dry beans, eggs, and nuts)	Protein, fat, thiamin, riboflavin, niacin, folacin, vitamin B_{12}, iron, zinc, magnesium	2 to 3 servings	◆ 2 to 3 oz (50 to 100 g) cooked meat, fish or poultry ◆ $\frac{1}{2}$ cup (125 mL) beans or tofu ◆ 2 tbsp (30 mL) peanut butter ◆ 2 to 3 tbsp (30 to 45 mL) nuts

Appropriate for children and adults over 4 years of age. Based on:
- ◆ Canada's Food Guide to Healthy Eating (www.hc-sc.gc.ca/hpfb-dgpsa/onpp-bppn/food_guide_rainbow_e.html);
- ◆ US Food Guide Pyramid (www.nal.usda.gov/fnic/Fpyr/pyramid.html); and
- ◆ *Becoming Vegan: The Complete Guide to Adopting a Healthy Plant-Based Diet*, Brenda Davis and Vesanto Melina (Summertown, TN: Book Publishing Company, 2000).

understanding nutrients

There are two major groups of nutrients: macronutrients, including carbohydrates, fat and protein; and micronutrients, which include the full range of vitamins and minerals. The macronutrients provide energy, or calories, which your body uses to function and for physical activity. Micronutrients are involved in helping your body use energy and in various structural and regulatory functions. Presently there is much confusion about what constitutes a healthy diet and the proper amount or ratio of the macronutrients. The amount of carbohydrates, fat and protein necessary for an optimal diet has become an intense point of discussion, and there are varying opinions as to what is deemed correct. The following sections help set some direction for planning the best diet.

carbohydrates

Carbohydrate foods, specifically whole grains, vegetables and fruit, are an important part of a healthy diet. These foods provide essential vitamins, minerals and fiber, as well as energy. Whole grains, vegetables and fruit also provide antioxidant nutrients and other phytochemicals, which are associated with health benefits such as reduced risk of heart disease and cancer. More highly processed carbohydrate choices, including many baked goods and snack foods, and high-protein or high-fat foods do not offer the same benefits.

A healthy diet should provide 45% to 65% of calories from carbohydrates. At least 130 g of carbohydrate is recommended each day to provide adequate energy (glucose) for the brain and body to function. Many low-carbohydrate diets limit carbohydrate intake to much less than this. If, over the course of a day, you have one cup (250 mL) of spaghetti (42 g), 1 cup (250 mL) of orange juice (28 g), 1 apple (21 g), ¾ cup (175 mL) low-fat fruit yogurt (19 g), 1 cup (250 mL) of 1% or 2% milk (12 g), and 10 baby carrots (8 g), you will have eaten 130 g of carbohydrate.

Carbohydrates are found in most foods as sugars, starches and fiber. Complex carbohydrate foods include bread, pasta, vegetables, fruit and beans. Eating more complex carbohydrate foods, especially whole grains rather than refined products, is recommended for a healthy diet. Simple carbohydrate foods such as table sugar, candy, and honey contribute calories, but little in the way of important nutrients. These foods can be included in small amounts in a healthy diet.

It was previously thought that only sugary foods caused blood sugar levels to spike, but research now shows that some higher-nutrient carbohydrate foods, such as potatoes, can also cause blood sugar levels to rise quickly. Foods that break down quickly in the blood are considered high glycemic foods. Diets containing a lot of high glycemic foods are now believed to be linked to an increased risk of diabetes and heart disease. This association has resulted in a great interest in diets based on the glycemic index of foods.

the glycemic index

The glycemic index (GI) is a system used to classify carbohydrate foods. It measures the speed at which blood sugar (glucose) rises after eating a carbohydrate food. The faster a food breaks down, the more quickly it releases sugar into the bloodstream and the higher its GI. Eating a lot of high-GI foods can cause very rapid increases in blood sugar levels. Therefore, the goal is to eat a diet consisting of mostly low-GI foods, which are absorbed more slowly into the blood stream.

foods and GI

Lower-GI foods	Higher-GI foods
◆ Whole wheat, oat, bran, rye breads and cereals	◆ Refined breakfast cereals
◆ Brown rice, barley, bulgur	◆ White pasta, bread and rice
◆ Beans, dried peas, and lentils	◆ Cake, muffins, croissants, donuts and waffles
◆ Milk, cheese, yogurt	◆ Potatoes, French fries, parsnips
◆ Fresh whole fruit (e.g., cherries, grapefruit, apples, pears, plums)	◆ Bananas, raisins, watermelon, pineapple
◆ Meat, fish, poultry, eggs, nuts	◆ Soft drinks
	◆ Sugar and most candies

In general, most highly processed foods, such as white bread and pasta, have a high GI, while most high-fiber foods, such as whole grains, beans and legumes, have a low GI. Meats, milk and cheese also tend to have a low GI.

It sounds simple: eating a diet that is high in foods with a low GI is one route to health. The problem is that following a GI diet can be quite challenging and not very practical. The glycemic response to foods is influenced by many factors, including how much food is eaten, the way the food is processed or prepared and the ripeness of vegetables and fruits. In addition, any other foods eaten at a meal also influence the GI response.

Consider, for instance, that pasta cooked al dente has a lower GI than overcooked pasta, and that ripe fruits or vegetables have a higher GI than those that are less ripe. Moreover, meat or fat can lower the glycemic response of high-GI foods when included in the same meal. Finally, because most people eat a combination of foods in any given meal, the GIs of single foods will be affected by the GI of other foods eaten, thus changing the GI of the entire meal. Consequently, following a diet based solely on the GI of certain foods can be complicated. The bottom line is that you don't need to follow a GI diet to eat well. You can, however, work toward including more low-GI foods in your diet.

the best advice about carbohydrates

◆ Choose complex carbohydrate foods, such as whole-grain bread, cereals and pasta and brown rice over highly processed white bread, cereals and pasta to reduce glycemic response.

◆ Eat more bulgur, barley and legumes such as lentils, kidney beans, chickpeas and other beans, which are digested slowly and add fiber to your diet.

◆ Include plenty of fruits and vegetables in your diet to take advantage of their beneficial nutrients and fiber.

◆ Cut back on sweets and baked goods to control your calorie intake and blood sugar levels.

◆ Eat carbohydrate foods at intervals throughout the day, in small meals or snacks that also include foods containing some protein and fat to help control blood sugar levels.

Fat is part of a healthy diet as it helps to keep you optimally nourished. Not only does fat provide energy, it helps your body absorb the fat-soluble vitamins A, D, E and K and carotenoids such as beta carotene. Fat also provides essential fatty acids, including linoleic acid (n-6 polyunsaturates including vegetable oils) and alpha-linolenic acid (n-3 polyunsaturates found in fish and flaxseeds), which your body doesn't make.

One problem with fat is that it can contribute to weight gain. Fat provides more calories per gram (9 calories) than protein or carbohydrates (4 calories). Eating too many high-fat foods may cause you to consume more calories than you need on a daily basis, and that can make it difficult to maintain an optimum weight. However, the connection between fat and obesity is far from clear. Recent reports on the eating habits of North Americans show that although fat intakes have declined over the past two to three decades, the number of overweight or obese individuals has climbed steadily. The influx of low-fat foods into the marketplace has not had a positive impact on controlling weight gain. Inactivity and larger serving sizes may be more significant contributors to the obesity epidemic than fat.

how much fat do you need?

The amount of fat required in a healthy diet ranges from 20% to 35% of calories per day. This range accommodates different lifestyle needs and variations in daily food choices. For heart health it's generally best to aim for a lower intake of fat, especially saturated fat. People who have high blood cholesterol levels and diabetes are at increased risk of heart disease and may need to monitor their fat intakes more rigorously. These individuals, as well as those with other health conditions, should follow the advice of their physician and dietitian regarding the quantity of fat that is right for them.

measuring fat in food

To meet a dietary objective of 30% of calories from fat, you should be consuming about 65 g of fat if you normally eat 2,000 calories a day (suitable for a woman) or about 90 grams of fat if you normally eat 2,700 calories a day (suitable for a man). It is very easy to use up or exceed your daily limit in one fast-food meal. A meal consisting of a double burger with cheese (36 g), a large order of fries (27 g) and a large shake (25 g) provides 88 grams of fat! If you are a woman, you have exceeded your limit. If you are a man, you have little room left for other fat-containing foods throughout the rest of the day.

From a health perspective, the amount of fat may not be as important as the kind of fat you eat on a regular basis. Although diets high in saturated and trans fat are linked to increased blood cholesterol levels and heart disease, eating the right kinds of fat can actually have significant health benefits.

sample daily intakes of fat

A daily intake of 65 g for a woman could include:

- ◆ 2 tsp (10 mL) butter or margarine (8 g)
- ◆ ¼ cup (50 mL) almonds (19 g)
- ◆ 1 tbsp (15 mL) regular salad dressing (10 g)
- ◆ 1 tbsp (15 mL) peanut butter (9 g)
- ◆ 2 cups (500 mL) 2% milk (10 g)
- ◆ 1 egg (5 g)
- ◆ ½ chicken breast (4 g)

If you are a man, you can add a 3 oz (90 g) serving of sirloin steak (8 g) and 2 slices of pepperoni pizza (14 g) to total 87 g of fat.

the different types of fat

Two types of fat are found naturally in food: unsaturated and saturated. Most foods contain a mixture of these fats, but are typically higher in one type.

unsaturated fats

Unsaturated fats fall into two categories, polyunsaturated and monounsaturated. These fats provide many of the essential fatty acids we need to stay healthy. Among their health benefits, they lower total and LDL (bad cholesterol) and increase HDL (good cholesterol), which reduces the risk of heart disease.

Polyunsaturated fats are found in nuts and seeds, soybeans, fish and oils made from corn, safflower and sunflower.

Monounsaturated fats are found in olives, olive oil, canola oil, soft margarine containing these oils, peanuts, peanut oil, peanut butter, most other nuts and avocados.

omega-3 fats

Omega-3s are a type of polyunsaturated fat found in fish oils, some fatty fish, flaxseeds and their oil, walnuts and their oil and omega-3 enriched eggs. These fats have been shown to reduce the risk of coronary heart disease and stroke and may also play a role in preventing cancer. Eating 2 or 3 fish meals a week along with other omega-3 containing foods may be beneficial to your health.

saturated fats

Saturated fats are found in meat, poultry skin, whole milk, cheese, butter, ice cream, egg yolks, tropical oils, coconuts and coconut milk.

Although diets high in saturated fats are linked to heart disease and cancer, there is some evidence that these fats are okay in moderate quantities.

trans fats

Trans fats are found naturally in some foods, such as dairy products and meats. However, the trans fats found in processed foods have been identified as a serious health concern. Trans fats are made when manufacturers add extra hydrogen to highly polyunsaturated vegetable oils to make them more solid and extend their shelf life. They are found in some margarines, vegetable shortenings and partially hydrogenated vegetable oils. They are also found in foods containing these ingredients, including most commercial bakery products, snack foods and deep-fried foods. The problem with trans fats is that they have unknown health risks and no redeeming health benefits. You should aim to reduce your intake of trans fats as much as possible. That means cutting down on most commercially prepared foods.

avoiding trans fats

- ◆ Check the fine print on ingredient lists for the words "hydrogenated" or "partially hydrogenated oils" or "vegetable oil shortening." Eat these foods less often.
- ◆ Study the "Nutrition Facts" panel on labels to find the amount of trans fat in a product. To be considered "trans fat free" it must contain less than 0.2 g trans fat per serving, and must also be low in saturated fat (less than 2 g per serving).
- ◆ If the label does not show the amount of trans fat, add up all the fats listed (mono-, polyunsaturated) and subtract from the total fat. What's left is mostly trans fat.
- ◆ Most of the trans fat in our diet comes from soft tub margarines, commercial baked foods, deep-fried foods and snack foods, so limit these in your diet.

good cholesterol/bad cholesterol

High intakes of saturated and trans fat can contribute to high blood cholesterol, which is a risk factor for heart disease. If you've had your blood cholesterol checked, it's also important to know the ratio of lipoproteins in your blood. High levels of low-density lipoprotein (LDL) or "bad cholesterol" and low levels of high-density lipoprotein (HDL) or "good cholesterol" also increase risk of heart disease.

Low-density lipoproteins carry cholesterol from the liver through the blood to the rest of the body. If there is too much LDL cholesterol in the blood, it can be deposited on artery walls and cause blockages or atherosclerosis, which in turn can cause heart attacks or stroke. Decreasing LDL cholesterol levels is good for your heart health. Cutting back on saturated and trans fats can help decrease LDL cholesterol levels.

High-density lipoproteins take cholesterol from the blood back to the liver, and then get rid of it from the body. HDLs help reduce excess cholesterol in the blood, so that less will be deposited in the coronary arteries. Increasing HDL cholesterol levels is good for your heart health. Eating more polyunsaturated and monounsaturated fats in place of saturated and trans fats can help increase HDL cholesterol levels.

Being physically active and having alcohol in moderation can also increase HDL cholesterol levels. Other strategies for controlling and lowering total blood cholesterol levels include losing weight and eating more fiber.

fat and blood cholesterol levels

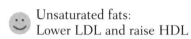 Unsaturated fats:
Lower LDL and raise HDL

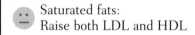 Saturated fats:
Raise both LDL and HDL

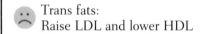 Trans fats:
Raise LDL and lower HDL

dietary cholesterol

The cholesterol you get from eating foods is known as dietary cholesterol. It is not strongly linked to blood cholesterol levels, but some individuals, particularly those with heart disease or diabetes, may still need to monitor their intake of high-cholesterol foods.

Although some foods such as eggs, milk and nuts, contain high levels of dietary cholesterol or fat, they are also very nutritious, and healthy people should enjoy them in moderation as part of a balanced diet.

eggs

Eggs are a source of important nutrients, including protein, vitamins A, E, and B_{12}, folate, niacin, riboflavin, zinc and phosphorus. One egg also provides 5 g of fat and 215 mg of cholesterol. While eggs are a higher-cholesterol food, the cholesterol from food has been found to have only a slight impact on blood cholesterol levels for normal, healthy individuals. A recent study of more than 80,000 female nurses found that moderate egg consumption (up to one a day) did not increase heart disease risk in healthy individuals. However, people with heart disease or diabetes should follow the recommendations of their physician or dietitian regarding egg consumption.

READ THE LABEL "A healthy diet low in saturated and trans fats may reduce the risk of heart disease."
To make this health claim, a food must be low in saturated and trans fats and the amount of saturated and trans fats must be included on the label.

milk

Milk products provide important nutrients, including protein, riboflavin, vitamin B_{12}, vitamin A, vitamin D, calcium, zinc and magnesium. They can also be high in fat. One cup (250 mL) constitutes a serving of milk. Whole milk contains the most fat (9 g/serving) and cholesterol (35 mg/serving). A serving of 2% milk provides 5 g of fat and only 19 mg of cholesterol; 1% milk provides 3 g of fat and 10 mg of cholesterol, and skim milk provides only a trace of fat and 5 mg of cholesterol.

Most of the fat in milk is in the form of saturated fat, but there are other substances in milk that appear to play a role in preventing insulin resistance and hypertension and that may help with weight control. Research has found that overweight individuals with low milk consumption (less than $1\frac{1}{2}$ servings per day) were at greater risk of developing insulin resistance than those who consumed more than five servings a day. Also, a diet that included 2 to 3 servings a day of low-fat milk products and 8 to 10 servings a day of fruits and vegetables lowered blood pressure better than medication. Eating a diet containing milk products and high amounts of dietary calcium (about 1,200 mg from food, not supplements) has been associated with weight loss and fat loss.

nuts

Nuts are nutritious. They are rich in fiber and vitamin E, and supply B vitamins, magnesium, zinc and selenium. They are also cholesterol-free, but they should be consumed in moderation because they are high in fat. However, most of the fat in nuts is monounsaturated or polyunsaturated, which can help to lower blood cholesterol levels, including LDL bad cholesterol, while maintaining HDL good cholesterol.

nut alert

Watch the quantity of Brazil nuts, coconuts and coconut products you eat, as these are higher in saturated fat.

getting the right fats in your diet

◆ Replace the saturated and trans fats in your diet with monounsaturated and polyunsaturated fats by using soft margarine made without trans fat (look for "non-hydrogenated" and "low in saturated and trans fat" on the label) and using liquid oils (safflower, sunflower, canola and olive) instead of solid fats (lard, solid margarine) for cooking.

◆ Use salad oils made with olive or canola oil, which contain monounsaturated fat.

◆ Avoid deep-frying, which adds more saturated and trans fat to foods.

◆ Include 2 to 4 servings of milk products per day in your diet, including milk or yogurt with 2% or less milk fat and cheese in moderation (a serving of cheese is 50 g or 2 oz).

◆ Trim the fat from meat and the skins from poultry. Bake, broil or grill, and avoid deep-frying.

◆ Have omega-3 rich fish (salmon, sardines, tuna, herring, mackerel, rainbow trout) 2 to 3 times a week.

◆ Eat nuts in small amounts (2 to 3 tbsp/30 to 45 mL).

◆ Eat fewer high-fat snacks such as cookies, snack crackers and chips, which are high in trans fat. Check the ingredient list and avoid those made with hydrogenated oils. The higher they are on the list, the higher the trans fat content.

protein

Protein is a major structural component of every body cell. In addition to being a source of energy for your body, it is necessary for the growth, repair and maintenance of skin, muscles, bones and organs. It also plays important roles in the functioning of membranes, enzymes and hormones.

Most North Americans get enough protein in their diet — some, especially those following a high-protein diet, may be getting more than they really need. About 10% to 30% of your calories should come from protein. This range varies depending on how much carbohydrate and fat is in your diet. Adults over 19 require 0.8 g of protein per kg of body weight per day. That works out to a daily requirement of about 56 g of protein for men and 46 g of protein for women. If you have 1 egg (6 g), 1 tbsp (15 mL) peanut butter (4 g), ½ cup (125 mL) cooked beans or lentils (8 g), ½ chicken breast (16 g), and 1 cup (250 mL) 2% milk (20 g), you will have eaten 54 g of protein.

protein sources

To make the protein your body needs, you must get essential amino acids in sufficient amounts from the foods you eat. Protein from animal foods such as meat, poultry, fish, eggs, milk, cheese and yogurt supplies all of the essential amino acids, as does the protein from soy products. These foods are typically referred to as "complete" proteins. Other plant foods provide varying amounts of protein, but do not provide all the essential amino acids. These are often referred to as "incomplete" proteins.

plant protein

Legumes (beans, dried peas and lentils), seeds and nuts are much higher in protein than grain products and many vegetables. To get the full range of essential amino acids from a primarily plant-based vegetarian diet, you will have to eat a wide variety of foods. It is not necessary to combine specific foods at each meal to get a complete source of protein, as once thought. Eating an assortment of plant foods (legumes, nuts, seeds, grains, vegetables and fruit) with soy products over the course of a day can provide the essential amino acids you need. You also need to make sure you are getting enough calories to meet your energy needs.

best ways to get the protein you need in your diet

◆ Eat a variety of protein-rich foods, including meat, fish, poultry, eggs, milk, cheese, yogurt, legumes (beans, dried peas and lentils), peanut or almond butter, nuts, seeds, tofu and soy alternatives.

◆ If you don't eat meat, fish, eggs or dairy products, choose soy alternatives such as soy meat substitutes or products made with soy to get some complete proteins in your diet.

◆ Consume the recommended serving sizes (see chart, page 5) to control your calorie intake and weight.

10 best strategies for healthy eating

1. Eat a variety of foods.

2. Pay attention to portion sizes; use those recommended in the food guide to control the amount of food and calories you consume.

3. Eat more whole grains such as whole-wheat, bran and oat breads and cereals, whole-wheat pasta and brown rice to increase the fiber in your diet.

4. Include a variety of vegetables and fruits, especially dark red, orange and green varieties, to get more antioxidant nutrients like beta carotene and lycopene.

5. Have fruit or vegetables more often than their juice to control calories and get more fiber.

6. Keep your meals moderate in total fat and low in saturated and trans fats to promote a healthy heart by eating low-fat dairy products, lean meats and foods prepared without added fat.

7. Balance the amount of food you eat with the amount of physical activity you do to maintain or improve your weight.

8. Limit your consumption of salty foods to keep your blood pressure in a healthy range.

9. If you drink alcohol, have it in moderate amounts, which may help promote a healthy heart (1 drink a day for women, 2 drinks a day for men) or eliminate it altogether, as too much alcohol is linked with liver disease and increased rates of breast cancer in women.

10. Cut back on high-caffeine beverages, which may interfere with bone health and are dehydrating.

losing weight and keeping it off

More than half of North American adults are presently considered overweight or obese, which puts them at risk for a variety of health problems, such as heart disease, some types of cancer, type-2 diabetes, gallbladder disease, respiratory disease, sleep apnea and osteoarthritis. Obesity in children has also become a disturbing trend, as it puts children at risk for adult health problems, including adult-onset diabetes.

Studies show that overweight individuals who reduce their body weight by 5% to 10% reap numerous health benefits, including lower LDL (bad cholesterol), higher HDL (good cholesterol), better blood glucose levels, lower blood pressure (high blood pressure is linked to heart disease), and lower triglycerides (high triglycerides in the blood are linked to heart disease and diabetes). A 160-pound woman who loses 8 to 16 pounds or a 200-pound man who loses 10 to 20 pounds can expect real health benefits.

Being physically active is likely the best way to maintain a healthy weight. Regular exercise also helps to control blood cholesterol, diabetes and high blood pressure. And the good news is that it is never too late to become active. In fact, studies show that sedentary individuals who begin to exercise actually reap the greatest benefits from physical activity. Becoming more physically active on a regular basis even protects people who are already overweight or obese.

Being active helps you burn calories and maintain lean muscle, which burns more calories than body fat. Ideally, you should get aim for an hour or more of activity each day to maintain a healthy body weight. This doesn't mean working out at the gym for an hour every day. It could involve two ten-minute walks to do your errands, twenty minutes of dancing, cycling or home exercise, and twenty minutes playing actively with the kids.

---

is your weight a health concern?

To determine if your weight puts you at risk for health problems, find your Body Mass Index or BMI. A BMI greater than 25 increases the risk for health problems, a BMI of 30 or greater puts you at an even higher risk. You should also take a waist measurement, as excess weight carried around the middle is another indicator of health risk. A waist measurement equal to or greater than 40 inches (102 cm) for men and equal to or greater than 35 inches (88 cm) for women increases risk for type-2 diabetes, heart disease and hypertension.

To find your BMI, visit:
http://www.hc-sc.gc.ca/hpfb-dgpsa/onpp-bppn/bmi_chart_java_e.html.

---

the skinny on diets

It's hard to pick up a newspaper or magazine today without reading about the latest diet. We're obsessed with losing weight, and can choose from a variety of methods to do so, ranging from eating a very low-fat/high-carbohydrate diet to eating one that is high in protein and low in carbs. The problem is, there's little evidence to show that these jazzy new diets work better than any other low-calorie diet as far as weight loss is concerned. The trick to rapid weight loss diets is that they're typically very low in calories, and as such may be limited in essential nutrients, which is not the best for your health. Some people can benefit from going on a kick-start diet to help them lose some weight initially, but it's important to assess the diet to ensure that it provides adequate calories and the full range of vitamins and minerals you need. If an entire food group is missing, you can be sure you are missing out some key nutrients.

very low-fat/high-carbohydrate diets

Some diets are very low in fat and high in carbohydrate (10% fat; 70% to 80% carbohydrate). This type of diet, which has been promoted for heart health and lowering blood cholesterol, is very restricted in fat, making it difficult for most people to follow. It seems outdated now because we know that switching to the healthier types of fat is more important than strictly limiting fat.

There are also some negatives associated with eating too much carbohydrate. A diet that's too high in carbohydrates, particularly sugars, can increase blood triglyceride levels. This puts individuals at higher risk for type-2 diabetes and heart disease. People who follow this type of diet may turn to fat-free and reduced-fat foods as a way to reduce fat, but may not realize that these products often provide a significant amount of calories and carbohydrates. For example, fat-free cookies or low-fat ice cream are not calorie-free. These foods still provide a lot of calories in the form of simple carbohydrates, and need to be eaten in moderation, not liberally, to help control calorie intake.

Another problem with very low-fat diets is that they are not very satisfying. Fat-containing foods provide satiety (a feeling of fullness). Followers of low-fat diets may overeat high-carbohydrate foods to fill the void. These diets are also very difficult to stick with for a long time because they are not satisfying and exclude many foods people normally eat.

Rather than following on a strict low-fat diet, it is better to work on changing your current eating habits. You can cut down on your usual fat intake, but focus on changing the type of fat in your diet by replacing saturated and trans fats with polyunsaturated and monounsaturated fats. It's also important to eat more high-fiber foods, such as whole grains, fruits, vegetables and beans, instead of processed white flour or sugary foods.

---

know the risks

Very low-fat/high-carbohydrate diets may:

✦ increase blood triglyceride levels, increasing your risk for type-2 diabetes and heart disease;

✦ increase your consumption of fat-free and reduced-fat foods, which are likely to be high in calories and carbohydrates;

✦ induce cravings for fat, or food in general, which you are likely to satisfy by overindulging in carbs if you follow the diet rigorously.

---

high-protein/low-carbohydrate diets

High-protein/low-carbohydrate diets (55% fat; less than 20% carbohydrate) include foods such as red meat, bacon, sausages, whole milk and cheese. People initially enjoy following these diets because they include higher-fat foods that are typically forbidden on other diets, and that helps them to feel more satisfied. However, some people find it difficult to stay on this diet for long, as they miss the foods that provide them with a quick source of energy, namely carbohydrates.

People are often successful at losing weight on these diets because, overall, they tend to be low in calories (about 1,500 calories). Even though these diets are high in fat, a lot of the foods people typically eat are missing, and the net result is fewer calories consumed. These diets are also very encouraging, as during the first few weeks on the diet, people lose weight rapidly. Unfortunately this is due to water loss — one result of reducing carbohydrate consumption, as carbs hold more water than protein and fat.

The main concern with a high-protein/low-carbohydrate diet is that it is high in saturated fat. As discussed earlier, too much saturated fat can increase the level of LDL cholesterol in the blood, which increases the risk of heart disease. These diets also restrict grain products, vegetables and fruits, which mean they lack some important vitamins and minerals. Although preliminary research suggests such diets may not be detrimental to blood cholesterol and triglyceride levels, the studies have been conducted on a limited number of people who have followed the diet for 12 months or less. Another concern is that following a high-protein diet for a long time may increase the risk for osteoporosis and kidney disease, but we won't know this for sure until further studies have been conducted. Until more is known about the real risks and benefits of high-protein/low-carbohydrate diets, they should be viewed with caution.

know the risks

High-protein/low-carbohydrate diets:

✦ may increase LDL cholesterol levels;

✦ lack important vitamins and minerals;

✦ may increase risk for osteoporosis and kidney disease.

high-carbohydrate/moderate-fat diet

A recent review of all diets, conducted by the United States Department of Agriculture (USDA), concluded that a high-carbohydrate/moderate-fat diet (20% to 30% fat; 55% to 60% carbohydrate), which follows the eating pattern outlined in the Canadian and American food guides, promotes healthier calorie and fat intakes than other diets. The study compared the diets, calorie intakes and body mass index (BMI) of more than 10,000 adults. It found that a high-carbohydrate/moderate-fat diet was lower in calories and higher in nutritional quality compared to a high-protein/low-carbohydrate diet. Saturated fat intakes were almost twice as high in the high-protein/low-carbohydrate diet. BMIs were also found to be lower in those consuming a high-carbohydrate diet.

know the benefits

High-carbohydrate/moderate-fat diets:

✦ lower saturated fat intakes;

✦ lower BMI;

✦ are more likely to keep weight off.

the best advice about weight-loss diets

The best advice about diets is that they don't guarantee weight loss. And most people who need to lose weight don't need to follow any particular diet, they simply need to eat fewer calories and exercise more. Calories *do* count!

Any diet that causes you to eat fewer calories than you usually consume will contribute to weight loss. For example, most popular weight loss diets provide around 1,500 calories per day, which is roughly 500 fewer calories than a sedentary woman might consume to maintain her weight. Losing 1 pound a week requires losing 3,500 less calories over the week, or eating roughly 500 fewer calories per day.

Alternatively, burning up 500 calories a day in exercise can also result in a pound of weight loss. When a reduced-calorie diet is accompanied by exercise, additional calories are burned, which helps to speed weight loss.

Unfortunately, most people who are trying to lose weight do not typically reduce calories while increasing physical activity for an adequate period of time. Individuals who don't keep their calories in check and who don't keep physically active are likely to regain any weight they have lost after returning to their usual eating and exercise habits. A long-term commitment to eating right and keeping active is necessary to achieve and maintain a healthy weight.

keeping weight off

The National Weight Control Registry has kept track of the weight-control behaviors of more than 3,000 American adults who have lost an average of 60 pounds and kept it off for an average of six years. Four common behaviors were associated with weight loss:

◆ eating a lower-fat (20% to30% fat), higher-carbohydrate diet;

◆ monitoring themselves by weighing in frequently;

◆ being physically active; and

◆ eating breakfast.

pay attention to portions

Eating food in portions that are larger than you need sneaks in extra calories and unwanted weight gain over the years. If you are wondering how you gained an extra 10 to 20 pounds over the past decade, take a look at how much you are eating. As we age, our metabolisms slow down and we actually need fewer calories. The problem is, most of us don't make the adjustment and switch to smaller serving sizes.

a calorie is a calorie

As far as the body is concerned, one calorie is the same as another, no matter where they came from. Eat too many calories (whether from fat, carbohydrates or protein) and you'll gain weight.

Studies show that people of all ages are eating larger portions, not only when they eat out, but also at home. Super-sizing foods and offering more food for just a few extra cents is common practice in fast-food restaurants. While it is important to watch what you eat in restaurants, controlling portions at home can be more effective over the long term because the food you eat on a regular basis has the greatest impact on your weight over time.

tips for managing quantities

◆ Take notice of the size of the plates, bowls and cups you commonly use at home. If you are serving meals on a dinner plate or drinking from a 16-ounce (500 mL) glass, switch to a luncheon plate and use a smaller glass.

◆ Measure out your usual servings of cereal, pasta, vegetables, juice, milk and so on using a measuring cup. Notice the size of your typical serving of meat or cheese. Compare this quantity to the Guide to Food Choices and Amounts chart on page 5. It might surprise you to find you are eating much more than you really need.

◆ Watch out for high-calorie beverages. A single serving of 100% juice in a bottle can provide up to 2 cups (500 mL), which is equivalent to 4 food guide servings! Most people don't realize that even "real" juice can be a source of significant calories. If you are thirsty, cut back on the juice and sugary beverages and have water instead.

◆ Check the serving sizes on food package labels. These provide a guide as to how much to eat and the calories per serving. If you eat twice the serving size, don't forget to double the calories too.

◆ Cut back, not out. Eating smaller servings means you can have your cake and eat it too. Have two cookies instead of four. Share a large muffin or rich dessert with a friend. Savor one scoop of ice cream instead of devouring a whole bowl.

---

watch those calories

Drinking fruit juices and other sweetened beverages several times a day can add a lot of calories to your daily diet. Here are the calories contained in a serving (1 cup/250 mL) of some popular drinks:

◆ freshly squeezed orange juice: 118 calories

◆ apple juice: 123 calories

◆ grape juice: 136 calories

◆ citrus fruit drinks: 121 calories

◆ cranberry cocktail: 155 calories

◆ ice teas and soda pop: 104 to 126 calories

10 best strategies for managing your weight

1. Eat breakfast every day! Reduce the amount of fat by using skim or 1% milk or low-fat yogurt. Include high-fiber foods such as whole-wheat bread or bagels, bran or oat cereals, and dried or fresh fruit.

2. Eat 3 to 5 meals or snacks, spaced evenly throughout the day to keep you energized. Avoid skipping meals to reduce the temptation to snack or eat more than you need later in the day.

3. If you eat a high-calorie and/or high-fat meal, balance it with smaller, lower-calorie and/or lower-fat snacks or meals during the day.

4. Watch how much you eat. Try smaller portions of food consistent with the serving sizes recommended on the food guide. If you are still hungry, add vegetables and fruits.

5. Cut back on sugars and sweets and high-calorie and/or high-fat foods that don't offer key nutrients, such as chips, cookies and donuts.

6. Be aware that low-fat foods are not a panacea. Many low-fat foods are actually high in sugar and calories and won't help you lose weight.

7. Fill up on foods that are naturally high in fiber, such as vegetables, fruits, whole grains and legumes such as cooked beans, dried peas and lentils.

8. Get moving! Gradually work up to 60 minutes a day of physical activity — brisk walking, cycling, swimming, strength training or aerobic dancing. Adding a half-hour brisk walk each day is an easy way to start. Once you get into the routine, mix and match your other activities.

9. Set realistic goals — aim to lose 5% to 10% of your body weight. After you achieve that goal, aim for another 5% to 10%. Keep going until you achieve a healthy weight. Breaking weight loss into manageable chunks may take time, but the long-term effort will be easier to manage.

10. Keep track of your weight loss and physical activity on your calendar or in a journal. Reward yourself for achieving your goals and keep going. Set new goals to keep you motivated.

other essentials

In addition to carbohydrates, fats and proteins, you need many other important vitamins and minerals to look and feel your best. Remember, you need over 50 different nutrients to be healthy, and no single one is a magic bullet for health. Here's a rundown of some of the key nutrients you need to function optimally.

vitamins

vitamin A and beta carotene

Vitamin A is a fat-soluble vitamin that promotes good vision and helps maintain healthy skin, teeth and skeletal and soft tissue. Some animal foods contain vitamin A, but most vitamin A comes from plant foods, especially dark green and orange vegetables and fruit. Beta carotene is the component found in these foods that converts to vitamin A in the body. Beta carotene is also an important antioxidant nutrient that may play a role in cancer prevention.

> **sources:**
> Carrots, sweet potatoes, pumpkin, cantaloupe, pink grapefruit, tomatoes and tomato products, broccoli and dark green leafy vegetables including spinach, beet greens, Swiss chard and kale.

vitamin C

Vitamin C is a water-soluble vitamin that aids in iron absorption, helps to heal cuts and wounds and maintain connective tissue, which holds muscles, bones and tissues together, and maintains strong blood vessel walls. Vitamin C also acts as an antioxidant, helping to reduce oxidation in cells and cell damage, thereby playing a role in preventing disease processes from starting.

> **sources:**
> Oranges and orange juice, grapefruit and grapefruit juice, apple juice, kiwi fruit, strawberries, red, yellow and green peppers, broccoli, Brussels sprouts, potatoes and tomatoes.

vitamin E

Vitamin E is a fat-soluble vitamin that acts as an antioxidant to help reduce oxidation in cells. Vitamin E, especially as a supplement, has been promoted widely as a way to improve heart health. It is also being studied for its potential role in cataract prevention. However, the research on supplements is not conclusive, and high intakes are not recommended. The best way to get vitamin E is to eat foods containing vitamin E.

> **sources:**
> Nuts, seeds, vegetable oils, wheat germ, sweet potatoes and papaya.

vitamin B_6

Vitamin B_6 is a water-soluble vitamin involved in many of the chemical reactions of protein and amino acids. It also helps maintain normal brain function and is involved in forming red blood cells. Vitamin B_6 has been found to help reduce symptoms of PMS, but high intakes are neither necessary nor desirable. High doses of vitamin B_6 from supplements, not food, can cause numbness and other neurological disorders. For adults, the safe upper limit is 100 mg of vitamin B_6 per day.

> **sources:**
> Meat, fish, poultry, organ meats, legumes (beans and lentils), peanut butter, fortified breads and cereals, bananas and watermelon.

vitamin B₁₂

Vitamin B_{12} plays an important role in helping your body function. It works in combination with folate to make DNA and helps form red blood cells. Vitamin B_{12} also helps maintain the central nervous system. A deficiency of Vitamin B_{12} can cause a disease called pernicious anemia. Older people (we lose our ability to absorb Vitamin B_{12} as we age) and strict vegetarians who do not consume any animal products are at greater risk of deficiency.

sources:
Milk and milk products, meat, poultry, fish and eggs, and foods fortified with Vitamin B_{12}. Strict vegetarians should look for foods fortified with vitamin B_{12}, such as soy and rice beverages and soy-based meat substitutes.

folate

Folate is a B vitamin that works with Vitamin B_{12} to make DNA and red blood cells. It plays an important role in preventing fetal neural tube defects. A lack of folate, along with a lack of vitamin B_6 and vitamin B_{12}, can increase blood homocysteine levels, which are associated with increased risk of heart attack and stroke.

Folic acid is the form of folate used in vitamin supplements. Women who may become pregnant are advised to take a folic acid supplement (0.4 mg or 400 µg per day), as it is difficult to get enough folate in the diet.

sources:
Liver, legumes (beans, dried peas, lentils), dark leafy greens, asparagus, broccoli, corn, green peas, oranges and orange juice, canned pineapple juice, honeydew melon, cantaloupe, strawberries, nuts and sunflower seeds, wheat germ and fortified breads, cereals and pasta.

vitamin D

Vitamin D works with calcium to help build and maintain strong bones. Vitamin D also helps the body maintain normal levels of calcium in the blood. A deficiency of Vitamin D, especially in older adults, is linked to an increased risk of bone fractures and osteoporosis.

how much vitamin D do you need?
19–50 years of age: 5 µg (200 IU)
51–70 years of age: 10 µg (400 IU)
Over 70 years: 15 µg (600 IU)

(Source: National Academy of Sciences, 1997)

Vitamin D is made in the body when the skin is exposed to sunlight. Older individuals who don't get enough dietary vitamin D and who have a limited exposure to sunlight are most at risk of a deficiency. Also, people who live in northern climates (all of Canada and the northern United States) don't get enough sunlight during the winter months to make the vitamin D their bodies need. A vitamin D supplement during the winter months can be beneficial to people who don't get adequate sun exposure.

sources:
Milk, eggs, fatty fish (salmon, mackerel, sardines, tuna, rainbow trout), fish liver oils, margarine, soy and rice beverages enriched with vitamin D.

calcium

Calcium helps with many important body functions, including regulating heart and muscle contractions, nerve transmission, blood clotting and numerous enzyme functions. Calcium is best known for its role in building strong bones and teeth, which it does in conjunction with the other bone-building nutrients, specifically, vitamin D, phosphorus and magnesium. An adequate intake of calcium and vitamin D, as well as regular weight-bearing exercise throughout life helps prevent osteoporosis.

You can get 1,000 mg of calcium in a day by consuming, for example, 2 cups (500 mL) of 1% or 2% milk (630 mg), ¾ cup (175 g) of 1% to 2% yogurt (215 mg), ¼ cup (50 mL) of almonds (75 mg) and ½ cup (125 mL) of cooked bok choy (85 mg).

how much calcium do you need?
19–50 years of age: 1,000 mg/day
51–70 years of age: 1,200 mg/day

(Source: National Academy of Sciences, 1997)

sources:
Milk, cheese, yogurt, calcium-fortified beverages (soy, rice and orange juice), canned salmon and sardines with bones, sesame seeds, cooked beans, tofu containing calcium sulfate, almonds, bok choy, kale and broccoli.

READ THE LABEL
"A healthy diet with adequate calcium and vitamin D, and regular physical activity, helps to achieve strong bones and may reduce the risk of osteoporosis."
To make this health claim, a food must be a good, high or excellent source of calcium.

phosphorus

Phosphorus is a major component of bones and teeth. It also helps the body produce and regulate energy and form the membranes and genetic material in cells. Phosphorus is widely distributed throughout the food supply. It is found in high amounts in most animal foods and in some plant foods. Phosphorus is also found in food additives and soft drinks.

sources:
Meat, fish, poultry, eggs, milk products, legumes and nuts.

magnesium

Magnesium helps to build and maintain strong bones. It also plays a role in energy production and is involved in many enzyme functions, which maintain normal muscle and nerve function as well as a normal heart rhythm.

sources:
Legumes (beans, dried peas and lentils), nuts and seeds, whole grains such as wheat and oat bran, brown rice, meat and milk products.

potassium

Potassium works with sodium, calcium and magnesium to maintain proper water balance in the body and to help regulate blood pressure. Potassium also helps nerves, muscles, heart and kidneys function properly. A diet high in potassium may help reduce the risk of hypertension and stroke.

sources:

Oranges and orange juice, bananas, melon, papaya, pears, figs, prunes and other dried fruit, tomatoes and tomato juice, potatoes, meat, poultry, milk and yogurt.

READ THE LABEL

"A healthy diet containing foods high in potassium and low in sodium may reduce risk of high blood pressure, a risk factor for stroke and heart disease."

To make this health claim, the food must be low in sodium or sodium-free.

---

sodium

Sodium is required to regulate blood pressure and water balance in your body. Too much sodium in the diet can cause increased blood pressure in individuals who are sensitive to sodium. High blood pressure in a risk factor for heart disease. Sodium is pervasive in our food supply, especially in processed foods such as canned goods, packaged foods and cured and pickled products. Most North Americans eat more sodium than they really need, which is not a good thing for heart health.

sources:

Table salt, salted processed foods (chips, crackers, pickles, sauerkraut, dry soup and pasta and seasoning mixes, canned soups and foods with added salt) and salt-cured meats such as bacon and many luncheon meats.

tips for lowering blood pressure

✦ Lower sodium intake by eating fewer salty foods and choosing foods that are labeled "low in sodium" or "sodium reduced." Aim to consume less than 2,400 mg of sodium per day.

✦ Eat a diet that contains 8 to 10 servings of fruits and vegetables and 2 to 3 servings of low-fat dairy products.

✦ Maintain a healthy weight, keep physically active and have alcohol in moderation.

(Source: DASH Diet — NEJM 336:1117-1124, 1997. www.nhlbi.nih.gov)

the best ways to cut back on sodium

✦ Read food labels and choose those labeled "salt-free" or "sodium-free" or "low in sodium/salt."

✦ Prepare foods without adding salt to the cooking water and omit the salt in recipes.

✦ Season foods with herbs, spices, lemon juice or garlic instead of salt or mixtures containing salt such as seasoning salt, garlic salt or onion salt.

✦ Avoid canned, bottled or dehydrated soups, sauces and pasta and rice mixes.

✦ Limit salty snack foods such as chips, pretzels, crackers and salted nuts.

✦ Cut back on processed, smoked or salt-cured meats, such as bacon, hot dogs, sausages and luncheon meats.

✦ Avoid salty vegetable and tomato juices.

✦ Limit processed cheeses and cheese spreads and pickled foods such as pickles, relish, sauerkraut.

iron

Iron is an essential component of hemogloblin, which carries oxygen to all cells in the body. Inadequate iron intakes can lead to depleted iron stores and iron-deficiency anemia. Women and adolescent girls need to pay special attention to their iron needs, since iron is lost each month during menstruation. This group needs to eat plenty of iron-rich foods, and some individuals may need a supplement.

sources:

Red meat, dark meat poultry, other meat and poultry, clams, oysters, legumes (beans, dried peas and lentils), iron-fortified breakfast cereals, oat and wheat bran, tofu, flaxseeds, blackstrap molasses, eggs, pasta, bread, nuts and seeds, dried fruit and prune juice.

There are two kinds of iron: heme and non-heme. Heme iron, found in meat, poultry, fish and seafood, is absorbed readily by the body. Non-heme iron, found in eggs, grains, beans, vegetables and dried fruit is less well absorbed by the body. Eating non-heme iron foods with heme iron foods (e.g., beef chili with beans), increases overall iron absorption. Having vitamin C–rich foods (e.g., oranges or tomatoes) with an iron-containing food (e.g., spinach) also increases iron absorption.

zinc

Zinc has various structural and regulatory roles in the body. It controls many enzyme functions and helps with the growth and maintenance of cells. It is also needed for taste and smell acuity. A deficiency of zinc can retard growth, impair immune function, reduce appetite and cause hair loss and skin lesions. Strict vegetarians (who may get less zinc from a plant-based diet) and heavy alcohol consumers (who may have impaired zinc absorption) are at greater risk for a deficiency.

sources:

Meats, seafood (especially oysters), whole grains, wheat germ, eggs, milk, cheese and yogurt.

---

is a vegetarian diet better than a meat diet?

Vegetarian diets offer a number of advantages, including lower levels of saturated fat, cholesterol and animal protein and higher levels of carbohydrates, fiber, magnesium, folate, phytochemicals and antioxidants such as vitamins C and E and carotenoids.

A vegetarian diet can be just as healthy as a meat containing diet, but careful planning is required. To get the necessary nutrients, vegetarians need to eat plenty of whole-grain breads and cereals, vegetables, fruits, legumes, nuts, soy products and calcium alternatives. Some supplements might also be necessary, for example, calcium and vitamin D (if no milk products are consumed), iron (for women with low iron stores) and vitamin B_{12} (which is only found in animal products and meat alternatives fortified with vitamin B_{12}).

---

beyond vitamins and minerals

Some substances in food go beyond what basic vitamins and minerals can do in terms of promoting health. Substances called phytochemicals, for instance, are chemicals found in plants that are essential to good health. They include flavonoids and carotenoids that have various functions. Some act as antioxidants, protecting cells from damage, others may have a role in preventing cancer or heart disease. Fiber is another non-nutritive substance that carries out functions that are very important for your health. Finally, fluids are crucial for keeping your body hydrated and working properly. Making the right choices with these substances in mind can help you achieve better health.

plant powerhouses

Some plant foods contain biologically active components called phytochemicals, which can affect certain risk factors for disease. These foods should not be considered magic bullets for better health, but rather part of a balanced diet that includes a variety of other healthful food choices.

---

foods rich in phytochemicals

+ Blueberries are high in antioxidants, which help reduce oxidative stress in cells and may help protect against cancer and heart disease.

+ Cranberries are a rich source of procyanidins, which help prevent urinary tract infections.

+ Dark red, yellow or orange fruits and vegetables contain carotenoids (alpha and beta carotene, lycopene and luetin), which are being studied for their potential role in preventing heart disease, cancer, macular degeneration and cataracts.

+ Tomato products, such as ketchup and pizza or pasta sauces, and tomato juice contain lycopene, which has been found to help reduce certain types of cancer, particularly prostate cancer.

+ Red grapes and purple grape juice contain some of the same flavonoids as red wine, and resveratrol, which may be good for heart health.

+ Flax seeds (not flaxseed oil) contain lignins, which convert to a form of estrogen and are thought to have some protective effect against cancer.

+ Soy foods contain isoflavonoids and lignins, which are converted to a form of estrogen in the body. Some women find soy foods help reduce symptoms of menopause.

+ Tea (green and black) contains antioxidants, including flavonoids, which may protect against certain cancers and heart disease.

---

fiber

Fiber is a non-nutritive substance that is not completely broken down by the body. It plays an important role in keeping your digestive system healthy and maintaining regularity. Eating high-fiber foods can also help control blood sugar and blood cholesterol levels. Diets low in fat and high in fruits, vegetables and grain products that contain fiber are associated with a reduced risk of some types of cancers and heart disease.

There are two kinds of fiber — soluble and insoluble. Insoluble fiber, found in whole grains, wheat bran, vegetables and fruits with edible skins and seeds, helps maintain regularity and keep the digestive system healthy. Soluble fiber, found in fruits, legumes, barley, psyllium and oats (oatmeal), helps lower blood cholesterol and control blood sugar levels. A high-fiber diet is also beneficial for weight control, as high-fiber foods are generally low in fat and help to make you feel full.

Most North Americans don't get nearly enough total fiber in their diet. A typical daily intake is about 15 g. Ideally, women should consume 25 g and men 38 g of total fiber per day.

the best ways to add fiber to your diet

◆ Add fiber-rich foods to your diet gradually to reduce the chances of bloating, gas or cramps.

◆ Try to eat foods high in both insoluble and soluble fiber at every meal.

◆ Include 5 to 12 servings of whole-grain products in your diet every day. Choose whole-wheat, bran, oat or rye cereals and breads instead of white bread and processed cereals, and whole-wheat pasta and brown rice instead of white pasta and rice.

◆ Eat 5 to 10 servings of vegetables and fruit every day. Leave the skins on and have whole fruits or vegetables instead of juice for added fiber.

◆ Include more legumes (beans, dried peas, lentils) in your meals as spreads or dips, soups, salads and main dishes.

◆ Read food labels and choose foods that are high in fiber, at least 4 g per serving.

fluids

To be in the best of health, you need to be properly hydrated. You could live for several weeks with no food, but only a few days without water. Over half of your body weight is water, and every cell and process in your body depends on water to function properly. Water is also essential to maintain a normal body temperature.

Dizziness, lightheadedness, muscle cramps, nausea and headaches are all warning signs of dehydration. If left unheeded, dehydration can cause a dangerous increase in body temperature, which can lead to heat exhaustion and, more seriously, heat stroke. Thirst is not a good indication of your body's need for fluids. You may not feel thirsty until you are already dehydrated.

A normal fluid requirement for most people living at moderate temperatures is about 8 cups (2 L) a day. In hot and humid conditions, daily fluid requirements may double or triple. Working strenuously or exercising outside in hot temperatures increases fluid requirements. Sweating helps keep the body cool, but results in lost fluids and electrolytes (sodium and potassium). Drinking adequate fluids and including sodium- and potassium-rich foods (e.g., a snack of orange juice, a banana or salted crackers) helps replace fluids and electrolytes. Eating high-fluid foods such as soup, lettuce, watermelon, cucumbers, tomatoes and oranges can also help keep you hydrated.

what to drink

◆ *Water:* While water has no calories, it also has no nutrients. Nevertheless, the majority of your fluid requirements should be met by drinking water because that's what your body needs most of all. There are a wide variety of waters on the market today and all — purified, tap or bottled — will meet your fluid needs.

◆ *Juice:* The best choice is freshly made juice, from fruits or vegetables, with no added sugar or salt. Freshly made juice contains all the nutrients of the plants from which it is made, except for fiber. If you are purchasing juice in a bottle, the kind labeled "100% pure" or "reconstituted" is best for providing more of the important nutrients you need.

◆ *Fruit juice beverages and cocktails:* These are not to be confused with "real" juice. Although fruit juice beverages often contain added vitamin C, they are higher in sugar than pure or reconstituted juice. Also, most fruit juice beverages contain less than 25% real juice, which means they have fewer nutrients.

◆ *Fruit-flavored beverages and soft drinks:* These include lemonade, ice tea and other fruit-flavored or soda beverages that are mostly water with sugar and flavorings added. They are lower in nutrients than 100% juice and contain significant calories unless they are calorie-reduced. All of these beverages can help keep you hydrated, but most come in serving sizes that are bigger than one needs. Research conducted by the World Health Organization has found that individuals, including children, who consume a lot of sugary drinks are at risk of excess weight gain. Soft drinks and ice tea also contain caffeine, which can be dehydrating.

◆ *Coffee and tea:* Drinks that contain caffeine are not good choices for keeping you hydrated because they cause the body to lose water. When these beverages are consumed, intake of other fluids should be increased to compensate for fluid losses. Studies show that coffee is okay in moderation, if you can tolerate it, and can help get you going in the morning. Tea, green or black, contains antioxidants that have been shown to have health benefits. Herbal teas can help increase fluid intake, as most don't contain caffeine. Decaffeinated choices are better for people who may feel jittery or nervous after drinking regular coffee or tea.

◆ *Sports drinks:* These drinks contain water, carbohydrates (glucose) for energy and the electrolytes sodium and potassium. They are a helpful fluid choice for physically active people. However, these drinks do not contain many nutrients and shouldn't be used to replace more nutrient-dense juices in a daily meal plan. They are higher in sodium and calories than most people, particularly children, need on a daily basis. These beverages are particularly problematic for children who choose them over more nutritious milk and juice and consume them in larger quantities than they really need.

top up your fluids

When you are adding more fiber to your diet, be sure to drink plenty of fluids. Extra fluid is required to help the fiber work properly and to help move high-fiber foods effectively through your digestive system.

shopping for the best nutrition

Getting the best nutrition begins at the grocery store. To make sure you bring home the products that will help you eat well, start by reading labels. Labels can help you choose foods that are higher in fiber, lower in saturated fat, free of trans fat, low in sodium, or packed with more nutrients. Here how labels can help you get the best nutrition.

using food labels

Food labels can help you to make the best food choices to suit your needs, whether you are looking for foods that are low in fat or salt or high in fiber. Food labels can also help you avoid ingredients that might trigger an allergic reaction or find foods that are culturally appropriate, such as kosher foods.

The ingredient list is a good place to start your research. Ingredients are listed by weight, from most to least. Those with the highest weight are listed first. If you are looking for whole-wheat bread, whole-wheat flour, not white flour, should be listed first on the ingredient list.

Food labels also include a nutrition facts table. This tells you about the nutrients you will get from eating the amount of food specified on the label. The % Daily Value is a simple benchmark for assessing the nutrient content of foods quickly. It shows you if the food has a lot or a little of a nutrient. The Daily Values are based on recommendations for a healthy diet. For example, a food that has a % Daily Value of 5% or less for fat, sodium or cholesterol would be low in these nutrients. A food that has a % Daily Value of 15% or more for calcium, iron or fiber would be high in these nutrients.

Nutrition claims on food labels can also help you decide what food is best for you. For example a label can help you find foods that are "lower in sodium or salt," "free of sugars," "free of trans fatty acids," or "a source of omega-3 polyunsaturated fatty acids." Government rules must be met before a nutrition claim can be made on a label or advertisement.

---

claims for vitamins or minerals

✦ **"A source of" or "contains":** provides greater than 5% of the recommended daily intake (RDI) of that vitamin or mineral per serving.

✦ **"A good source of" or "high in":** provides greater than or equal to 15% RDI (except for vitamin C, for which greater than or equal to 30% RDI must be provided).

✦ **"An excellent source of" or "very high in":** provides greater than or equal to 25% RDI (except for vitamin C, for which greater than or equal to 50% RDI must be provided).

---

understanding nutrition claims on labels

◆ **Fat-free:** contains less than 0.5 g fat per serving.

◆ **Low-fat:** contains 3 g or less fat per serving.

◆ **Saturated fat-free:** contains less than 0.2 g saturated fatty acids and less than 0.2 g trans fatty acids per serving.

◆ **Low in saturated fat:** contains 2 g or less saturated fatty acids and trans fatty acids combined per serving.

◆ **Free of trans fatty acids:** contains less than 0.2 g of trans fatty acids per serving and is low in saturated fat.

◆ **Source of omega-3 polyunsaturated fatty acids:** contains 0.3 g or more omega-3 fatty acids per serving.

◆ **Cholesterol-free:** contains less than 2 mg of cholesterol per serving and is low in saturated fat.

◆ **Low in cholesterol:** contains 20 mg or less of cholesterol per serving and is low in saturated fat.

◆ **Salt- or sodium-free:** contains less than 5 mg sodium per serving.

◆ **Low in sodium/salt:** contains 140 mg or less sodium per serving.

◆ **Sugar-free:** contains less than 0.5 g of sugars per serving.

◆ **Source of fiber:** contains 2 g or more fiber per serving.

◆ **High in fiber:** contains 4 g or more fiber per serving.

◆ **Very high in fiber:** contains 6 g or more fiber per serving.

◆ **Light (in energy or fat):** food must be reduced in energy or fat.

◆ **Lean:** contains 10% or less fat per serving of meat or poultry (*not* ground) or fish; for ground meat, not more than 17% fat per serving.

◆ **Extra lean:** contains 7.5% or less fat per serving of meat or poultry (*not* ground) or fish; for ground meat, not more than 10% fat per serving.

what's better — fresh, frozen, canned or organic?

What kinds of food you choose to buy depends on a number of factors: your personal preferences, availability, price and how fast you can use them. Here are some quick tips to help you choose what's best for you.

fresh

When buying fruits and vegetables, fresh is usually your best choice for nutrients — but only if fruit or vegetables are bought soon after they are picked, look good and haven't spoiled. You must also eat them within a reasonable amount of time. If you let your leafy greens wilt or take more than a few days to eat perishable fruit or vegetables you might be better off with frozen or even canned versions. That's because food loses nutrients as it begins to spoil.

Nutrient loss varies depending on the fruit or vegetable, as well as on how it is stored and how it is prepared and cooked. For example, if you keep asparagus at room temperature rather than in the refrigerator, about half its vitamin C content is lost within a couple of days. Vegetables and fruits lose nutrients when they are cut or shredded ahead of serving, stored in water in the refrigerator, overcooked or cooked in too much water. The more you cook, cut or mix fresh produce, the more you increase its exposure to oxygen and the greater the chances of losing valuable nutrients.

frozen

Frozen vegetables and fruits are a good alternative to fresh. Most vegetables and fruits are flash-frozen soon after they are picked, and therefore retain most of their nutrients, except for small amounts of vitamin C and other water-soluble vitamins.

Frozen vegetables are convenient and easy to use because most of the preparation work has been done. Like fresh vegetables, they need to be cooked properly to reduce nutrient losses. The best way to cooked frozen vegetables is to steam them. They can also be cooked in the microwave. To retain nutrients, add a couple of tablespoons of water, cover and cook at medium heat (60% to 80%). Cooking vegetables at extremely high temperatures, which is a problem with many new microwaves, can cause nutrient losses. Boiling them for too long or in too much water also increases nutrient losses.

Fruits such as strawberries and blueberries that are frozen whole, without sugar, are a good buy, especially when fresh varieties are not in season.

canned

Canned vegetables undergo a heating process that can destroy some of the vitamin C and B vitamins. Some canned vegetables contain a lot of sodium, so it's a good idea to check the label and buy sodium-reduced versions. Canned fruits do not lose as many nutrients as vegetables because they are processed at lower temperatures. Many fruits are packed in juice, which is a source of nutrients if eaten. Fruit packed in syrup is higher in sugar.

organic

Organic foods are increasingly available in food markets and mainstream grocery stores. Certified organic foods are meant to be free of pesticides, fertilizers and genetically engineered plants. But you should be aware that the majority of conventional fruits and vegetables produced today also have very little or no pesticide residues (certainly well below safety standards set by government agriculture and food regulations). Studies show that organic foods provide the same amount of nutrients as conventional foods, but they are not necessarily safer. The potential for microbial contamination during food production exists for both organic and conventional foods, and that depends on good growing, shipping, preparation and storage practices. Organic foods tend to cost more than conventional ones, so the choice is yours.

Starters

Chunky Artichoke Dip

1	can (19 oz/398 mL) artichoke hearts, drained	1
¼ cup	5% ricotta cheese	50 mL
¼ cup	light sour cream or 2% yogurt	50 mL
¼ cup	chopped fresh parsley	50 mL
¼ cup	chopped green onions, about 2 medium	50 mL
3 tbsp	light mayonnaise	45 mL
3 tbsp	grated Parmesan cheese	45 mL
1 tsp	minced garlic	5 mL

Serves 8

1. Put artichoke hearts, ricotta, sour cream, parsley, green onions, mayonnaise, Parmesan and garlic in food processor; process until slightly chunky.

Tips

✦ Serve with vegetables or crackers.

✦ To make tortilla or pita crisps for this or any other dip, cut tortilla or pita into wedges and put on a sprayed baking sheet. Brush lightly with oil and bake at 350°F (180°C) for 5 to 10 minutes, or until lightly browned.

✦ Serve either at room temperature or chilled.

Make Ahead

✦ Prepare up to a day in advance; stir before serving.

Nutritional Analysis (Per Serving)
✦ Calories: 56 ✦ Protein: 3 g ✦ Cholesterol: 6 mg
✦ Sodium: 198 mg ✦ Fat, total: 3 g ✦ Carbohydrates: 5 g
✦ Fiber: 0 g ✦ Fat, saturated: 0.9 g

Artichoke and Blue Cheese Dip

¾ cup	drained canned artichokes	175 mL
¼ cup	chopped green onions	50 mL
½ tsp	crushed garlic	2 mL
2 oz	blue cheese	50 g
1 tbsp	chopped fresh parsley	15 mL
¼ cup	2% yogurt	50 mL
	Salt and pepper	

Serves 4 to 6 or makes 1¼ cups (300 mL)

1. In food processor, combine artichokes, onions, garlic, cheese, parsley, yogurt, and salt and pepper to taste; process until smooth. Transfer to serving bowl.

Tips

✦ If a more subtle flavor is desired, cut back on the blue cheese, using only 1½ oz (40 g).

✦ Other strong cheeses, such as grated Parmesan or Swiss, can replace the blue cheese.

Make Ahead

✦ Make and refrigerate up to a day before. Stir just before serving.

Nutritional Analysis (Per Serving)
✦ Calories: 53 ✦ Protein: 3 g ✦ Cholesterol: 7 mg
✦ Sodium: 160 mg ✦ Fat: 3 g ✦ Carbohydrates: 4 g
✦ Fiber: 1 g

Hot Three-Cheese Dill Artichoke Bake

1	can (14 oz/398 mL) artichoke hearts, drained and halved	1
½ cup	shredded part-skim mozzarella cheese (about 2 oz/50 g)	125 mL
⅓ cup	shredded Swiss cheese (about 1½ oz/35 g)	75 mL
⅓ cup	minced fresh dill (or 1 tsp/5 mL dried)	75 mL
¼ cup	light sour cream	50 mL
3 tbsp	light mayonnaise	45 mL
1 tbsp	freshly squeezed lemon juice	15 mL
1 tsp	minced garlic	5 mL
Pinch	cayenne pepper	Pinch
1 tbsp	grated Parmesan cheese	15 mL

This tastes like the traditional hot artichoke dip loaded with fat and calories, but has less than half the fat.

Serves 6 to 8
Preheat oven to 350°F (180°C)
Small casserole dish

1. In a food processor, combine artichoke hearts, mozzarella and Swiss cheeses, dill, sour cream, mayonnaise, lemon juice, garlic and cayenne. Process on and off just until combined but still chunky. Place in a small casserole dish. Sprinkle with Parmesan cheese.
2. Bake uncovered 10 minutes. Broil 3 to 5 minutes just until top is slightly browned. Serve warm with crackers.

Tip
✦ Serve over French bread or with vegetables.

Make Ahead
✦ Prepare up to 1 day in advance. Bake just before serving.

Nutritional Analysis (Per Serving)
✦ Calories: 79 ✦ Protein: 5 g ✦ Cholesterol: 10 mg
✦ Sodium: 271 mg ✦ Fat, total: 5 g ✦ Carbohydrates: 6 g
✦ Fiber: 2 g ✦ Fat, saturated: 2 g

Avocado, Tomato and Chili Guacamole

Half	avocado, peeled	Half
¾ tsp	crushed garlic	4 mL
2 tbsp	chopped green onions	25 mL
1 tbsp	lemon juice	15 mL
¼ cup	finely diced sweet red pepper	50 mL
½ cup	chopped tomato	125 mL
Pinch	chili powder	Pinch

Serves 4 to 6 or makes ¾ cup (175 mL)

1. In bowl, combine avocado, garlic, onions, lemon juice, red pepper, tomato and chili powder; mash with fork, mixing well.

Tips
✦ Adjust the chili powder to your taste.
✦ Serve with pita bread, vegetables or crackers.

Make Ahead
✦ Make early in day and squeeze more lemon juice over top to prevent discoloration. Refrigerate. Stir just before serving.

Nutritional Analysis (Per Serving)
✦ Calories: 30 ✦ Protein: 0.5 g ✦ Cholesterol: 0 mg
✦ Sodium: 4 mg ✦ Fat: 2 g ✦ Carbohydrates: 2 g
✦ Fiber: 1 g

Avocado Tomato Salsa

2 cups	finely chopped plum tomatoes	500 mL
1/2 cup	finely chopped ripe but firm avocado (about 1/2 avocado)	125 mL
1/3 cup	chopped fresh coriander	75 mL
1/4 cup	chopped green onions (about 2 medium)	50 mL
1 tbsp	olive oil	15 mL
1 tbsp	lime or lemon juice	15 mL
1 tsp	minced garlic	5 mL
1/8 tsp	chili powder	1 mL

Serves 8

1. In serving bowl, combine tomatoes, avocado, coriander, green onions, olive oil, lime juice, garlic and chili powder; let marinate 1 hour before serving.

Tips

✦ Serve with crackers or tortilla crisps.

✦ For an authentic, intense flavor, use 1/2 tsp (2 mL) finely diced chili pepper, or more chili powder.

Make Ahead

✦ Prepare up to 4 hours ahead; stir before serving.

Nutritional Analysis (Per Serving)
✦ Calories: 53 ✦ Protein: 1 g ✦ Cholesterol: 0 mg
✦ Sodium: 8 mg ✦ Fat, total: 4 g ✦ Carbohydrates: 4 g
✦ Fiber: 1 g ✦ Fat, saturated: 0.6 g

Tuna and White Bean Spread

1 cup	canned, cooked white kidney beans, drained	250 mL
1	can (6.5 oz/184 g) tuna in water, drained	1
1 1/2 tsp	minced garlic	7 mL
2 tbsp	lemon juice	25 mL
2 tbsp	light mayonnaise	25 mL
1/4 cup	5% ricotta cheese	50 mL
3 tbsp	minced red onions	45 mL
1/4 cup	minced fresh dill (or 1 tsp/5 mL dried)	50 mL
1 tbsp	grated Parmesan cheese	15 mL
1/4 cup	diced red pepper	50 mL

Serves 8

1. Place beans, tuna, garlic, lemon juice, mayonnaise and ricotta in food processor; pulse on and off until combined but still chunky. Place in serving bowl.

2. Stir onions, dill, Parmesan and red pepper into bean mixture.

Tip

✦ White navy pea beans can also be used. If you cook your own dry beans, 1/2 cup (125 mL) dry yields approximately 1 1/2 cups (375 mL) cooked beans.

Make Ahead

✦ Prepare up to a day ahead; keep covered and refrigerated. Stir before using.

Nutritional Analysis (Per Serving)
✦ Calories: 73 ✦ Protein: 8 g ✦ Cholesterol: 6 mg
✦ Sodium: 188 mg ✦ Fat, total: 2 g ✦ Carbohydrates: 7 g
✦ Fiber: 2 g ✦ Fat, saturated: 0.5 g

White Bean and Roasted Pepper Bruschetta

1 cup	canned white kidney beans, rinsed and drained	250 mL
1/4 cup	chopped fresh basil (or 1/2 tsp/2 mL dried)	50 mL
1 1/2 tsp	freshly squeezed lemon juice	7 mL
1/2 tsp	minced garlic	2 mL
1/2 tsp	sesame oil	2 mL
1	baguette or thin French loaf	1
2 tbsp	chopped roasted red peppers	25 mL

Tired of garlic bread? This is a great alternative.

Serves 6 to 8
Preheat oven to 425°F (220°C)
Baking sheet

1. In a food processor, purée beans, basil, lemon juice, garlic and sesame oil until smooth.
2. Slice baguette into 1-inch (2.5 cm) slices. In a toaster oven or under a preheated broiler, toast until golden; turn and toast opposite side. Spread each slice with approximately 1 1/2 tsp (7 mL) bean mixture. Top with chopped red peppers.
3. Bake until warm, approximately 5 minutes.

Tips
✦ Double recipe and use as a dip.
✦ If fresh basil is not available, substitute parsley.
✦ Roast your own red bell peppers or buy water-packed roasted red peppers.

Make Ahead
✦ Prepare bean mixture up to 1 day in advance.

Nutritional Analysis (Per Serving)
✦ Calories: 197   ✦ Protein: 7 g   ✦ Cholesterol: 0 mg
✦ Sodium: 185 mg   ✦ Fat, total: 2 g   ✦ Carbohydrates: 37 g
✦ Fiber: 3 g   ✦ Fat, saturated: 0.4 g

Hummus (Chickpea Pâté)

1/4 cup	water	50 mL
1 cup	drained canned chickpeas	250 mL
3/4 tsp	crushed garlic	4 mL
2 tbsp	lemon juice	25 mL
4 tsp	olive oil	20 mL
1/4 cup	tahini	50 mL
1 tbsp	chopped fresh parsley	15 mL

Tahini is a Middle Eastern condiment found in the specialty section of some supermarkets. If not available, use smooth peanut butter.

Serves 4 to 6 or makes 1 cup (250 mL)

1. In food processor, combine water, chickpeas, garlic, lemon juice, oil and tahini; process until creamy and smooth.
2. Transfer to serving dish; sprinkle with parsley.

Tip
✦ Surround the dip with crackers, fresh vegetable sticks or pita bread pieces.

Make Ahead
✦ Prepare dip up to a day before. Stir just before serving and garnish with parsley.

Nutritional Analysis (Per Serving)
✦ Calories: 134   ✦ Protein: 4 g   ✦ Cholesterol: 0 mg
✦ Sodium: 80 mg   ✦ Fat: 9 g   ✦ Carbohydrates: 10 g
✦ Fiber: 2 g

Tofu and Chickpea Garlic Dip

1 cup	canned chickpeas, rinsed and drained	250 mL
8 oz	soft (silken) tofu, drained	250 g
2 tbsp	tahini	25 mL
2 tbsp	freshly squeezed lemon juice	25 mL
1 tsp	minced garlic	5 mL
1/4 cup	chopped fresh dill (or 1 tsp/5 mL dried)	50 mL
1/4 cup	chopped green onions	50 mL
1/4 cup	chopped green olives	50 mL
1/4 cup	chopped red bell peppers	50 mL
1/4 tsp	freshly ground black pepper	1 mL

Serves 6 to 8

1. In a food processor, combine chickpeas, tofu, tahini, lemon juice and garlic; purée. Stir in dill, green onions, olives, red peppers and pepper.
2. Chill. Serve with vegetables, crackers or bread.

Tip

✦ Be sure to buy soft (silken) tofu to ensure a creamy dip. Firm or pressed tofu will result in a granular texture.

Make Ahead

✦ Prepare up to 1 day in advance. Mix before serving.

Nutritional Analysis (Per Serving)
✦ Calories: 86 ✦ Protein: 5 g ✦ Cholesterol: 0 mg
✦ Sodium: 153 mg ✦ Fat, total: 4 g ✦ Carbohydrates: 8 g
✦ Fiber: 2 g ✦ Fat, saturated: 1 g

Spinach and Ricotta Dip

Half	package (10 oz/284 g) fresh spinach	Half
1/2 cup	2% yogurt	125 mL
3/4 cup	ricotta cheese	175 mL
1/2 tsp	crushed garlic	2 mL
2 tbsp	chopped fresh parsley	25 mL
2 tbsp	grated Parmesan cheese	25 mL
	Salt and pepper	

An interesting way to serve this is to hollow out a small round bread or roll. Fill with dip and use bread chunks as dippers. Or serve in a decorative bowl with vegetable sticks or crackers.

Serves 4 to 6 or makes 1 1/2 cups (375 mL)

1. Rinse spinach and shake off excess water. With just the water clinging to leaves, cook until wilted; drain and squeeze out excess moisture.
2. In food processor, combine spinach, yogurt, ricotta, garlic, parsley, Parmesan cheese, and salt and pepper to taste; process just until still chunky. Do not purée.

Tip

✦ You can cook half a package (5 oz/150 g) frozen spinach instead of the fresh, then continue with recipe.

Make Ahead

✦ Prepare and refrigerate up to a day before. Stir just before serving. (If filling bread, do so just prior to serving.)

Nutritional Analysis (Per Serving)
✦ Calories: 20 ✦ Protein: 1 g ✦ Cholesterol: 4 mg
✦ Sodium: 23 mg ✦ Fat: 1 g ✦ Carbohydrates: 1 g
✦ Fiber: 0 g

Ricotta and Blue Cheese Appetizers

2 oz	blue cheese	50 g
1/2 cup	ricotta cheese	125 mL
2 tbsp	2% yogurt	25 mL
2 tbsp	chopped fresh dill (or 1 tsp/5 mL dried dillweed)	25 mL
2	Belgian endives	2

Serves 4 to 6 or makes 25 hors d'oeuvres

1. In food processor, combine blue cheese, ricotta, yogurt and dill; process until creamy and smooth.
2. Separate Belgian endive leaves. Spoon 2 tsp (10 mL) cheese mixture onto stem end of each.

Tips

✦ For blue cheese lovers, increase to 3 oz (75 g).
✦ Instead of endive leaves, fill empty mushroom caps, or serve as a dip with crackers or vegetables.

Make Ahead

✦ Prepare dip and refrigerate up to a day before. Spoon onto endive leaves just before serving.

Nutritional Analysis (Per Serving)
- ✦ Calories: 87   ✦ Protein: 6 g   ✦ Cholesterol: 13 mg
- ✦ Sodium: 190 mg ✦ Fat: 4 g   ✦ Carbohydrates: 6 g
- ✦ Fiber: 3 g

Asparagus Wrapped with Ricotta Cheese and Ham

12	medium asparagus, trimmed	12
4 oz	ricotta cheese	125 g
1/4 tsp	crushed garlic	1 mL
1 tbsp	finely chopped green onion or chives	15 mL
	Salt and pepper	
4	thin slices cooked ham (about 4 oz/125 g)	4

Choose the greenest asparagus, with straight firm stalks. The tips should be tightly closed and firm.

Serves 4
Preheat oven to 400°F (200°C)
Baking sheet sprayed with nonstick vegetable spray

1. Steam or microwave asparagus just until tender-crisp; drain and let cool. Set aside.
2. In small bowl, combine cheese, garlic, onion, and salt and pepper to taste; mix well.
3. Spread evenly over each slice of ham. Top each with 3 asparagus and roll up. Place on baking sheet and bake for 3 to 4 minutes or until hot.

Tip

✦ Prosciutto, a salt-cured meat, can replace the ham.

Make Ahead

✦ Assemble rolls early in day and refrigerate. Serve cold or hot.

Nutritional Analysis (Per Serving)
- ✦ Calories: 94   ✦ Protein: 10 g   ✦ Cholesterol: 23 mg
- ✦ Sodium: 378 mg ✦ Fat: 4 g   ✦ Carbohydrates: 4 g
- ✦ Fiber: 1 g

Mushrooms Stuffed with Spinach and Ricotta Cheese

2 cups	fresh spinach	500 mL
16	medium mushrooms	16
1 tbsp	vegetable oil	15 mL
2 tsp	crushed garlic	10 mL
1/4 cup	finely chopped onions	50 mL
1/3 cup	ricotta cheese	75 mL
1 tbsp	grated Parmesan cheese	15 mL
	Salt and pepper	

Don't throw out those mushroom stems — use them in salads or soups, or sauté in a nonstick skillet and serve as a side vegetable dish.

Serves 8
Preheat oven to 400°F (200°C)
Baking sheet

1. Rinse spinach and shake off excess water. With just the water clinging to leaves, cook until wilted. Drain and squeeze out excess moisture; chop finely and set aside.

2. Remove stems from mushrooms. Place caps on baking sheet. Dice half of the stems and reserve. Use remaining stems for another use (see sidebar at left).

3. In small nonstick saucepan, heat oil; sauté garlic, onions and diced stems until softened. Add spinach and cook for 1 minute. Remove from heat.

4. Add ricotta, half the Parmesan, and salt and pepper to taste; mix well and carefully fill mushroom caps. Sprinkle with remaining Parmesan. Bake for 8 to 10 minutes or just until mushrooms release their liquid.

Tips

✦ Instead of fresh spinach, you can use 1/3 cup (75 mL) frozen spinach, cooked and well drained.

✦ Cherry tomatoes can replace the mushrooms.

✦ Serve as an appetizer or side dish.

Make Ahead

✦ Prepare early in day and refrigerate. Bake just before serving.

Nutritional Analysis (Per Serving)
✦ Calories: 51   ✦ Protein: 2 g   ✦ Cholesterol: 5 mg
✦ Sodium: 33 mg   ✦ Fat: 3 g   ✦ Carbohydrates: 3 g
✦ Fiber: 1 g

Brie-Stuffed Mushrooms

16 to 20	medium mushrooms	16 to 20
2 oz	Brie cheese	50 g
1/4 cup	chopped roasted red peppers	50 mL
1/4 cup	chopped green onions	50 mL
3 tbsp	dried bread crumbs	45 mL
1 tsp	minced garlic	5 mL
1/2 tsp	dried basil	2 mL

Roast your own red bell peppers or buy water-packed roasted red peppers.

Use another soft cheese of your choice to replace the Brie.

Serves 4
Preheat oven to 400°F (200°C)
Baking sheet

1. Wipe mushrooms; remove stems and reserve for another use (see sidebar, page 38.) Place caps on baking sheet.
2. In a small bowl, stir together Brie, red peppers, green onions, bread crumbs, garlic and basil. Divide mixture among mushroom caps, approximately 1½ tsp (7 mL) per cap.
3. Bake 15 minutes, or until mushrooms release their liquid. Serve warm or at room temperature.

Make Ahead
✦ Fill mushroom caps up to 1 day in advance. Bake just before serving.

Nutritional Analysis (Per Serving)
✦ Calories: 86 ✦ Protein: 5 g ✦ Cholesterol: 13 mg
✦ Sodium: 205 mg ✦ Fat, total: 4 g ✦ Carbohydrates: 9 g
✦ Fiber: 1 g ✦ Fat, saturated: 2 g

Marinated Greek Mushrooms

1 lb	button mushrooms, cleaned	500 g
1/2 cup	chopped fresh coriander	125 mL
1/2 cup	chopped red onions	125 mL
1/3 cup	sliced black olives	75 mL
1/3 cup	balsamic vinegar	75 mL
2 tbsp	water	25 mL
2 tbsp	olive oil	25 mL
1 tbsp	freshly squeezed lemon juice	15 mL
1 tsp	minced garlic	5 mL
1/2 to 3/4 tsp	chili powder or ½ tsp (2 mL) minced fresh jalapeño pepper	2 to 4 mL
1/4 tsp	freshly ground black pepper	1 mL
2 oz	feta cheese, crumbled	50 g

To make this a vegan dish, just eliminate the cheese.

Serves 6 to 8

1. In a large bowl, stir together mushrooms, coriander, red onions, olives, vinegar, water, olive oil, lemon juice, garlic, chili powder, pepper and feta.
2. Cover and chill 1 hour or overnight, mixing occasionally.

Tips
✦ The longer the mushrooms marinate, the more flavorful they will be.
✦ If you can't find small button mushrooms, use larger mushrooms, and cut into quarters.

Make Ahead
✦ Prepare 1 day in advance. Stir before serving.

Nutritional Analysis (Per Serving)
✦ Calories: 71 ✦ Protein: 2 g ✦ Cholesterol: 6 mg
✦ Sodium: 125 mg ✦ Fat, total: 5 g ✦ Carbohydrates: 5 g
✦ Fiber: 1 g ✦ Fat, saturated: 2 g

Sautéed Mushrooms on Toast Rounds

2 tsp	vegetable oil	10 mL	
1 tsp	crushed garlic	5 mL	
2 tbsp	finely chopped onions	25 mL	
½ lb	mushrooms, chopped	250 g	
1 tbsp	chopped fresh parsley	15 mL	
2 tbsp	white wine	25 mL	
2 tbsp	chopped green onions or chives	25 mL	
1 tsp	soya sauce	5 mL	
2 tbsp	dry bread crumbs	25 mL	
2 tbsp	grated Parmesan cheese	25 mL	
	Salt and pepper		
16	slices small rye bread or French baguette	16	

This mixture can also be served in whole mushroom caps.

Serves 4 to 6 or makes 16 hors d'oeuvres
Preheat broiler

1. In small nonstick saucepan, heat oil; sauté garlic, onions and mushrooms until softened, approximately 5 minutes.

2. Add parsley, wine, green onions, soya sauce, bread crumbs, 1 tbsp (15 mL) of the Parmesan, and salt and pepper to taste; cook for 2 minutes. Set aside.

3. On baking sheet, toast bread in oven just until browned on both sides, approximately 2 minutes (or brown in toaster). Divide mushroom mixture over bread; sprinkle with remaining Parmesan. Broil for 5 minutes or until hot, being careful not to burn.

Make Ahead

✦ Prepare mushroom mixture early in day and keep at room temperature. Assemble and broil just before serving.

Nutritional Analysis (Per Serving)
✦ Calories: 75   ✦ Protein: 2 g   ✦ Cholesterol: 1 mg
✦ Sodium: 193 mg ✦ Fat: 2 g   ✦ Carbohydrates: 11 g
✦ Fiber: 2 g

Roasted Garlic Sweet Pepper Strips

4	large sweet peppers (combination of green, red and yellow)	4
2 tbsp	olive oil	25 mL
1½ tsp	crushed garlic	7 mL
1 tbsp	grated Parmesan cheese	15 mL

When shopping, be critical of the foods you put in your cart. Stick to the freshest and healthiest foods possible. Keep the sweet and salty treats out of your cart — if they're not in the house, you're less likely to eat them.

Serves 4
Preheat oven to 400°F (200°C)

1. On baking sheet, bake whole peppers for 15 to 20 minutes, turning occasionally, or until blistered and blackened. Place in paper bag; seal and let stand for 10 minutes.
2. Peel off charred skin from peppers; cut off tops and bottoms. Remove seeds and ribs; cut into 1 inch (2.5 cm) wide strips and place on serving platter.
3. Mix oil with garlic; brush over peppers. Sprinkle with cheese.

Tip
✦ Add a sprinkle of fresh herbs such as parsley or basil to oil mixture.

Make Ahead
✦ These peppers can be prepared ahead of time and served cold.

Nutritional Analysis (Per Serving)
✦ Calories: 95   ✦ Protein: 1 g   ✦ Cholesterol: 1 mg
✦ Sodium: 26 mg   ✦ Fat: 7 g   ✦ Carbohydrates: 7 g
✦ Fiber: 2 g

Spicy Mexican Dip

1 cup	canned refried beans	250 mL
⅓ cup	minced red onion	75 mL
⅓ cup	finely diced sweet red pepper	75 mL
¾ tsp	crushed garlic	4 mL
2 tsp	chili powder	10 mL
2 tbsp	chopped fresh parsley	25 mL
2 tbsp	2% yogurt	25 mL
2 tsp	lemon juice	10 mL
3 tbsp	crushed bran cereal*	45 mL
	Parsley sprigs	

* Use a wheat bran breakfast cereal

Serves 6 to 8 or makes 2 cups (500 mL)

1. In bowl, combine beans, onion, red pepper, garlic, chili powder, parsley, yogurt, lemon juice and cereal; stir until blended. Place in serving bowl and garnish with parsley sprigs.

Tips
✦ Serve with crackers, vegetables or pita bread.
✦ This dip can also be placed in a flour tortilla and slightly warmed.

Make Ahead
✦ Make and refrigerate up to a day before. Stir before garnishing.

Nutritional Analysis (Per Serving)
✦ Calories: 11   ✦ Protein: 0.6 g   ✦ Cholesterol: 0 mg
✦ Sodium: 37 mg   ✦ Fat: 0 g   ✦ Carbohydrates: 2 g
✦ Fiber: 0.5 g

Creamy Pesto Dip

1 cup	well-packed basil leaves	250 mL
2 tbsp	toasted pine nuts	25 mL
2 tbsp	grated Parmesan cheese	25 mL
2 tbsp	olive oil	25 mL
2 tsp	lemon juice	10 mL
1 tsp	minced garlic	5 mL
1/2 cup	5% ricotta cheese	125 mL
1/4 cup	light sour cream	50 mL

Toast pine nuts in nonstick skillet over medium-high heat for 3 minutes, stirring occasionally. Or put them on a baking sheet and toast in a 400°F (200°F) oven for 5 minutes. Whichever method you choose, watch carefully — nuts burn quickly.

Serves 6 to 8

1. Put basil, pine nuts, Parmesan, olive oil, lemon juice and garlic in food processor; process until finely chopped, scraping sides of bowl down once. Add ricotta and sour cream and process until smooth. Serve with pita or tortilla crisps, or fresh vegetables.

Tip

✦ If basil is not available, use parsley or spinach leaves.

Make Ahead

✦ Prepare early in the day and keep covered and refrigerated.

Nutritional Analysis (Per Serving)
✦ Calories: 67 ✦ Protein: 4 g ✦ Cholesterol: 8 mg
✦ Sodium: 53 mg ✦ Fat, total: 5 g ✦ Carbohydrates: 2 g
✦ Fiber: 0 g ✦ Fat, saturated: 2 g

Creamy Sun-Dried Tomato Dip

4 oz	dry-packed sun-dried tomatoes	125 g
3/4 cup	5% ricotta cheese	175 mL
1/2 cup	chopped fresh parsley	125 mL
1/3 cup	Basic Vegetable Stock (see recipe, page 52) or water	75 mL
3 tbsp	chopped black olives	45 mL
2 tbsp	olive oil	25 mL
2 tbsp	toasted pine nuts (see sidebar, above)	25 mL
2 tbsp	grated Parmesan cheese	25 mL
1 tsp	minced garlic	5 mL

Avoid sun-dried tomatoes packed in oil; these have a lot extra calories and fat.

Serves 8

1. In a small bowl, pour boiling water to cover over sun-dried tomatoes. Let stand 15 minutes. Drain and chop.

2. In a food processor combine sun-dried tomatoes, ricotta, parsley, stock, olives, olive oil, pine nuts, Parmesan and garlic; process until well combined but still chunky. Makes 1¾ cups (425 mL).

Tips

✦ Great as a topping with crackers or baguettes or as a dip for vegetables or baked tortilla chips.

✦ Use as a topping for cooked vegetables or on non-vegetarian days for fish or chicken.

Make Ahead

✦ Prepare and refrigerate up to 3 days before.

Nutritional Analysis (Per Serving)
✦ Calories: 113 ✦ Protein: 7 g ✦ Cholesterol: 7 mg
✦ Sodium: 413 mg ✦ Fat, total: 6 g ✦ Carbohydrates: 10 g
✦ Fiber: 3 g ✦ Fat, saturated: 2 g

Eggplant, Tomato and Fennel Appetizer

2 tsp	vegetable oil	10 mL
2 tsp	minced garlic	10 mL
1 cup	chopped fennel	250 mL
1 cup	chopped onions	250 mL
1 cup	chopped red bell peppers	250 mL
3 cups	diced unpeeled eggplant	750 mL
2 cups	chopped plum tomatoes	500 mL
1/4 cup	sliced green olives	50 mL
1 1/2 tbsp	balsamic vinegar	22 mL
4 tsp	drained capers	20 mL
2 tsp	dried basil	10 mL

For an interesting salad, omit Step 2, then serve chilled on top of green beans.

Serves 6

1. In a nonstick saucepan, heat oil over medium-high heat. Add garlic, fennel, onions and red peppers; cook, stirring occasionally, 4 minutes. Add eggplant; cook 5 minutes longer, stirring occasionally. Stir in tomatoes, olives, vinegar, capers and basil; reduce heat to medium-low and simmer 15 minutes.
2. Transfer to a food processor; pulse on and off until chunky. Chill.

Make Ahead

✦ Prepare and refrigerate up to 2 days before.

Nutritional Analysis (Per Serving)
- ✦ Calories: 69
- ✦ Sodium: 529 mg
- ✦ Fiber: 4 g
- ✦ Protein: 2 g
- ✦ Fat, total: 3 g
- ✦ Fat, saturated: 0.3 g
- ✦ Cholesterol: 0 mg
- ✦ Carbohydrates: 11 g

Eggplant and Tuna Antipasto Appetizer

1 tbsp	olive oil	15 mL
1 1/2 cups	peeled, chopped eggplant	375 mL
1 cup	sliced mushrooms	250 mL
3/4 cup	chopped red peppers	175 mL
1/2 cup	chopped onions	125 mL
2 tsp	minced garlic	10 mL
1 tsp	dried basil	5 mL
1/2 tsp	dried oregano	2 mL
1/2 cup	chicken stock or water	125 mL
1/2 cup	crushed tomatoes (canned or fresh)	125 mL
1/3 cup	sliced pimiento-stuffed green olives	75 mL
1/3 cup	bottled chili sauce	75 mL
2 tsp	drained capers	10 mL
1	can (6.5 oz/184 g) tuna in water, drained	1

This antipasto is also delicious as a sauce over 8 oz (250 g) of pasta.

Serves 8 to 10

1. Spray a nonstick pan with vegetable spray. Heat oil in pan over medium-high heat; add eggplant, mushrooms, red peppers, onions, garlic, basil and oregano. Cook for 8 minutes, stirring occasionally, or until vegetables are softened.
2. Add stock, tomatoes, olives, chili sauce and capers; simmer uncovered for 6 minutes, stirring occasionally until most of the liquid is absorbed.
3. Transfer to bowl of food processor and add tuna; process for 20 seconds or until combined but still chunky.

Make Ahead

✦ Prepare up to 2 days before and keep refrigerated. Stir before serving cold or reheating to serve with crackers or French bread.

Nutritional Analysis (Per Serving)
- ✦ Calories: 65
- ✦ Sodium: 411 mg
- ✦ Fiber: 2 g
- ✦ Protein: 5 g
- ✦ Fat, total: 2 g
- ✦ Fat, saturated: 0.4 g
- ✦ Cholesterol: 3 mg
- ✦ Carbohydrates: 6 g

Leek Mushroom Cheese Pâté

2 tsp	vegetable oil	10 mL
1½ tsp	minced garlic	7 mL
1½ cups	chopped leeks	375 mL
½ cup	finely chopped carrots	125 mL
12 oz	oyster or regular mushrooms, thinly sliced	375 g
2 tbsp	sherry or white wine	25 mL
2 tbsp	chopped fresh dill (or 2 tsp/10 mL dried)	25 mL
1½ tsp	dried oregano	7 mL
¼ tsp	coarsely ground black pepper	1 mL
2 oz	feta cheese, crumbled	50 g
2 oz	light cream cheese	50 g
½ cup	5% ricotta cheese	125 mL
2 tsp	freshly squeezed lemon juice	10 mL
2 tbsp	chopped fresh dill	25 mL

If using wild mushrooms, try shiitake or cremini.

Serves 8 to 10
9- by 5-inch (2 L) loaf pan lined with plastic wrap

1. In a large nonstick frying pan sprayed with vegetable spray, heat oil over medium-high heat. Add garlic, leeks and carrots; cook 3 minutes, stirring occasionally. Stir in mushrooms, sherry, dill, oregano and pepper; cook, stirring occasionally, 8 to 10 minutes or until carrots are tender and liquid is absorbed. Remove from heat.

2. Transfer vegetable mixture to a food processor. Add feta, cream cheese, ricotta and lemon juice; purée until smooth. Spoon into prepared loaf pan. Cover and chill until firm.

3. Invert onto serving platter; sprinkle with chopped dill. Serve with crackers, bread or vegetables.

Make Ahead
+ Prepare and refrigerate up to 2 days before.

Nutritional Analysis (Per Serving)
+ Calories: 75   + Protein: 4 g   + Cholesterol: 11 mg
+ Sodium: 17 mg   + Fat, total: 3 g   + Carbohydrates: 6 g
+ Fiber: 1 g   + Fat, saturated: 2 g

Sautéed Vegetable Feta Cheese Spread

½ cup	chopped carrots	125 mL
2 tsp	vegetable oil	10 mL
2 tsp	minced garlic	10 mL
¾ cup	chopped red bell peppers	175 mL
¾ cup	chopped leeks	175 mL
½ cup	chopped onions	125 mL
¼ cup	sliced black olives	50 mL
2 tbsp	light sour cream	25 mL
2 tbsp	light mayonnaise	25 mL
1 tbsp	freshly squeezed lemon juice	15 mL
½ tsp	dried oregano	2 mL
2 oz	feta cheese, crumbled	50 g

Serves 6 to 8

1. Boil or steam carrots just until tender, about 5 minutes. Drain, and set aside.

2. In a saucepan heat oil over medium-low heat. Add garlic, red peppers, leeks, onions and carrots; cook, stirring occasionally, for 5 minutes or until tender. Cool.

3. In a food processor combine cooled vegetables, black olives, sour cream, mayonnaise, lemon juice, oregano and feta. Process to desired consistency. Serve with crackers or vegetables.

Make Ahead
+ Prepare and refrigerate up to 2 days before.

Nutritional Analysis (Per Serving)
+ Calories: 72   + Protein: 2 g   + Cholesterol: 6 mg
+ Sodium: 134 mg   + Fat, total: 4 g   + Carbohydrates: 8 g
+ Fiber: 1 g   + Fat, saturated: 1 g

Fettuccine Baskets with Zucchini Parmesan

6 oz	fettuccine (regular or spinach), broken into pieces	175 g
1	large egg	1
2 tbsp	grated low-fat Parmesan cheese	25 mL
1/2 tsp	dried basil	2 mL
2 tsp	vegetable oil	10 mL
Half	small zucchini, thinly sliced	Half
1/2 cup	tomato pasta sauce	125 mL
1/2 cup	shredded low-fat mozzarella cheese	125 mL

Watching your fat and cholesterol intake? A large whole egg has 75 calories, 5 g fat and 213 mg of cholesterol. The yolk accounts for 59 of the calories and all of the fat and cholesterol. Egg whites, on the other hand, are pure protein and zero fat. So just substitute 2 egg whites for 1 whole egg and you'll never know the difference. Of course, you can still use whole eggs in moderation — as we do here, dividing one between 6 servings.

Serves 6
Preheat oven to 400°F (200°C)
12 muffin cups sprayed with vegetable spray
Baking sheet

1. In a pot of boiling water, cook fettuccine for 8 to 10 minutes or until tender but firm; drain. In a bowl combine pasta, egg, 1 tbsp (15 mL) Parmesan cheese, basil and oil. Spoon mixture into prepared muffin cups. Bake in preheated oven for 20 minutes. Transfer pasta baskets to baking sheet.

2. Meanwhile, in a nonstick frying pan sprayed with vegetable spray, cook zucchini over medium-high heat for 5 minutes or until golden and tender.

3. Spoon tomato sauce over pasta baskets. Top with zucchini slices; sprinkle with mozzarella cheese and remaining Parmesan cheese. Bake in preheated oven for 5 minutes or until cheese melts.

Tip

✦ For a totally different flavor and texture, try replacing the fettuccine with linguine or spaghetti and the zucchini with diced red or green bell peppers. In place of the tomato sauce, try 1/3 cup (75 mL) pesto or sun-dried tomato pesto and replace the mozzarella cheese with 1 oz (25 g) goat cheese. Mmmm — these new flavors are fantastic!

Nutritional Analysis (Per Serving)
✦ Calories: 188   ✦ Protein: 8 g   ✦ Cholesterol: 32 mg
✦ Sodium: 197 mg   ✦ Fat, total: 6 g   ✦ Carbohydrates: 26 g
✦ Fiber: 1 g   ✦ Fat, saturated: 1.9 g

Bruschetta with Basil and Oregano

2	small tomatoes, diced	2
2 tbsp	olive oil	25 mL
1 tsp	crushed garlic	5 mL
2 tbsp	chopped fresh basil (or 1 tsp/5 mL dried)	25 mL
1 tbsp	chopped fresh oregano (or 1/2 tsp/2 mL dried)	15 mL
1 tbsp	chopped green onion	15 mL
12	slices (1/2 inch/1 cm thick) French bread	12
1 tbsp	grated Parmesan cheese	15 mL

Vary the bruschetta by adding 3 tbsp (45 mL) finely diced yellow or red pepper or red onion to mixture. Or sprinkle 2 tbsp (25 mL) diced sun-dried tomatoes over slices just before broiling.

Serves 4 to 6 or makes 12 slices
Preheat broiler

1. In small bowl, combine tomatoes, oil, garlic, basil, oregano and onion. Let stand for at least 20 minutes.
2. Toast bread on baking sheet under broiler, turning once, until brown on both sides. Divide tomato mixture over bread; sprinkle with cheese. Broil for 2 minutes or until heated through.

Make Ahead
+ Prepare tomato mixture early in day and marinate to allow flavors to blend well. Bake just before serving.

Nutritional Analysis (Per Serving)
+ Calories: 93
+ Protein: 2 g
+ Cholesterol: 0 mg
+ Sodium: 148 mg
+ Fat: 2 g
+ Carbohydrates: 15 g
+ Fiber: 1 g

Double Salmon and Dill Pâté

1 cup	5% ricotta cheese	250 mL
1	can (7.5 oz/213 g) salmon, drained and skin removed	1
1/4 cup	chopped green onions (about 2 medium)	50 mL
3 tbsp	chopped fresh dill (or 1 tsp/5 mL dried dillweed)	45 mL
2 tbsp	lemon juice	25 mL
4 oz	smoked salmon, cut into thin shreds	125 g

Serves 8

1. Place ricotta, canned salmon, green onions, dill and lemon juice in bowl of food processor; process for 20 seconds or until smooth.
2. Transfer mixture to serving bowl and fold in shredded smoked salmon. Serve with crackers.

Tips
+ Leaving in the bones from the canned salmon increases the calcium content.
+ Leftover cooked salmon can also be used instead of canned.
+ Also tastes great as a spread on French bread or served with vegetables.

Make Ahead
+ Prepare up to a day ahead and keep refrigerated.

Nutritional Analysis (Per Serving)
+ Calories: 91
+ Protein: 10 g
+ Cholesterol: 18 mg
+ Sodium: 237 mg
+ Fat, total: 4 g
+ Carbohydrates: 1 g
+ Fiber: 0 g
+ Fat, saturated: 2 g

Smoked Salmon and Goat Cheese Cucumber Slices

3 oz	smoked salmon, diced	75 g
3 oz	goat cheese	75 g
2 tbsp	2% yogurt	25 mL
1/2 tsp	lemon juice	2 mL
4 tsp	chopped fresh dill (or 1/2 tsp/2 mL dried dillweed)	20 mL
25	slices (1/4 inch/5 mm thick) cucumber	25

Goat cheese, also known as chèvre, comes in a variety of shapes, ranging from logs to pyramids to discs. Some are sprinkled with herbs and spices throughout. Use any variety. Serve also as a dip or serve on celery sticks or in hollow cherry tomatoes.

Serves 4 to 6 or makes 25 hors d'oeuvres

1. Reserve about 25 bits of salmon for garnish.
2. In bowl or using food processor, combine goat cheese, yogurt, remaining salmon, lemon juice and dill; mix with fork or using on/off motion just until combined but not puréed.
3. Place spoonful of filling on each cucumber slice. Garnish with bit of reserved salmon.

Make Ahead

✦ Prepare and refrigerate mixture up to a day before. Place on cucumber slices just before serving.

Nutritional Analysis (Per Serving)
- ✦ Calories: 14
- ✦ Protein: 1 g
- ✦ Cholesterol: 4 mg
- ✦ Sodium: 66 mg
- ✦ Fat: 1 g
- ✦ Carbohydrates: 0 g
- ✦ Fiber: 0 g

Crab Celery Sticks

1	can (4.2 oz/120 g) crabmeat, well drained	1
1/4 cup	sliced green onions	50 mL
1/4 tsp	crushed garlic	1 mL
3 tbsp	chopped fresh dill (or 1 tsp/5 mL dried dillweed)	45 mL
1 tbsp	lemon juice	15 mL
1/4 cup	chopped celery	50 mL
1/4 cup	chopped sweet red or green pepper	50 mL
2 tbsp	2% yogurt	25 mL
1/4 cup	light mayonnaise	50 mL
	Salt and pepper	
24	pieces (2 inch/5 cm) celery stalks	24
	Paprika	

Serves 4 to 6 or makes 24 hors d'oeuvres

1. In food processor, combine crabmeat, onions, garlic, dill, lemon juice, chopped celery, red pepper, yogurt and mayonnaise. Using on/off motion, process just until combined but still chunky. Season with salt and pepper to taste.
2. Stuff each celery stalk evenly with mixture. Sprinkle with paprika to taste.

Tips

✦ Serve as a dip with vegetables or broiled on top of pitas or English muffins.

✦ For a less expensive version, use imitation crab, often called Surimi.

Make Ahead

✦ Make and refrigerate filling early in day. Stir well and pour off any excess liquid before filling celery.

Nutritional Analysis (Per Serving)
- ✦ Calories: 15
- ✦ Protein: 1 g
- ✦ Cholesterol: 5 mg
- ✦ Sodium: 35 mg
- ✦ Fat: 1 g
- ✦ Carbohydrates: 0.6 g
- ✦ Fiber: 0 g

Fresh Mussels with Tomato Salsa

24	mussels	24
½ cup	water or wine	125 mL
¾ cup	finely chopped onions	175 mL
1½ tsp	crushed garlic	7 mL
1 cup	coarsely chopped tomato	250 mL
4 tsp	chopped fresh basil (or ½ tsp/2 mL dried)	20 mL
2 tbsp	chopped fresh parsley	25 mL
2 tsp	olive oil	10 mL
¼ tsp	chili powder	1 mL
	Salt and pepper	

You can't change the shape you were born with, but you can change your food and activity habits to achieve a healthier weight. Set small goals for eating better and being more active — goals you can achieve and live with.

Serves 4 to 6 or makes 24 hors d'oeuvres

1. Scrub mussels under cold running water; remove any beards. Discard any mussels that do not close when tapped.

2. In saucepan, combine mussels, water, ¼ cup (50 mL) of the onions and 1 tsp (5 mL) of the garlic; cover and steam just until mussels open, approximately 5 minutes. Discard any that do not open. Let cool then remove mussels from shells, reserving half of shell. Place mussels in bowl.

3. In food processor, combine remaining ½ cup (125 mL) onions and ½ tsp (2 mL) garlic, tomatoes, basil, parsley, oil, chili powder, and salt and pepper to taste; process using on/off motion just until chunky. Do not purée. Add to mussels and stir to mix. Refrigerate until chilled.

4. Divide mussel mixture evenly among reserved shells and arrange on serving plate.

Tips

+ Substitute fresh coriander for the parsley for a change.
+ This recipe can also be made with fresh clams.
+ Serve as a salad over lettuce.

Make Ahead

+ Prepare and refrigerate mixture early in day to allow flavors to blend. Spoon into shells a couple of hours prior to serving and keep chilled.

Nutritional Analysis (Per Serving)
+ Calories: 18
+ Protein: 2 g
+ Cholesterol: 5 mg
+ Sodium: 47 mg
+ Fat: 0.5 g
+ Carbohydrates: 1 g
+ Fiber: 0 g

Fettuccine Baskets with Zucchini Parmesan (page 45) ➤

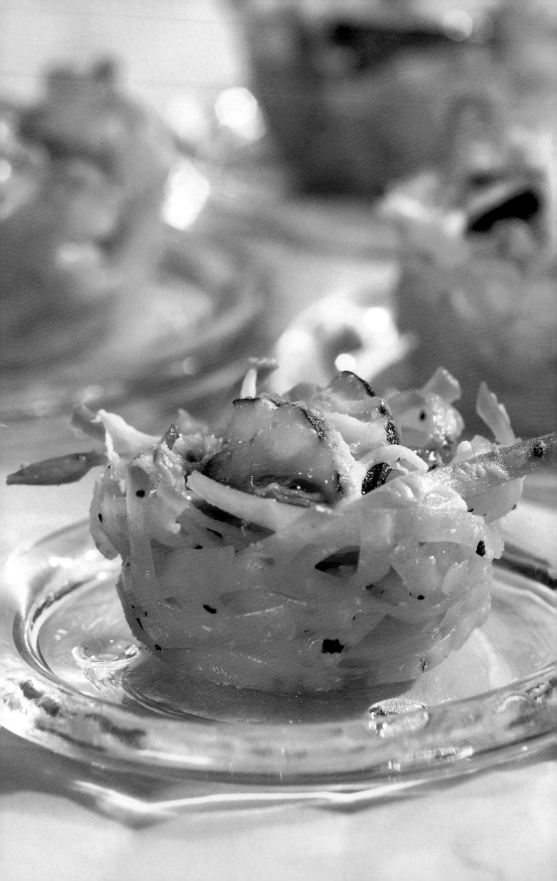

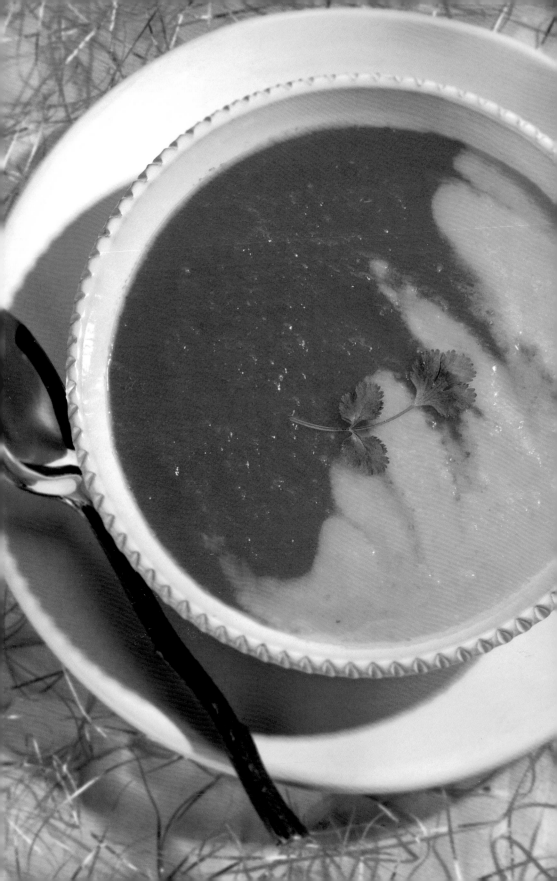

Oriental Chicken Wrapped Mushrooms

1 tbsp	rice wine vinegar	15 mL
1 tbsp	vegetable oil	15 mL
2 tbsp	soya sauce	25 mL
1 tsp	crushed garlic	5 mL
2 tbsp	finely chopped onion	25 mL
1 tsp	sesame oil	5 mL
2 tbsp	water	25 mL
2 tbsp	brown sugar	25 mL
1/2 tsp	sesame seeds (optional)	2 mL
3/4 lb	boneless skinless chicken breast	375 g
18	medium mushroom caps (without stems)	18

Soya sauce is a big flavor booster in recipes. But if you're concerned about sodium, watch out — soya sauce is like bottled salt! What to do? Well, you can buy light soya sauce (which has 50% less sodium) or you can just dilute 2 parts regular soya sauce with 1 part water.

Serves 4 to 6 or makes 18 hors d'oeuvres
Preheat broiler
Baking sheet sprayed with nonstick vegetable spray

1. In bowl, combine vinegar, oil, soya sauce, garlic, onion, sesame oil, water, sugar, and sesame seeds (if using); mix well.
2. Cut chicken into strips about 3 inches (8 cm) long and 1 inch (2.5 cm) wide to make 18 strips. Add to bowl and marinate for 20 minutes, stirring occasionally.
3. Wrap each chicken strip around mushroom; secure with toothpick. Place on baking sheet. Broil for approximately 5 minutes or until chicken is no longer pink inside. Serve immediately.

Tip
✦ Tender beef is delicious with this sweet oriental sauce.

Make Ahead
✦ Refrigerate chicken in marinade early in day.
✦ Wrap chicken around mushroom caps and broil just before serving.

Nutritional Analysis (Per Serving)
✦ Calories: 131 ✦ Protein: 14 g ✦ Cholesterol: 31 mg
✦ Sodium: 376 mg ✦ Fat: 5 g ✦ Carbohydrates: 8 g
✦ Fiber: 1 g

◄ Red and Yellow Bell Pepper Soup (page 67)

Chicken Satay with Peanut Sauce

1 lb	skinless, boneless chicken breasts	500 g
Peanut Sauce		
2 tbsp	peanut butter	25 mL
2 tbsp	chicken stock	25 mL
2 tbsp	chopped fresh coriander	25 mL
1 tbsp	rice wine vinegar	15 mL
1 tbsp	honey	15 mL
2 tsp	sesame oil	10 mL
2 tsp	soya sauce	10 mL
1 tsp	minced garlic	5 mL
1 tsp	minced gingerroot	5 mL
1 tsp	sesame seeds, toasted	5 mL

Eat only as much as you need. Avoid temptations to overeat. A little bit is good, a lot is not. If you eat more than you need to on a regular basis, weight gain is sure to follow.

Serves 5
Preheat oven to 425°F (220°C)
Baking pan sprayed with vegetable spray

1. In small bowl or food processor, combine peanut butter, chicken stock, coriander, vinegar, honey, sesame oil, soya sauce, garlic, ginger and sesame seeds. Set 3 tbsp (45 mL) aside.

2. Cut chicken into 1-inch (2.5 cm) cubes. Thread onto 10 small bamboo or barbecue skewers. Place skewers in prepared pan. Brush with half of the peanut sauce that has been set aside. Bake approximately 5 minutes. Turn over and brush the remaining 1½ tbsp (20 mL) sauce and bake 5 more minutes or just until chicken is done. Serve with remaining peanut sauce.

Tip

✦ These satays can be barbecued for approximately 10 minutes or until chicken is cooked.

✦ Chicken can be replaced with fresh salmon, pork or beef.

✦ This sauce can be used as a marinade for beef or fish.

✦ These appetizers have a fair amount of protein. Have a main course with less protein.

✦ Toast sesame seeds in nonstick skillet over high heat for 2 to 3 minutes.

Make Ahead

✦ Prepare sauce up to 2 days in advance. Keep refrigerated.

Nutritional Analysis (Per Serving)
✦ Calories: 167   ✦ Protein: 23 g   ✦ Cholesterol: 553 mg
✦ Sodium: 218 mg   ✦ Fat, total: 6 g   ✦ Carbohydrates: 5 g
✦ Fiber: 1 g   ✦ Fat, saturated: 1 g

Soups

Basic Vegetable Stock

8 cups	fresh water or cooking water	2 L
2	stalks celery, chopped	2
2	large onions, chopped	2
2	large carrots, washed and chopped	2
4	cloves garlic, chopped	4
4	bay leaves	4
4	whole cloves (or pinch ground)	4
10	peppercorns, crushed	10
1/4 cup	chopped fresh parsley (or 1/4 tsp/1 mL dried)	50 mL
1/4 tsp	salt (optional)	1 mL

Makes 8 cups (2 L)

1. Combine all ingredients in a large pot. Bring to simmer and cook, uncovered, for 45 minutes.
2. Remove from heat; let cool. Strain, discarding solids. Store in a container with tight-fitting lid. Stock will keep 1 week in refrigerator and several months if frozen.

Stock Tips

✦ Use vegetable bouillon cubes, powder or canned vegetable bouillon.

✦ Freeze in 1-cup (250 mL) portions; label and date.

✦ Substitute other vegetables of your choice. Try fennel, mushrooms, leeks, potatoes, yams or lettuce.

If you're looking for a snack to keep you going until dinner, try heating a mug of broth. One cup (250 mL) chicken or vegetable stock contains only 31 calories and zero fat. (Beef broth has just 1 g fat.)

Vegetable Stock

6 cups	water	1.5 L
1	large sweet potato, diced	1
2	large celery stalks, chopped	2
2	large leeks, cleaned and sliced	2
1	large onion, chopped	1
1/2 cup	chopped parsley	125 mL
2	large cloves garlic	2
2	bay leaves	2
1/4 tsp	freshly ground black pepper	1 mL
1/8 tsp	salt	0.5 mL

Makes 6 cups (1.5 L)

1. In a saucepan over medium-high heat, combine water, potato, celery, leeks, onion, parsley, garlic, bay leaves, pepper and salt; bring to a boil. Reduce heat to low; simmer, covered, for 1 1/2 hours.
2. Pour mixture through a strainer; discard solids. Refrigerate stock until cold. Stock can be kept, refrigerated, for up to 3 days or frozen in an air-tight container.

Tip

✦ The advantage of making your own stock is that the flavor is richer. As well, there is virtually no sodium compared to commercially prepared bouillon, which contains about 780 mg sodium per 1 cup (250 mL) serving!

Here's the perfect stock for all you vegetarians out there. It keeps for up to 6 months if frozen in air-tight containers.

Super Stocks for Chicken, Beef or Seafood

6 cups	water	1.5 L
2	large chicken pieces (breasts or thighs) or 1½ lbs (750 g) beef bones or 1½ lbs (750 g) fish or seafood pieces	2
1	large carrot, peeled and chopped	1
1	medium onion, quartered	1
1	large celery stalk, chopped	1
3	large cloves garlic	3
¼ tsp	freshly ground black pepper	1 mL
⅛ tsp	salt	0.5 mL
½ cup	chopped parsley	125 mL
2	bay leaves	2

Makes 6 cups (1.5 L)

1. In a saucepan over medium-high heat, combine water, chicken pieces (or beef bones or fish/seafood pieces), carrot, onion, celery, garlic, pepper, salt, parsley and bay leaves. Bring to a boil, skimming any foam that rises to the top. Cover, reduce heat to low; simmer for 1½ hours.

2. Pour mixture through a strainer; discard solids. Refrigerate stock until cold; skim fat off surface. Stock can be refrigerated for up to 3 days or frozen in an air-tight container.

Tips

✦ For chicken and beef stocks, refrigerate overnight, remove any layers of fat and freeze in containers for later use.

✦ For fish or seafood stock, use whatever pieces you can find — including fish heads and bones, shrimp shells, or unused pieces of flesh.

Cold Two-Melon Soup

6 cups	cubed ripe honeydew or other green melon	1.5 L
2 tsp	grated lime zest	10 mL
¼ cup	freshly squeezed lime juice	50 mL
¼ cup	granulated sugar	50 mL
3 cups	cubed ripe cantaloupe	750 mL
1 tbsp	orange juice concentrate	15 mL
1 tsp	grated orange zest	5 mL
	Mint sprigs	

This is a terrific summer soup.

Serves 4

1. In a food processor purée honeydew melon, lime zest, lime juice, and 2 tbsp (25 mL) of the sugar until smooth. Transfer to a bowl.

2. Rinse out bowl of food processor. Add cantaloupe, orange juice concentrate, orange zest and remaining sugar; purée until smooth. Transfer to a separate bowl.

3. Chill both soups 30 minutes or until cold.

4. To serve, ladle 1 cup (250 mL) green soup into each of 4 individual serving bowls. Carefully pour ½ cup (125 mL) orange soup into the center. Garnish with mint sprigs and serve.

Make Ahead

✦ Prepare early in day and chill.

Nutritional Analysis (Per Serving)

✦ Calories: 170   ✦ Protein: 3 g   ✦ Cholesterol: 0 mg
✦ Sodium: 41 mg   ✦ Fat, total: 1 g   ✦ Carbohydrates: 44 g
✦ Fiber: 3 g   ✦ Fat, saturated: 0 g

Cold Mango Soup

2 tsp	vegetable oil	10 mL
½ cup	chopped onions	125 mL
2 tsp	minced garlic	10 mL
2 cups	basic vegetable stock	500 mL
2½ cups	chopped ripe mango (about 2 large)	625 mL

Garnish (optional)

| | 2% plain yogurt | |
| | Coriander leaves | |

Try to ensure that the mango is ripe. If not, add some sugar to taste. This soup can be frozen for up to 3 weeks.

Serves 4

1. In a nonstick saucepan, heat oil over medium heat. Add onions and garlic; cook, stirring, 4 minutes or until browned.
2. Add stock. Bring to a boil; reduce heat to medium-low and cook 5 minutes or until onions are soft.
3. Transfer mixture to a food processor. Add 2 cups (500 mL) of the mango. Purée until smooth. Stir in remaining chopped mango.
4. Chill 2 hours or until cold. Serve with a dollop of yogurt and garnish with coriander, if desired.

Make Ahead

✦ Prepare and refrigerate up to 2 days before.

Nutritional Analysis (Per Serving)
✦ Calories: 99   ✦ Protein: 1 g   ✦ Cholesterol: 0 mg
✦ Sodium: 7 mg   ✦ Fat, total: 3 g   ✦ Carbohydrates: 20 g
✦ Fiber: 3 g   ✦ Fat, saturated: 0.2 g

Madeira Mushroom and Leek Soup

1½ tsp	vegetable oil	7 mL
2 tsp	crushed garlic	10 mL
1 cup	chopped onion	250 mL
1	leek, thinly sliced	1
2½ cups	beef stock	625 mL
1 cup	diced peeled potatoes	250 mL
1½ tsp	margarine	7 mL
12 oz	mushrooms, sliced	375 g
⅓ cup	Madeira wine	75 mL
½ cup	2% milk	125 mL

Madeira wine gives this soup a subtle sweetness. If unavailable, use a sweet red wine.

When using margarine, choose a soft (non-hydrogenated) version to limit consumption of trans fats.

Serves 4

1. In nonstick medium saucepan, heat oil; sauté garlic, onion and leek until softened, approximately 10 minutes.
2. Add stock and potatoes; cover and simmer for 20 to 25 minutes or until softened. Purée in food processor until smooth. Return to saucepan and set aside.
3. In nonstick skillet, melt margarine; sauté mushrooms until softened, approximately 5 minutes. Add Madeira and cook for 2 minutes. Add to soup and stir until combined. Stir in milk.

Make Ahead

✦ Prepare and refrigerate early in the day and reheat before serving, adding more stock if too thick.

Nutritional Analysis (Per Serving)
✦ Calories: 150   ✦ Protein: 6 g   ✦ Cholesterol: 2 mg
✦ Sodium: 444 mg   ✦ Fat: 4 g   ✦ Carbohydrates: 18 g
✦ Fiber: 2 g

Onion Soup with Mozzarella

1 tbsp	vegetable oil	15 mL
1 tsp	crushed garlic	5 mL
5 cups	thinly sliced onions	1.25 L
1½ tsp	granulated sugar	7 mL
1½ tsp	all-purpose flour	7 mL
3 cups	beef stock	750 mL
¼ cup	sherry (optional)	50 mL
2	thin slices whole wheat bread, crusts removed	2
½ cup	shredded mozzarella cheese	125 mL

The sweeter the onion, the better. Vidalia onions are fabulous and are available during May and June.

Serves 4
Preheat broiler

1. In medium nonstick saucepan, heat oil; sauté garlic and onions until softened, approximately 5 minutes. Stir in sugar and flour; cover and simmer for 20 minutes, stirring occasionally.
2. Add beef stock, and sherry (if using); cover and simmer for 20 minutes. Pour into individual ovenproof soup bowls.
3. On baking sheet, broil bread until toasted on both sides, 2 to 3 minutes. Cut in half and float on each soup.
4. Sprinkle cheese over toast; broil just until melted and golden. Serve immediately.

Make Ahead
✦ Make and refrigerate the soup up to a day before. Gently reheat and add bread and cheese prior to serving.

Nutritional Analysis (Per Serving)
✦ Calories: 236 ✦ Protein: 12 g ✦ Cholesterol: 8 mg
✦ Sodium: 638 mg ✦ Fat: 6 g ✦ Carbohydrates: 30 g
✦ Fiber: 5 g

Fresh Tomato Dill Soup

1 tbsp	olive oil	15 mL
1 tsp	crushed garlic	5 mL
1	medium carrot, chopped	1
1	celery stalk, chopped	1
1 cup	chopped onion	250 mL
2 cups	chicken stock	500 mL
5 cups	chopped ripe tomatoes	1.25 L
3 tbsp	tomato paste	45 mL
2 tsp	granulated sugar	10 mL
3 tbsp	chopped fresh dill	45 mL

A dollop of light sour cream enhances each soup bowl.

Serves 6

1. In large nonstick saucepan, heat oil; sauté garlic, carrot, celery and onion until softened, approximately 5 minutes.
2. Add stock, tomatoes and tomato paste; reduce heat, cover and simmer for 20 minutes, stirring occasionally.
3. Purée in food processor until smooth. Add sugar and dill; mix well.

Make Ahead
✦ Prepare and refrigerate early in day, then serve cold or reheat gently.

Nutritional Analysis (Per Serving)
✦ Calories: 95 ✦ Protein: 4 g ✦ Cholesterol: 0 mg
✦ Sodium: 347 mg ✦ Fat: 3 g ✦ Carbohydrates: 14 g
✦ Fiber: 3 g

Sweet Pea Soup

1½ tsp	vegetable oil	7 mL
¾ cup	chopped onion	175 mL
1 tsp	crushed garlic	5 mL
1	carrot, chopped	1
¼ lb	mushrooms, sliced	125 g
3 cups	chicken stock	750 mL
1	medium potato, peeled and chopped	1
1	package (350 g) frozen sweet peas	50 mL
½ cup	corn niblets	125 mL
2 tsp	dried tarragon (or 3 tbsp/45 mL chopped fresh), optional	10 mL

If you do not enjoy tarragon, omit it; the soup is delicious either way.

Serves 4

1. In large nonstick saucepan, heat oil; sauté onion, garlic, carrot and mushrooms until softened, approximately 5 minutes.
2. Add stock, potato and all but ¼ cup (50 mL) of the peas; reduce heat, cover and simmer for 20 to 25 minutes or until potato is tender.
3. Purée soup in food processor until creamy and smooth. Return to pan and add reserved peas and corn niblets. Season with tarragon (if using).

Make Ahead

✦ Prepare and refrigerate early in day and reheat gently before serving.

Nutritional Analysis (Per Serving)
- ✦ Calories: 174
- ✦ Protein: 10 g
- ✦ Cholesterol: 0 mg
- ✦ Sodium: 658 mg
- ✦ Fat: 3 g
- ✦ Carbohydrates: 28 g
- ✦ Fiber: 7 g

Curried Carrot Orange Soup

1 tsp	vegetable oil	5 mL
1½ tsp	minced garlic	7 mL
1 tsp	curry powder	5 mL
1 cup	chopped onions or sliced leeks	250 mL
1 lb	carrots, peeled and sliced	500 g
3¾ cups	chicken stock	925 mL
1 cup	peeled, diced sweet potatoes	250 mL
½ cup	orange juice	125 mL
2 tbsp	honey	25 mL
1 tbsp	grated orange zest (1 large orange)	15 mL

Leeks can have a lot of hidden dirt — to clean thoroughly, slice in half lengthwise and wash under cold running water, getting between the layers, where dirt hides.

Serves 6

1. In nonstick saucepan sprayed with vegetable spray, heat oil over medium heat. Add garlic, curry, onions and carrots; cook for 5 minutes or until onions are softened. Add stock and sweet potatoes; bring to a boil. Cover, reduce heat to low and simmer for 25 minutes or until carrots and sweet potatoes are tender.
2. Transfer soup to food processor or blender; purée. Return to saucepan and stir in orange juice, honey and zest.

Make Ahead

✦ Prepare and refrigerate up to a day ahead and reheat gently before serving, adding more stock if too thick.

Nutritional Analysis (Per Serving)
- ✦ Calories: 119
- ✦ Protein: 2 g
- ✦ Cholesterol: 0 mg
- ✦ Sodium: 624 mg
- ✦ Fat, total: 1 g
- ✦ Carbohydrates: 26 g
- ✦ Fiber: 3 g
- ✦ Fat, saturated: 0.1 g

Dill Carrot Soup

1 lb	carrots, sliced (6 to 8 medium)	500 g
2 tsp	vegetable oil	10 mL
2 tsp	crushed garlic	10 mL
1 cup	chopped onion	250 mL
3½ cups	chicken stock	875 mL
¾ cup	2% milk	175 mL
2 tbsp	chopped fresh dill (or 1 tsp/5 mL dried dillweed)	25 mL
2 tbsp	chopped fresh chives or green onions	25 mL

A dollop of yogurt on each bowlful enhances both the appearance and flavor.

Serves 4 to 6

1. In large saucepan of boiling water, cook carrots just until tender. Drain and return to saucepan; set aside.
2. In nonstick skillet, heat oil; sauté garlic and onion until softened, approximately 5 minutes. Add to carrots along with stock; cover and simmer for 25 minutes.
3. Purée in food processor until smooth, in batches if necessary. Return to saucepan; stir in milk, dill and chives.

Tip
+ This soup can be served hot or cold.

Make Ahead
+ Make and refrigerate up to a day before. If serving warm, reheat gently.

Nutritional Analysis (Per Serving)
+ Calories: 96 + Protein: 5 g + Cholesterol: 2 mg
+ Sodium: 494 mg + Fat: 3 g + Carbohydrates: 12 g
+ Fiber: 3 g

Carrot, Sweet Potato and Parsnip Soup

2 tsp	vegetable oil	10 mL
1 tsp	crushed garlic	5 mL
1 cup	chopped onion	250 mL
3½ cups	chicken stock	825 mL
1	small potato, peeled and chopped	1
¾ cup	chopped carrots	175 mL
¾ cup	chopped peeled sweet potato	175 mL
½ cup	chopped peeled parsnip	125 mL
2 tbsp	chopped fresh dill (or 1 tsp/5 mL dried dillweed)	25 mL

You can substitute all carrots for the parsnips or vice versa.

Serves 4

1. In medium nonstick saucepan, heat oil; sauté garlic and onion for approximately 5 minutes or until softened.
2. Add stock, potato, carrots, sweet potato and parsnip; reduce heat, cover and simmer for 30 to 40 minutes or until vegetables are tender.
3. Purée in food processor until creamy and smooth. Stir in dill.

Make Ahead
+ Make and refrigerate up to a day before and reheat before serving, adding more stock if too thick.

Nutritional Analysis (Per Serving)
+ Calories: 149 + Protein: 6 g + Cholesterol: 0 mg
+ Sodium: 692 mg + Fat: 4 g + Carbohydrates: 23 g
+ Fiber: 4 g

Squash and Carrot Soup

2 tsp	vegetable oil	10 mL
1½ tsp	minced garlic	7 mL
1½ cups	sliced leeks	375 mL
6 cups	chopped butternut squash (about 1¾ lb/875 g)	1.5 L
3½ to 4½ cups	basic vegetable stock	875 mL to 1.125 L
1 cup	diced carrots	250 mL
½ tsp	dried thyme	2 mL

Garnish (optional)

| | 2% plain yogurt or light sour cream | |

For easier preparation, look for squash that has been pre-cut at your grocery store.

Start with the smaller amount of stock, adding more if soup is too thick.

Serves 4 to 6

1. In a nonstick saucepan sprayed with vegetable spray, heat oil over medium-low heat. Stir in garlic and leeks; cook, covered, for 5 minutes or until softened.
2. Stir in squash, stock, carrots and thyme. Bring to a boil; reduce heat to medium-low, cover and cook 12 to 15 minutes or until vegetables are tender.
3. Transfer soup to a food processor or blender. Purée until smooth. Serve with a dollop of yogurt or sour cream, if desired.

Make Ahead

+ Prepare up to 2 days in advance. Reheat, adding extra stock if necessary. Freeze up to 4 weeks.

Nutritional Analysis (Per Serving)
+ Calories: 106   + Protein: 2 g   + Cholesterol: 0 mg
+ Sodium: 23 mg   + Fat, total: 2 g   + Carbohydrates: 23 g
+ Fiber: 1 g   + Fat, saturated: 0.2 g

Curried Squash and Sweet Potato Soup

2 tsp	vegetable oil	10 mL
1 tsp	crushed garlic	5 mL
1	small onion, chopped	1
1 cup	sliced mushrooms	250 mL
1	butternut squash (8 oz/250 g), peeled, seeded and chopped	1
1½ cups	chopped peeled sweet potato	375 mL
3¼ cups	chicken stock	800 mL
½ tsp	ground ginger	2 mL
1 tsp	curry powder	5 mL
1 tbsp	honey	15 mL
½ cup	2% milk	125 mL

Other spices that pair with curry are cumin, cardamom, coriander and tumeric; experiment with what you have on hand.

Serves 4

1. In large nonstick saucepan, heat oil; sauté garlic, onion and mushrooms until softened, approximately 5 minutes.
2. Add squash, sweet potato, stock, ginger and curry powder; reduce heat, cover and simmer for 30 minutes or until vegetables are tender.
3. Purée in food processor until creamy and smooth. Return to saucepan; stir in honey and milk, blending well.

Make Ahead

+ Make and refrigerate up to a day before and reheat gently before serving, adding more stock if too thick.

Nutritional Analysis (Per Serving)
+ Calories: 188   + Protein: 7 g   + Cholesterol: 2 mg
+ Sodium: 652 mg   + Fat: 4 g   + Carbohydrates: 30 g
+ Fiber: 4 g

Sweet Potato Orange Soup with Maple Syrup

1 tsp	vegetable oil	5 mL
1¹/₂ tsp	minced garlic	7 mL
³/₄ cup	chopped onions	175 mL
1³/₄ lbs	sweet potatoes, peeled and chopped (about 6 cups/1.5 L)	875 g
3¹/₂ cups	basic vegetable stock	875 mL
2	bay leaves	2
1 tbsp	grated orange zest	15 mL
¹/₂ cup	orange juice	125 mL
3 tbsp	maple syrup	45 mL

Freshly squeezed juice is the best to use. Use the orange from which you obtained the zest. When grating orange zest, be careful not to scrape the white underneath the zest. It is bitter.

Serves 4 to 6

1. In a nonstick saucepan sprayed with vegetable spray, heat oil over medium heat. Add garlic and onions; cook 4 minutes or until softened.
2. Stir in sweet potatoes, stock and bay leaves. Bring to a boil; reduce heat to medium-low, cover and cook 20 minutes or until sweet potatoes are tender. Remove bay leaves.
3. In a food processor or blender, purée soup along with orange zest, orange juice and maple syrup until smooth.

Make Ahead
+ Prepare up to 2 days in advance, adding more stock when reheating.
+ Freeze up to 3 weeks.

Nutritional Analysis (Per Serving)
+ Calories: 203   + Protein: 3 g   + Cholesterol: 0 mg
+ Sodium: 25 mg   + Fat, total: 1 g   + Carbohydrates: 46 g
+ Fiber: 5 g   + Fat, saturated: 0.2 g

Creamy Pumpkin Soup

2 tsp	vegetable oil	10 mL
1 tsp	minced garlic	5 mL
1¹/₂ cups	chopped onions	375 mL
1¹/₂ cups	chopped carrots	375 mL
3¹/₂ cups	chicken stock	875 mL
1 tsp	cinnamon	5 mL
¹/₂ tsp	ground ginger	2 mL
¹/₈ tsp	nutmeg	0.5 mL
1¹/₂ cups	canned pumpkin purée	375 mL
1 cup	2% milk	250 mL
2 tbsp	honey	25 mL

In season, fresh cooked pumpkin is great in this soup.

Serves 4

1. In nonstick saucepan sprayed with vegetable spray, heat oil over medium-high heat. Add garlic, onions and carrots; cook for 10 minutes, stirring frequently, or until onions are browned and softened. Add stock, cinnamon, ginger, nutmeg and pumpkin; bring to a boil. Cover, reduce heat to low and simmer for 20 minutes or until carrot is tender.
2. Transfer soup to food processor or blender; purée until smooth. Return soup to saucepan. Stir in milk and honey and heat gently.

Make Ahead
+ Prepare and refrigerate up to a day ahead and reheat gently before serving, adding more stock if too thick.

Nutritional Analysis (Per Serving)
+ Calories: 174   + Protein: 5 g   + Cholesterol: 5 mg
+ Sodium: 871 mg   + Fat, total: 4 g   + Carbohydrates: 32 g
+ Fiber: 4 g   + Fat, saturated: 1 g

Corn, Tomato and Zucchini Soup

2 tsp	vegetable oil	10 mL
1 tsp	minced garlic	5 mL
3 cups	diced zucchini	750 mL
1½ cups	chopped onions	375 mL
3 cups	basic vegetable stock	750 mL
1	can (19 oz/540 mL) whole tomatoes	1
1¼ cups	frozen or canned corn, drained	300 mL
2 tsp	dried basil	10 mL

Great soup in just under 30 minutes. Fresh basil is excellent as a garnish.

Serves 4 to 6

1. In a nonstick saucepan sprayed with vegetable spray, heat oil over medium-high heat. Add garlic, zucchini and onions; cook for 5 minutes or until softened.

2. Stir in stock, tomatoes, corn, and basil. Bring to a boil, reduce heat to low and simmer 20 minutes, breaking up whole tomatoes with the back of a spoon.

Tip
✦ Try grilling or barbecuing corn on the cob until charred. Remove kernels with a knife.

Make Ahead
✦ Prepare up to 2 days in advance or freeze for up to 3 weeks. Add more stock if necessary when reheating.

Nutritional Analysis (Per Serving)
✦ Calories: 106   ✦ Protein: 4 g   ✦ Cholesterol: 0 mg
✦ Sodium: 159 mg   ✦ Fat, total: 2 g   ✦ Carbohydrates: 22 g
✦ Fiber: 4 g   ✦ Fat, saturated: 0.2 g

Wild Mushroom and Barley Soup

2 tsp	vegetable oil	10 mL
2 tsp	minced garlic	10 mL
1 cup	chopped onions	250 mL
3½ cups	basic vegetable stock	875 mL
1	can (19 oz/540 mL) tomatoes, crushed	1
½ cup	barley	125 mL
½ tsp	dried thyme	2 mL
¼ tsp	freshly ground black pepper	1 mL
8 oz	wild mushrooms, sliced	250 g

Oyster or cremini mushrooms are the best to use here. If unavailable, substitute white common mushrooms.

Serves 4 to 6

1. In a nonstick saucepan, heat oil over medium heat. Add garlic and onions; cook 4 minutes or until softened.

2. Stir in stock, tomatoes, barley, thyme and pepper. Bring to a boil; reduce heat to medium-low, cover and simmer 40 to 50 minutes, or until barley is tender.

3. Meanwhile, in a nonstick frying pan sprayed with vegetable spray, cook mushrooms over high heat, stirring, 8 minutes or until browned.

4. Stir mushrooms into soup and serve.

Make Ahead
✦ Prepare up to 2 days in advance or freeze for up to 3 weeks. Add more stock when reheating if too thick.

Nutritional Analysis (Per Serving)
✦ Calories: 173   ✦ Protein: 6 g   ✦ Cholesterol: 0 mg
✦ Sodium: 236 mg   ✦ Fat, total: 3 g   ✦ Carbohydrates: 33 g
✦ Fiber: 7 g   ✦ Fat, saturated: 0.3 g

Red Onion and Grilled Red Pepper Soup

3	large red bell peppers	3
2 tsp	vegetable oil	10 mL
2 tsp	minced garlic	10 mL
1 tbsp	packed brown sugar	15 mL
5 cups	thinly sliced red onions	1.25 L
3 to 3½ cups	Basic Vegetable Stock (see recipe, page 52)	750 mL to 875 mL

Garnish

⅓ cup	chopped fresh basil or parsley	75 mL
	Light sour cream (optional)	

If you decide you need to lose weight, take it off slowly — the way you put it on! A safe and reasonable weight loss is about 1 to 2 pounds per week.

Serves 4
Preheat oven to broil
Baking sheet

1. Arrange oven rack 6 inches (15 cm) under element. Cook peppers on baking sheet, turning occasionally, 20 minutes or until charred. Cool. Discard stem, skin and seeds; cut peppers into thin strips. Set aside.

2. In a large nonstick saucepan, heat oil over medium-low heat. Add garlic, brown sugar and red onions; cook, stirring occasionally, 15 minutes or until onions are browned. Stir in stock and red pepper strips; cook 15 minutes longer.

3. In a blender or food processor, purée soup until smooth. Serve hot, garnished with chopped basil or parsley and a dollop of sour cream, if desired.

Tips

✦ Sweet bell peppers and red onions make this a naturally sweet-tasting soup. Sugar may not be necessary.

✦ Start with the lesser amount of stock, adding more to reach the consistency you prefer.

✦ This soup is a good source of fiber.

Make Ahead

✦ Prepare up to 2 days in advance. Add more stock if too thick.

✦ Freeze up to 4 weeks.

Nutritional Analysis (Per Serving)

✦ Calories: 129 ✦ Protein: 3 g ✦ Cholesterol: 0 mg
✦ Sodium: 15 mg ✦ Fat, total: 3 g ✦ Carbohydrates: 25 g
✦ Fiber: 5 g ✦ Fat, saturated: 0.2 g

Roasted Eggplant and Bell Pepper Soup

1	medium eggplant (about 1 lb/500 g), cut in half lengthwise	1
1	medium red or yellow bell pepper	1
2 tsp	vegetable oil	10 mL
2 tsp	minced garlic	10 mL
1½ cups	chopped leeks	375 mL
½ cup	chopped onions	125 mL
2½ to 3 cups	Basic Vegetable Stock (see recipe, page, 52)	625 to 750 mL
1 cup	diced tomatoes	250 mL
2 tbsp	tomato paste	25 mL
2	bay leaves	2
⅓ cup	2% milk or Basic Vegetable Stock	75 mL

Garnish

⅓ cup	chopped fresh basil or parsley	75 mL
¼ cup	light sour cream (optional)	50 mL

Want a great way to thicken a soup without using cream or butter? Try the lower-fat alternative — evaporated milk. One-half cup (125 mL) of 2% evaporated milk has only 2.5 g fat. Compare that with 31 g fat for an equal quantity of whipping (35%) cream. Scary! Evaporated milk also has more calcium than cream.

Serves 4 to 6
Preheat broiler
Baking sheet

1. Put eggplant and pepper on baking sheet. With rack 6 inches (15 cm) under broiler, cook about 20 minutes, turning occasionally, until pepper is charred. Remove pepper; continue cooking eggplant 10 minutes longer or until very soft. Cool. Peel, stem, seed and chop pepper; scoop pulp out of eggplant shell, including seeds. Set aside chopped pepper and eggplant pulp.

2. In a nonstick saucepan, heat oil over medium heat. Add garlic, leeks and onions; cook 5 minutes or until softened. Stir in stock, tomatoes, tomato paste and bay leaves. Bring to a boil; reduce heat to medium-low, cover and cook 10 minutes.

3. In food processor or blender, purée soup with roasted eggplant and pepper. Add milk or stock.

4. Serve hot, garnished with chopped basil and a dollop of sour cream, if desired.

Tips

✦ This combination of eggplant and sweet peppers is unusual and delicious.

✦ Start with the smaller amount of stock, adding more if soup is too thick.

Make Ahead

✦ Prepare up to 2 days in advance, adding more stock if necessary.

✦ Freeze up to 4 weeks.

Nutritional Analysis (Per Serving)

✦ Calories: 82   ✦ Protein: 3 g   ✦ Cholesterol: 1 mg
✦ Sodium: 26 mg   ✦ Fat, total: 2 g   ✦ Carbohydrates: 15 g
✦ Fiber: 4 g   ✦ Fat, saturated: 0.3 g

Roasted Tomato and Corn Soup

2½ lbs	plum tomatoes (about 10)	1.25 kg
1	can (12 oz/341 mL) corn, drained	1
2 tsp	vegetable oil	10 mL
2 tsp	minced garlic	10 mL
1 cup	chopped onions	250 mL
¾ cup	finely chopped carrots	175 mL
2½ cups	Basic Vegetable Stock (see recipe, page 52)	625 mL
3 tbsp	tomato paste	45 mL
½ cup	chopped fresh basil (or 2 tsp/10 mL dried)	125 mL

Wondering what to do with leftover tomato paste? Just spoon into ice cube trays and freeze; then transfer the cubes to freezer bags and keep frozen until needed.

Serves 4 to 6
Preheat broiler
Two baking sheets lined with aluminum foil and sprayed with vegetable spray

1. Put tomatoes on one baking sheet. With rack 6 inches (15 cm) under broiler, broil tomatoes about 30 minutes, turning occasionally, or until charred on all sides. Meanwhile, spread corn on other baking sheet and broil, stirring occasionally, about 15 minutes or until slightly browned. (Some corn kernels will pop.) When cool enough to handle, chop tomatoes.

2. In a nonstick saucepan, heat oil over medium-high heat. Add garlic, onions and carrots; cook 5 minutes or until softened and beginning to brown. Add roasted tomatoes, stock, tomato paste and, if using, dried basil. (If using fresh basil, wait until Step 3.) Bring to a boil; reduce heat to medium-low, cover and cook 20 minutes or until vegetables tender.

3. In food processor or blender, purée soup. Return to saucepan; stir in corn and, if using, fresh basil.

Tips

✦ Regular fresh tomatoes can replace plum.

✦ Dill or coriander can replace basil.

✦ In the summer, grill tomatoes and 2 whole cobs of corn on the barbecue.

Make Ahead

✦ Prepare soup up to 2 days in advance, adding more stock, if necessary, when reheating.

✦ Freeze up to 4 weeks.

Nutritional Analysis (Per Serving)
✦ Calories: 117 ✦ Protein: 4 g ✦ Cholesterol: 0 mg
✦ Sodium: 173 mg ✦ Fat, total: 3 g ✦ Carbohydrates: 23 g
✦ Fiber: 4 g ✦ Fat, saturated: 0.3 g

Roasted Vegetable Soup

2	heads garlic	2
2	medium carrots, peeled	2
1	medium zucchini	1
2	medium leeks, white parts only	2
1	large red bell pepper	1
12 oz	plum tomatoes	375 g
1	medium sweet potato, peeled	1
1	medium red onion, peeled	1
1 tbsp	olive oil	15 mL
5½ cups	Basic Vegetable Stock (approx.) (see recipe, page 52)	1.375 L
1 tsp	dried basil	5 mL
½ tsp	coarsely ground black pepper	2 mL

Think of any vegetables you love and chances are they will taste even better roasted. Just toss them in a pan, drizzle with olive oil and spices, and roast until tender and sweet. Simple, yes, but oh so good! And good for you, too. Roasted vegetables keep their nutrients and have more intense flavors. When roasting, cut vegetables into large chunks, leaving the skin on to maintain moisture. Cook in a 400°F (200°C) oven for about 1 hour.

Serves 6 to 8
Preheat oven to 425°F (220°C)
Roasting pan sprayed with vegetable spray

1. Slice top off each head of garlic. Cut carrots and zucchini in half lengthwise; cut into large pieces. Cut leeks in half lengthwise; wash carefully then cut into large pieces. Stem, seed and quarter red pepper. Cut tomatoes, sweet potato and onion into wedges. Put all vegetables in roasting pan; toss with olive oil.

2. Bake 1 hour, tossing occasionally, or until vegetables are tender.

3. Squeeze garlic out of skins. Put in a food processor with rest of roasted vegetables. Purée until finely chopped. Add stock, basil and black pepper; purée in 2 batches until smooth. Add extra stock until desired consistency is reached. Transfer to a large saucepan; heat gently until hot. Serve.

Tips

✦ Here's an easy, delicious soup using roasting as a great alternative to other methods of cooking. Roasting gives a smoky flavor to foods.

✦ Other vegetables can be substituted. Keep amounts the same.

✦ Start with smaller amount of stock, adding more if soup is too thick.

Make Ahead

✦ Prepare soup up to 2 days in advance. Add more stock if necessary.

✦ Freeze up to 4 weeks.

Nutritional Analysis (Per Serving)
✦ Calories: 98   ✦ Protein: 2 g   ✦ Cholesterol: 0 mg
✦ Sodium: 27 mg   ✦ Fat, total: 2 g   ✦ Carbohydrates: 19 g
✦ Fiber: 3 g   ✦ Fat, saturated: 0.3 g

Green Onion, Potato and Dill Soup

2 tsp	vegetable oil	10 mL
2 tsp	minced garlic	10 mL
2²/₃ cups	chopped green onions	650 mL
3 cups	chicken stock	750 mL
2¹/₃ cups	diced potatoes	575 mL
3 tbsp	chopped fresh dill	45 mL
1¹/₂ oz	blue cheese or other strong cheese, crumbled	45 g

The blue cheese really adds flavor to this soup. If you don't like it, substitute another strong-flavored cheese, such as Swiss or goat cheese.

Serves 4

1. In saucepan, heat oil over medium heat; add garlic and green onions. Cook for 4 minutes, stirring occasionally. Add stock and potatoes; bring to a boil. Cover, reduce heat to low and cook for 20 to 25 minutes or until potatoes are tender.
2. Transfer soup to a blender or food processor and purée. Return purée to saucepan and stir in chopped dill and blue cheese; cook for 2 minutes or until blue cheese melts.

Make Ahead

✦ Prepare and refrigerate up to a day ahead and reheat gently before serving, adding more stock if too thick.

Nutritional Analysis (Per Serving)
- ✦ Calories: 166
- ✦ Protein: 6 g
- ✦ Cholesterol: 8 mg
- ✦ Sodium: 854 mg
- ✦ Fat, total: 6 g
- ✦ Carbohydrates: 25 g
- ✦ Fiber: 3 g
- ✦ Fat, saturated: 2 g

Chunky Red Pepper and Tomato Soup

2 tsp	vegetable oil	10 mL
1¹/₂ tsp	minced garlic	7 mL
1 cup	chopped onions	250 mL
4¹/₂ cups	chopped tomatoes	1.125 L
1¹/₄ cups	chopped red peppers	300 mL
2 cups	chicken stock	500 mL
Pinch	chili flakes	Pinch
¹/₄ cup	chopped fresh basil or dill	50 mL

If using dried basil or dillweed, add 1 tsp (5 mL) during the cooking. For a spicier taste, use ¹/₂ tsp (2 mL) fresh chopped chili pepper.

Serves 4

1. Heat oil in nonstick saucepan over medium heat. Add garlic and onions; cook for 4 minutes or until softened.
2. Reserve ¹/₂ cup (125 mL) each of tomatoes and red peppers; set aside. Add remaining tomatoes and red peppers to saucepan; cook for 10 minutes, stirring often. Add stock and chili flakes; bring to a boil. Cover, reduce heat to low and simmer 20 minutes.
3. Transfer soup to food processor and purée. Return to saucepan and stir in reserved tomatoes, red peppers and basil.

Make Ahead

✦ Prepare and refrigerate up to a day ahead and reheat gently before serving, adding more stock if too thick.

Nutritional Analysis (Per Serving)
- ✦ Calories: 108
- ✦ Protein: 3 g
- ✦ Cholesterol: 0 mg
- ✦ Sodium: 492 mg
- ✦ Fat, total: 3 g
- ✦ Carbohydrates: 19 g
- ✦ Fiber: 4 g
- ✦ Fat, saturated: 0.3 g

Yellow Bell Pepper Soup with Red Pepper Swirl

1	red pepper	1
3	yellow peppers	3
2 tsp	vegetable oil	10 mL
2 tsp	minced garlic	10 mL
1³/₄ cups	chopped onions	425 mL
1¹/₂ cups	chopped carrots	375 mL
4 cups	chicken or vegetable stock	1 L
1¹/₂ cups	diced, peeled potatoes	375 mL
	Pepper to taste	
¹/₄ cup	chopped fresh basil	50 mL

Roasted peppers taste wonderful, but they require some time to prepare. So when a recipe calls for just a small amount, use bottled roasted peppers. Look for those packaged in water (not oil) to avoid excess fat. Use about 4 oz (125 g) peppers in a jar for each fresh pepper required. Once opened, a jar of these peppers does not keep for very long, so freeze any unused peppers in small air-tight containers.

Serves 6
Preheat oven to broil

1. Roast the peppers under the broiler for 15 to 20 minutes, turning several times until charred on all sides. Place in a bowl covered tightly with plastic wrap; let stand until cool enough to handle. Remove skin, stem and seeds.

2. In a nonstick saucepan sprayed with vegetable spray, heat oil over medium heat. Add garlic, onions and carrots; cook for 8 minutes or until vegetables are softened, stirring occasionally. Add stock and potatoes; bring to a boil. Reduce heat to low; cover, and let cook for 20 to 25 minutes or until carrots and potatoes are tender.

3. Put the red peppers in food processor and process until smooth. Add about 1 cup (250 mL) of the soup mixture to the red pepper purée and process until smooth. Season with pepper and pour into saucepan. Rinse out food processor. Put yellow peppers in food processor and process until smooth; add remaining soup to yellow pepper purée and process until smooth. Season with pepper and pour into a serving bowl. To serve, ladle some of the yellow pepper soup into individual bowls, and pour some of the red pepper purée in the center and swirl through with a knife. Add basil to soup and serve.

Tips
✦ Orange peppers can be used instead of red or yellow.
✦ Use another fresh herb if desired.
✦ If desired, basil can be added while puréeing for a more intense flavor.

Make Ahead
✦ Roast peppers up to one day ahead and refrigerate.
✦ Prepare both soups earlier in day, and keep them separate until serving. Reheat gently.

Nutritional Analysis (Per Serving)
✦ Calories: 99 ✦ Protein: 3 g ✦ Cholesterol: 0 mg
✦ Sodium: 644 mg ✦ Fat: 2 g ✦ Carbohydrates: 19 g
✦ Fiber: 3 g

Red and Yellow Bell Pepper Soup

2	red peppers	2
2	yellow peppers	2
2 tsp	vegetable oil	10 mL
2 tsp	minced garlic	10 mL
1½ cups	chopped onions	375 mL
1¼ cups	chopped carrots	300 mL
½ cup	chopped celery	125 mL
4 cups	chicken or vegetable stock	1 L
1½ cups	diced, peeled potatoes	375 mL
	Pepper to taste	
¼ cup	chopped fresh coriander, dill or basil	50 mL

Roasted peppers in a jar (packed in water) can replace fresh peppers. Use about 4 oz (125 g) peppers in a jar for each fresh pepper required.

Serves 6
Preheat oven to broil

1. Roast the peppers under the broiler for 15 to 20 minutes, turning several times until charred on all sides. Place in a bowl covered tightly with plastic wrap; let stand until cool enough to handle. Remove skin, stem and seeds.

2. In a nonstick saucepan sprayed with vegetable spray, heat oil over medium heat. Add garlic, onion, carrots and celery; cook for 8 minutes or until vegetables are softened, stirring occasionally. Add stock and potatoes; bring to a boil. Reduce heat to low; cover, and let cook for 20 to 25 minutes or until carrots and potatoes are tender.

3. Put the red peppers in food processor and process until smooth. Add half of the soup mixture to the red pepper purée and process until smooth. Season with pepper and pour into serving bowl. Rinse out food processor. Put yellow peppers in food processor and process until smooth; add remaining soup to yellow pepper purée and process until smooth. Season with pepper and pour into another serving bowl. To serve, ladle some of the red pepper soup into one side of individual bowl, at the same time ladling some of the yellow pepper soup into the other side of the bowl. Add coriander to soup and serve.

Tips

✦ If desired, coriander can be added before puréeing for a more intense flavor.

✦ Orange peppers can be used instead of red or yellow.

Make Ahead

✦ Roast peppers earlier in the day and set aside.

✦ Prepare both soups earlier in day, and keep them separate until serving.

Nutritional Analysis (Per Serving)
✦ Calories: 99   ✦ Protein: 3 g   ✦ Cholesterol: 0 mg
✦ Sodium: 644 mg   ✦ Fat, total: 2 g   ✦ Carbohydrates: 19 g
✦ Fiber: 3 g   ✦ Fat, saturated: 0.2 g

Roasted Corn and Red Pepper Chowder

2 cups	corn niblets (canned or fresh)	500 mL
1½ tsp	margarine or butter	7 mL
1 cup	chopped leeks	250 mL
1 tsp	crushed garlic	5 mL
1 cup	diced, peeled potatoes	250 mL
1¾ cups	chicken or vegetable stock	425 mL
½ cup	chopped, roasted sweet red peppers	125 mL
1½ tbsp	all-purpose flour	20 mL
1½ cups	2% milk	375 mL
¼ tsp	Worcestershire sauce	1 mL
	Pepper	

Corn is rich in lutein, an antioxidant compound related to the famous beta carotene. Research has linked a lutein-rich diet with reduced breast cancer risk: according to the Harvard Nurse's Health Study, higher intakes of lutein offered a strong protective effect for breast cancer in premenopausal women. Other good sources of lutein include kale, collard greens, spinach, Romaine lettuce and red bell peppers.

When using margarine, choose a soft (non-hydrogenated) version to limit consumption of trans fats.

Serves 4 or 5

1. On baking sheet sprayed with vegetable spray, spread out corn niblets and broil approximately 8 minutes or until roasted and slightly browned.
2. In food processor, process half of the corn until puréed; add to remaining corn and set aside.
3. In large nonstick saucepan, melt margarine; sauté leeks and garlic for 3 minutes. Add potatoes, stock and roasted peppers. Bring to a boil. Reduce heat to low; cover and simmer until potatoes are tender, approximately 15 minutes.
4. In a small bowl combine flour, milk and Worcestershire until smooth. Add to potato mixture along with corn; simmer for approximately 5 minutes, or just until thickened.

Tips

✦ Frozen corn niblets would be fine to use.
✦ The roasted vegetables give this soup a smoky flavor.
✦ Roasted yellow or orange peppers are also delicious.
✦ Use either roasted peppers in a jar (packed in water) or grill your own.

Make Ahead

✦ Make and refrigerate early in day and reheat gently, adding more stock or milk if too thick.

Nutritional Analysis (Per Serving)
✦ Calories: 164 ✦ Protein: 7 g ✦ Cholesterol: 5 mg
✦ Sodium: 467 mg ✦ Fat: 3 g ✦ Carbohydrates: 28 g
✦ Fiber: 3 g

Corn Chowder with Wild Rice and Roasted Peppers

1 cup	chopped onions	250 mL
1½ tsp	minced garlic	7 mL
4 cups	vegetable or chicken stock	1 L
⅓ cup	wild rice	75 mL
1 cup	diced peeled potatoes	250 mL
⅛ tsp	salt	0.5 mL
⅛ tsp	freshly ground black pepper	0.5 mL
¾ cup	low-fat evaporated milk	175 mL
1 tbsp	all-purpose flour	15 mL
1	can (12 oz/341 mL) corn, drained or 2 cups/500 mL frozen corn, thawed	1
⅓ cup	chopped roasted red bell peppers	75 mL
⅓ cup	chopped fresh coriander, basil or dill	75 mL

Serves 4

1. In a nonstick saucepan sprayed with vegetable spray, cook onions and garlic over medium-high heat for 4 minutes or until softened. Add stock and wild rice; bring to a boil. Reduce heat to medium-low; cook, covered, for 15 minutes. Add potatoes, salt and pepper; cook, covered, for 20 minutes or until rice and potatoes are tender.

2. In a bowl whisk together evaporated milk and flour; add to soup. Add corn and roasted red peppers; cook for 3 minutes or until slightly thickened. Serve garnished with coriander.

Nutritional Analysis (Per Serving)
- Calories: 218
- Protein: 10 g
- Cholesterol: 5 mg
- Sodium: 400 mg
- Fat, total: 3 g
- Carbohydrates: 42 g
- Fiber: 3 g
- Fat, saturated: 1 g

Alphabet Soup with Hearty Roasted Vegetables

2 lbs	plum tomatoes, cut crosswise into halves	1 kg
1	large red onion, cut into wedges	1
2	large carrots, thinly sliced	2
1	large potato, cut into eighths	1
1 tbsp	olive oil	15 mL
1	large head garlic, top ½ inch (1 cm) cut off, wrapped loosely in foil	1
3 cups	vegetable or chicken stock	750 mL
2 tbsp	low-fat evaporated milk	25 mL
½ tsp	salt	2 mL
⅓ cup	alphabet soup pasta or other small pasta	75 mL
½ cup	chopped fresh basil, dill or parsley	125 mL

Serves 4
Preheat oven to 425°F (220°C)
Large baking sheet sprayed with vegetable spray

1. In a bowl combine tomatoes, red onion, carrots, potato and olive oil; toss well. Place vegetables and garlic on baking sheet. Bake in preheated oven, turning at halfway point, for 50 minutes or until tender.

2. When cool enough to handle, squeeze skins off garlic head. In a food processor, combine garlic, vegetable mixture and any accumulated juices; purée. Transfer to a saucepan over medium-high heat. Add stock, evaporated milk and salt; bring to a boil. Add pasta; reduce heat to medium-low. Cook, stirring occasionally, for 10 minutes or until pasta is tender. Garnish with basil; serve.

Nutritional Analysis (Per Serving)
- Calories: 209
- Protein: 6 g
- Cholesterol: 1 mg
- Sodium: 350 mg
- Fat, total: 5 g
- Carbohydrates: 37 g
- Fiber: 6 g
- Fat, saturated: 1 g

Potato Corn Chowder

2 cups	corn niblets (canned or fresh)	500 mL
1½ tsp	margarine	7 mL
1 cup	chopped onions	250 mL
½ cup	chopped sweet red pepper	125 mL
1 tsp	crushed garlic	5 mL
1 cup	diced peeled potato	250 mL
1⅓ cups	chicken stock	325 mL
2 tbsp	all-purpose flour	25 mL
1½ cups	2% milk	375 mL
¼ tsp	Worcestershire sauce	1 mL
	Pepper	

Frozen corn niblets would be fine to use. If time is available, make your own stock for a really delicious chowder. (See page 53.)

When using margarine, choose a soft (non-hydrogenated) version.

Serves 4 or 5

1. In food processor, process 1 cup (250 mL) of the corn until puréed; add to remaining corn and set aside.
2. In large nonstick saucepan, melt margarine; sauté onions, red pepper and garlic for 5 minutes. Add potato and stock; simmer, covered, until potato is tender, approximately 15 minutes.
3. Add corn mixture to soup; cook for 5 minutes. Stir in flour and cook for 1 minute. Add milk, Worcestershire sauce, and pepper to taste; cook on medium heat for approximately 5 minutes or just until thickened.

Make Ahead
✦ Make and refrigerate early in day and reheat gently, adding more stock or milk if too thick.

Nutritional Analysis (Per Serving)
✦ Calories: 164 ✦ Protein: 7 g ✦ Cholesterol: 5 mg
✦ Sodium: 467 mg ✦ Fat: 3 g ✦ Carbohydrates: 28 g
✦ Fiber: 3 g

Cauliflower Potato Soup

1 tbsp	vegetable oil	15 mL
1 tsp	crushed garlic	5 mL
1 cup	chopped onions	250 mL
1	medium cauliflower, separated into florets	1
4 cups	chicken stock	1 L
2 small	potatoes, peeled and chopped	2
¼ cup	shredded Cheddar cheese	50 mL
2 tbsp	chopped fresh chives	25 mL

Buy cauliflower with bright, light-colored heads and tightly packed florets.

Serves 4 to 6

1. In large nonstick saucepan, heat oil; sauté garlic and onions until softened, approximately 5 minutes.
2. Add cauliflower, stock and potatoes; bring to boil. Cover, reduce heat and simmer for 25 minutes or until tender. Transfer to food processor and purée until creamy and smooth. Return to saucepan and thin with more stock if desired.
3. Ladle into bowls; sprinkle with cheese and chives.

Make Ahead
✦ Make and refrigerate up to a day before and reheat gently, adding more stock if too thick.

Nutritional Analysis (Per Serving)
✦ Calories: 99 ✦ Protein: 6 g ✦ Cholesterol: 5 mg
✦ Sodium: 560 mg ✦ Fat: 5 g ✦ Carbohydrates: 8 g
✦ Fiber: 2 g

Asparagus and Leek Soup

³⁄₄ lb	asparagus	375 g
1¹⁄₂ tsp	vegetable oil	7 mL
1 tsp	crushed garlic	5 mL
1 cup	chopped onion	250 mL
2	leeks, sliced	2
3¹⁄₂ cups	chicken stock	875 mL
1 cup	diced peeled potato	250 mL
	Salt and pepper	
2 tbsp	grated Parmesan cheese	25 mL

Choose the greenest asparagus, with straight, firm stalks. The tips should be tightly closed and firm.

Serves 4 to 6

1. Trim asparagus; cut stalks into pieces and set tips aside.
2. In large nonstick saucepan, heat oil; sauté garlic, onion, leeks and asparagus stalks just until softened, approximately 10 minutes.
3. Add stock and potato; reduce heat, cover and simmer for 20 to 25 minutes or until vegetables are tender. Purée in food processor until smooth. Taste and adjust seasoning with salt and pepper. Return to saucepan.
4. Steam or microwave reserved asparagus tips just until tender; add to soup. Serve sprinkled with Parmesan cheese.

Make Ahead

✦ Make and refrigerate up to a day before and serve cold or reheat gently before serving, adding more stock if too thick.

Nutritional Analysis (Per Serving)
- ✦ Calories: 98
- ✦ Protein: 6 g
- ✦ Cholesterol: 1 mg
- ✦ Sodium: 491 mg
- ✦ Fat: 3 g
- ✦ Carbohydrates: 13 g
- ✦ Fiber: 3 g

Curried Broccoli Sweet Potato Soup

2 tsp	vegetable oil	10 mL
1¹⁄₂ tsp	minced garlic	7 mL
1¹⁄₂ cups	chopped onions	375 mL
1 tsp	curry powder	5 mL
4 cups	chicken stock	1 L
4 cups	broccoli florets	1 L
3 cups	peeled, diced sweet potato	750 mL
2 tbsp	honey	25 mL

Increase curry to 1¹⁄₂ tsp (7 mL) for more intense flavor.

Serves 6

1. Heat oil in nonstick saucepan over medium heat. Add garlic, onions and curry; cook for 4 minutes or until softened. Add stock, broccoli and sweet potatoes; bring to a boil. Cover, reduce heat to low and simmer for 30 minutes or until vegetables are tender.
2. Transfer soup to food processor or blender; add honey and purée.

Make Ahead

✦ Prepare and refrigerate up to a day ahead and reheat gently before serving, adding more stock if too thick.

Nutritional Analysis (Per Serving)
- ✦ Calories: 150
- ✦ Protein: 4 g
- ✦ Cholesterol: 0 mg
- ✦ Sodium: 648 mg
- ✦ Fat, total: 2 g
- ✦ Carbohydrates: 31 g
- ✦ Fiber: 4 g
- ✦ Fat, saturated: 0.3 g

Tomato, Zucchini and Tortellini Soup

2 tsp	vegetable oil	10 mL
1½ tsp	crushed garlic	7 mL
1 cup	chopped onions	250 mL
⅓ cup	chopped carrots	75 mL
2 cups	chicken stock	500 mL
1	can (28 oz/796 mL) crushed tomatoes	1
2 tsp	dried basil	10 mL
1 tsp	dried oregano	5 mL
6 oz	cheese tortellini	150 g
1 cup	diced zucchini	250 mL

Serves 6

1. In large nonstick saucepan, heat oil; sauté garlic, onions and carrots until tender, approximately 5 minutes.
2. Add stock, tomatoes, basil and oregano. Simmer on medium heat for 15 minutes, stirring occasionally.
3. Add tortellini and zucchini and cook for 10 minutes or just until pasta is cooked.

Tip
✦ Small ravioli or gnocchi can replace tortellini.

Make Ahead
✦ Prepare early in day, but do not add pasta until 10 minutes before serving.

Nutritional Analysis (Per Serving)
✦ Calories: 151　✦ Protein: 6 g　✦ Cholesterol: 0.2 mg
✦ Sodium: 577 mg　✦ Fat, total: 4 g　✦ Carbohydrates: 25 g
✦ Fiber: 5 g　✦ Fat, saturated: 0.5 g

Six-Root Vegetable Soup with Maple Syrup

⅔ cup	chopped onions	150 mL
2 tsp	minced garlic	10 mL
4 cups	vegetable or chicken stock	1.125 L
1½ cups	chopped peeled sweet potatoes	375 mL
¾ cup	chopped peeled parsnips	175 mL
¾ cup	chopped peeled rutabaga	175 mL
¾ cup	chopped peeled turnips	175 mL
½ cup	chopped peeled carrots	125 mL
1 tsp	dried tarragon	5 mL
⅓ cup	small pasta (orzo, ditali, stelline or tubetti)	75 mL
1 tbsp	maple syrup	15 mL

Serves 4

1. In a nonstick saucepan sprayed with vegetable spray, cook onions and garlic over medium-high heat for 3 minutes or until softened. Add stock, sweet potatoes, parsnips, rutabaga, turnips, carrots and tarragon; bring to a boil. Reduce heat to low; cook, covered, for 20 minutes or until vegetables are tender. Transfer mixture to a food processor or blender; process until smooth.
2. Return soup to saucepan over medium-high heat; bring to a boil. Add pasta; reduce heat to medium. Cook for 8 minutes or until pasta is tender; add maple syrup. Serve.

Nutritional Analysis (Per Serving)
✦ Calories: 221　✦ Protein: 6 g　✦ Cholesterol: 0 mg
✦ Sodium: 50 mg　✦ Fat, total: 1 g　✦ Carbohydrates: 48 g
✦ Fiber: 6 g　✦ Fat, saturated: 0.2 g

> *Maple syrup adds a subtle sweetness, unlike sugar.*

Asparagus and Leek Soup (page 71) ➤
Overleaf: Oriental Vegetable Salad (page 98)

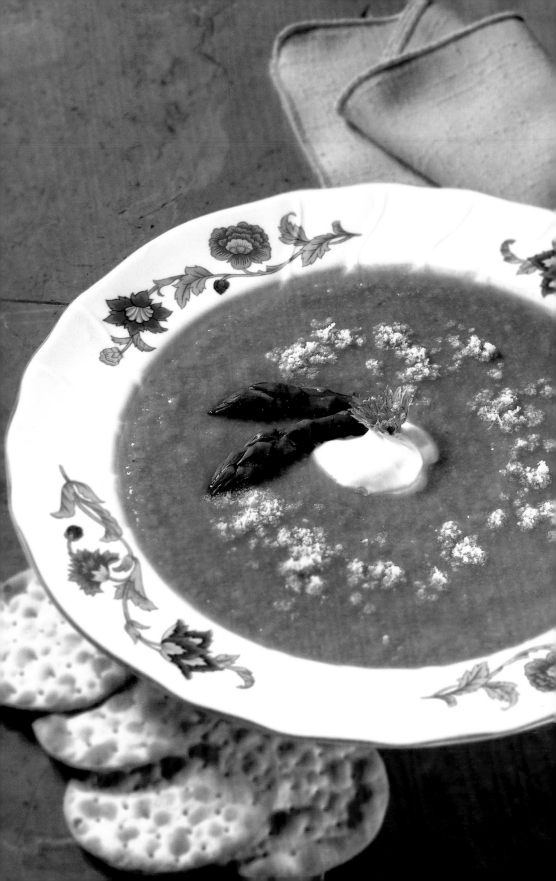

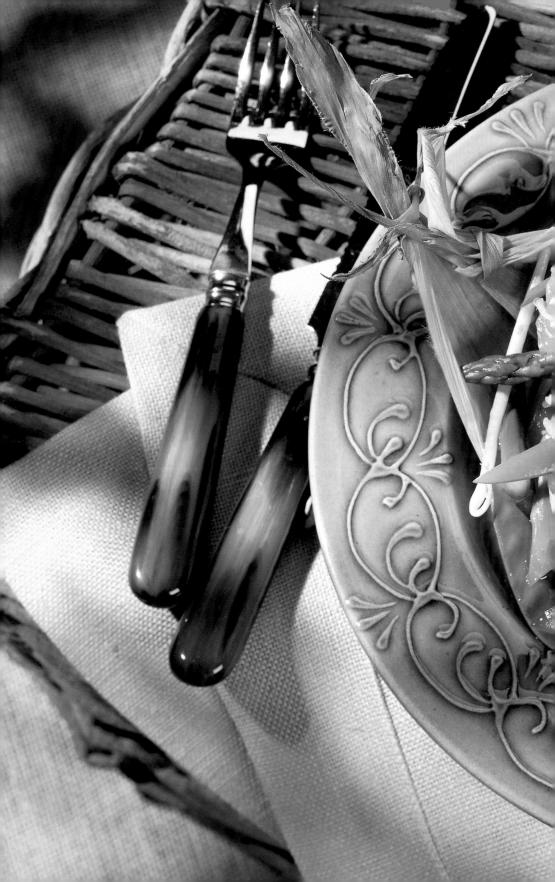

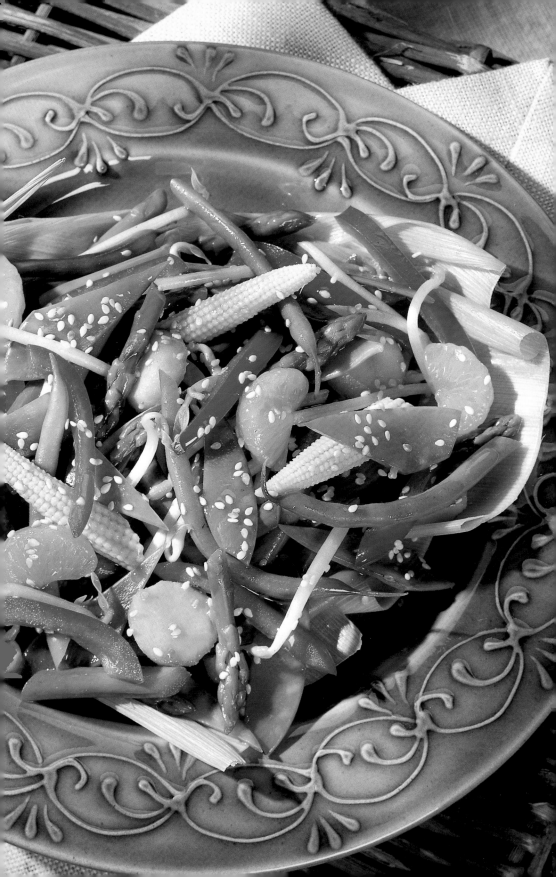

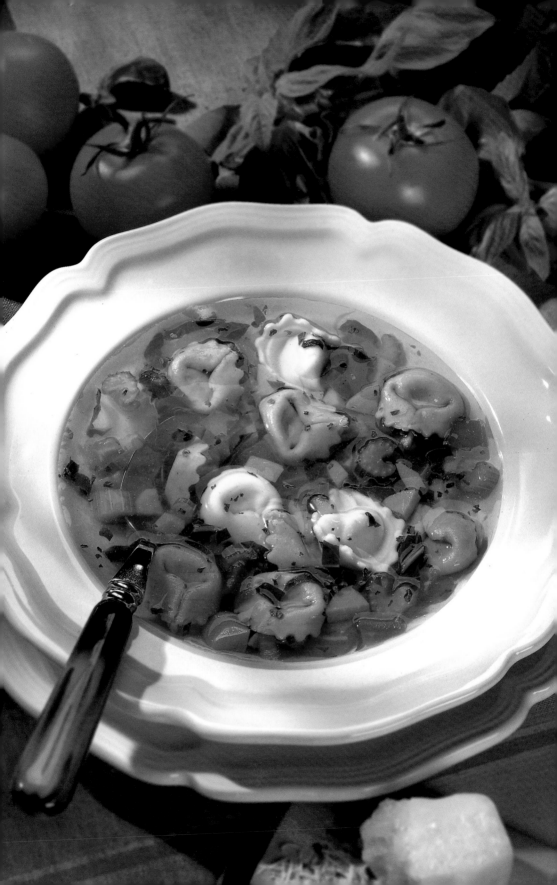

Roasted Vegetable Minestrone

2	ripe plum tomatoes, quartered	2
2	large carrots, peeled and thinly sliced	2
1	large red onion, cut into wedges	1
1	small zucchini, halved lengthwise	1
1	large sweet potato, peeled and cut into wedges	1
1	large red bell pepper, cored and quartered	1
1 tbsp	olive oil	15 mL
1	large head garlic, top $\frac{1}{2}$ inch (1 cm) cut off, wrapped loosely in foil	1
5 cups	vegetable or chicken stock	1.25 L
1$\frac{1}{2}$ tsp	dried basil	7 mL
1	bay leaf	1
$\frac{1}{4}$ tsp	freshly ground black pepper	1 mL
$\frac{1}{2}$ cup	elbow macaroni	125 mL
2 tbsp	grated low-fat Parmesan cheese	25 mL

Serves 6
Preheat oven to 425°F (220°C)
Large baking sheet sprayed with vegetable spray

1. In a bowl combine tomatoes, carrots, red onion, zucchini, sweet potato, red pepper and olive oil; toss well. Arrange in a single layer on baking sheet; add garlic. Roast in preheated oven, turning at halfway point, for 50 minutes or until tender. Set aside to cool.

2. When cool enough to handle, squeeze skins off garlic head. Chop tomatoes, carrots, red onion, zucchini, sweet potato and red pepper; transfer to a large saucepan over medium-high heat. Add stock, basil, bay leaf and black pepper; bring to a boil. Add macaroni; reduce heat to simmer. Cook for 10 minutes or until pasta is tender. Sprinkle with Parmesan cheese. Serve.

Tips

✦ Worried about what eating large amounts of fresh garlic will do to your breath — or stomach lining? Well, here's a solution: just roast that garlic and it will become deliciously sweet and mild. Squeeze cloves out of the skin after roasting and spread over fresh bread. So-o-o-o good!

✦ *Garlic may keep the cardiologist at bay:* Hailed by the ancient Egyptians for its miraculous healing properties, garlic is now recognized as having a protective effect against heart disease. In fact, studies have found that eating one clove a day can lower elevated cholesterol levels by up to 20%. This is attributed to a sulfur compound found in garlic called S-allyl cysteine, which increases in concentration when garlic is aged. If fresh garlic irritates your stomach, speak to your health practitioner about aged garlic extract.

Nutritional Analysis (Per Serving)
✦ Calories: 142 ✦ Protein: 4 g ✦ Cholesterol: 1 mg
✦ Sodium: 45 mg ✦ Fat, total: 4 g ✦ Carbohydrates: 24 g
✦ Fiber: 3 g ✦ Fat, saturated: 0.8 g

◄ Tortellini Minestrone with Spinach (page 76)

Barley Minestrone with Pesto

1 cup	chopped onions	250 mL
1½ tsp	minced garlic	7 mL
1½ cups	diced unpeeled zucchini	375 mL
1 cup	diced unpeeled eggplant	250 mL
½ cup	diced carrots	125 mL
4¾ cups	vegetable or chicken stock	1.175 L
1	can (19 oz/540 mL) whole tomatoes, with juice	1
1½ cups	diced peeled potatoes	375 mL
1 cup	canned cooked white kidney beans, rinsed and drained	250 mL
⅓ cup	pearl barley	75 mL
2½ tsp	dried basil	12 mL
1	bay leaf	1
2 tbsp	pesto (see recipe, page 128, or use store-bought variety)	25 mL
3 tbsp	grated low-fat Parmesan cheese	45 mL

Serves 8

1. In a large nonstick saucepan sprayed with vegetable spray, cook onions and garlic over medium-high heat for 2 minutes or until softened. Add zucchini, eggplant and carrots; cook for 5 minutes, stirring occasionally.

2. Add stock, tomatoes (with juice), potatoes, kidney beans, barley, basil and bay leaf. Bring to a boil, breaking tomatoes with back of a spoon. Reduce heat to medium-low; cook, covered, for 45 minutes or until barley is tender.

3. Ladle soup into bowls. Spoon a dollop of pesto in center of each serving; garnish with Parmesan cheese.

Nutritional Analysis (Per Serving)
- Calories: 153
- Protein: 7 g
- Cholesterol: 3 mg
- Sodium: 100 mg
- Fat, total: 3 g
- Carbohydrates: 26 g
- Fiber: 3 g
- Fat, saturated: 1.1 g

Hummus Soup with Couscous and Vegetables

¾ cup	chopped onions	175 mL
2 tsp	minced garlic	10 mL
4 cups	vegetable or chicken stock	1 L
2½ cups	canned chickpeas, rinsed and drained	625 mL
1 cup	diced peeled potatoes	250 mL
½ cup	chopped carrots	125 mL
2 tbsp	tahini (sesame paste)	25 mL
3 tbsp	couscous	45 mL
½ cup	chopped fresh coriander	125 mL

Serves 4

1. In a nonstick saucepan sprayed with vegetable spray, cook onions and garlic over medium-high heat for 5 minutes or until softened. Add stock, 2 cups (500 mL) chickpeas, potatoes, carrots and tahini; bring to a boil. Reduce heat to medium-low; cook, covered, for 15 minutes or until potatoes are tender.

2. In a food processor or blender, purée soup in batches until smooth. Return to saucepan; bring to a boil. Remove from heat; add couscous and remaining ½ cup (125 mL) chickpeas. Let stand, covered, for 5 minutes. Add coriander; serve immediately.

Nutritional Analysis (Per Serving)
- Calories: 314
- Protein: 15 g
- Cholesterol: 1 mg
- Sodium: 200 mg
- Fat, total: 6 g
- Carbohydrates: 53 g
- Fiber: 7 g
- Fat, saturated: 1.1 g

Sweet Potato, White Bean and Orzo Soup

2 tsp	vegetable oil	10 mL
1 tsp	crushed garlic	5 mL
1 cup	chopped onions	250 mL
1/2 cup	chopped celery	125 mL
3 cups	diced sweet potatoes	750 mL
1/2 cup	diced carrots	125 mL
4 cups	chicken stock	1 L
1 cup	canned white kidney beans, drained	250 mL
1/3 cup	orzo or small shell pasta	75 mL
1 cup	2% milk	250 mL
	Chopped parsley	

Orzo looks like large rice but is really a pasta. The texture is excellent for this soup. Be certain to stir after adding orzo, so it does not sink to bottom of pan.

Serves 6

1. In large nonstick saucepan, heat oil; sauté garlic, onions and celery until tender, approximately 4 minutes.
2. Add potatoes, carrots and stock. Cover and simmer on medium heat for 20 to 30 minutes or until potatoes are tender. Purée in food processor until smooth. Pour back into saucepan; add kidney beans and pasta. Cover and simmer for 10 minutes or until pasta is tender.
3. Add milk. Heat, then sprinkle with chopped parsley.

Make Ahead
✦ Prepare early in day, up to the point of adding orzo. Add orzo 10 minutes before serving.

Nutritional Analysis (Per Serving)
- ✦ Calories: 242
- ✦ Protein: 8 g
- ✦ Cholesterol: 3 mg
- ✦ Sodium: 799 mg
- ✦ Fat, total: 3 g
- ✦ Carbohydrates: 47 g
- ✦ Fiber: 8 g
- ✦ Fat, saturated: 0.7 g

Mexican Corn, Bean and Pasta Soup

2 tsp	vegetable oil	10 mL
2 tsp	crushed garlic	10 mL
1 cup	chopped onions	250 mL
1 1/2 cups	chopped sweet green peppers	375 mL
1	can (28 oz/796 mL) crushed tomatoes	1
2 1/2 cups	chicken stock	625 mL
2 cups	canned red kidney beans, drained	500 mL
1 cup	corn niblets	250 mL
1 tbsp	chili powder	15 mL
1/4 tsp	cayenne pepper	1 mL
1/2 cup	macaroni	125 mL
Dollop	yogurt	Dollop
	Coriander	

Chickpeas or other beans can replace kidney beans.

Serves 6 to 8

1. In large nonstick saucepan, heat oil; sauté garlic, onions and green peppers until soft, approximately 5 minutes.
2. Add tomatoes, stock, beans, corn niblets, chili powder and cayenne. Cover and simmer on low heat for 20 minutes.
3. Add pasta, simmer for 10 to 12 minutes or until pasta is "al dente" (firm to the bite). Garnish with yogurt and fresh coriander.

Tip
✦ Any small shell pasta can be used.

Make Ahead
✦ Prepare soup up to a day ahead, but do not add pasta until 10 minutes before serving.

Nutritional Analysis (Per Serving)
- ✦ Calories: 187
- ✦ Protein: 7 g
- ✦ Cholesterol: 0 mg
- ✦ Sodium: 682 mg
- ✦ Fat, total: 3 g
- ✦ Carbohydrates: 37 g
- ✦ Fiber: 7 g
- ✦ Fat, saturated: 0.2 g

Tortellini Minestrone with Spinach

2 tsp	vegetable oil	10 mL
2 tsp	minced garlic	10 mL
1 cup	chopped onions	250 mL
1/2 cup	chopped carrots	125 mL
1/2 cup	chopped celery	125 mL
4 cups	Basic Vegetable Stock (see recipe, page 52)	1 L
1 tsp	dried basil	5 mL
1/4 tsp	freshly ground black pepper	1 mL
1 1/2 cups	diced plum tomatoes	375 mL
2 cups	chopped fresh spinach	500 mL
2 cups	frozen cheese tortellini	500 mL
3 tbsp	grated Parmesan cheese	45 mL

If fresh spinach is not available, substitute one-quarter 10-oz (300 g) package frozen spinach. Thaw and drain excess liquid.

Serves 4 to 6

1. In a nonstick saucepan sprayed with vegetable spray, heat oil over medium-high heat. Add garlic, onions, carrots and celery; cook 4 minutes or until onions are softened.
2. Add stock, basil and pepper. Bring to a boil; reduce heat to medium and cook 8 minutes or until vegetables are tender-crisp.
3. Stir in tomatoes, spinach and tortellini. Cover and cook 5 minutes or until tortellini is heated through and vegetables are tender. Serve immediately, garnished with Parmesan cheese.

Make Ahead

✦ Prepare soup up to 2 days in advance, but do not add tortellini until ready to re-heat and serve.

✦ Can be frozen up to 3 weeks.

Nutritional Analysis (Per Serving)
✦ Calories: 157 ✦ Protein: 7 g ✦ Cholesterol: 3 mg
✦ Sodium: 234 mg ✦ Fat, total: 5 g ✦ Carbohydrates: 23 g
✦ Fiber: 3 g ✦ Fat, saturated: 1 g

Broccoli and Lentil Soup

1 1/2 tsp	vegetable oil	7 mL
2 tsp	crushed garlic	10 mL
1	medium onion, chopped	1
1	celery stalk, chopped	1
1	large carrot, chopped	1
4 cups	chicken stock	1 L
2 1/2 cups	chopped broccoli	625 mL
3/4 cup	dried green lentils	175 mL
2 tbsp	grated Parmesan cheese	25 mL

A dollop of light sour cream on top of each bowlful gives a great taste and sophisticated look.

Serves 4 to 6

1. In large nonstick saucepan, heat oil; sauté garlic, onion, celery and carrot until softened, approximately 5 minutes.
2. Add stock, broccoli and lentils; cover and simmer for 30 minutes, stirring occasionally, or until lentils are tender.
3. Purée in food processor until creamy and smooth. Serve sprinkled with Parmesan.

Make Ahead

✦ Prepare and refrigerate up to a day before and reheat gently, adding more stock if too thick.

Nutritional Analysis (Per Serving)
✦ Calories: 144 ✦ Protein: 11 g ✦ Cholesterol: 1 mg
✦ Sodium: 564 mg ✦ Fat: 3 g ✦ Carbohydrates: 18 g
✦ Fiber: 5 g

Vegetable and Bean Minestrone

1 tbsp	vegetable oil	15 mL
1 tsp	crushed garlic	5 mL
1½ cups	finely chopped onion	375 mL
1	medium carrot, finely chopped	1
1	small celery stalk, finely chopped	1
4½ cups	beef or chicken stock	1.125 L
1½ cups	finely chopped peeled potatoes	375 mL
1½ cups	chopped broccoli	375 mL
1	can (19 oz/540 mL) tomatoes, crushed	1
¾ cup	cooked chickpeas	175 mL
2	bay leaves	2
1½ tsp	dried basil	7 mL
1½ tsp	oregano	7 mL
	Pepper	
⅓ cup	broken spaghetti	75 mL
1 tbsp	grated Parmesan cheese	15 mL

Serves 6

1. In large nonstick saucepan, heat oil; sauté garlic, onion, carrot and celery until softened, approximately 5 minutes.
2. Add stock, potatoes, broccoli, tomatoes, chickpeas, bay leaves, basil and oregano; cover and simmer for approximately 40 minutes or until vegetables are tender, stirring occasionally. Remove bay leaves. Season with pepper to taste.
3. Add pasta; cook for 10 minutes, stirring often, or until spaghetti is firm to the bite. Sprinkle with cheese.

Make Ahead

✦ Make and refrigerate up to a day before and reheat gently before serving, adding more stock if too thick.

Nutritional Analysis (Per Serving)
- ✦ Calories: 194
- ✦ Protein: 10 g
- ✦ Cholesterol: 1 mg
- ✦ Sodium: 754 mg
- ✦ Fat: 3 g
- ✦ Carbohydrates: 32 g
- ✦ Fiber: 5 g

Red Lentil Soup with Cheese Tortellini

¾ cup	chopped onions	175 mL
2 tsp	minced garlic	10 mL
4 cups	vegetable or chicken stock	1 L
1½ cups	chopped peeled sweet potatoes	375 mL
1 cup	chopped red bell peppers	250 mL
½ cup	chopped carrots	125 mL
½ cup	red lentils	125 mL
1 tsp	dried basil	5 mL
4 oz	fresh or frozen cheese tortellini	125 g

This soup is perfect for the whole family. Because it's puréed, children can't identify specific vegetables they might otherwise object to eating!

Serves 4

1. In a nonstick saucepan sprayed with vegetable spray, cook onions and garlic over medium heat for 5 minutes or until golden. Add stock, sweet potatoes, red peppers, carrots, red lentils and basil; bring to a boil. Reduce heat to low; cook, covered, for 15 minutes or until lentils and vegetables are tender.
2. In a food processor or blender, purée soup in batches. Return to saucepan over medium-high heat; bring to a boil. Add tortellini; reduce heat to simmer. Cook for 5 minutes or until tortellini is tender.

Nutritional Analysis (Per Serving)
- ✦ Calories: 324
- ✦ Protein: 14 g
- ✦ Cholesterol: 12 mg
- ✦ Sodium: 127 mg
- ✦ Fat, total: 3 g
- ✦ Carbohydrates: 61 g
- ✦ Fiber: 9 g
- ✦ Fat, saturated: 1.7 g

Mushroom Split Pea Soup

1 tbsp	vegetable oil	15 mL
1	medium onion, chopped	1
1 tsp	crushed garlic	5 mL
1	celery stalk, chopped	1
1	medium carrot, chopped	1
1 cup	sliced mushrooms	250 mL
3½ cups	beef or chicken stock	875 mL
¾ cup	split peas	175 mL
4 tsp	2% yogurt (optional)	20 mL

Light sour cream can replace the yogurt for a thicker texture.

Serves 4 or 5

1. In large nonstick saucepan, heat oil; sauté onion, garlic, celery, carrot and mushrooms until softened, approximately 5 minutes.
2. Add stock and split peas; reduce heat, cover and simmer for 40 minutes or until split peas are tender, stirring occasionally. Purée in food processor until creamy and smooth.
3. Pour into soup bowls and garnish each with yogurt (if using).

Make Ahead
✦ Prepare and refrigerate up to a day before and reheat gently before serving, adding more stock if too thick.

Nutritional Analysis (Per Serving)
✦ Calories: 169   ✦ Protein: 12 g   ✦ Cholesterol: 0 mg
✦ Sodium: 499 mg   ✦ Fat: 3 g   ✦ Carbohydrates: 24 g
✦ Fiber: 4 g

Black Bean Soup

2 tsp	vegetable oil	10 mL
2 tsp	minced garlic	10 mL
1 cup	chopped onions	250 mL
1 cup	chopped carrots	250 mL
1	can (19 oz/540mL) black beans, drained (or 12 oz/375 g cooked beans)	1
3 cups	chicken stock	750 mL
¾ tsp	ground cumin	4 mL
¼ cup	chopped coriander or parsley	50 mL

Canned black beans can sometimes be difficult to find. Use 12 oz (375 g) cooked beans. One cup (250 mL) of dry beans yields approximately 3 cups (750 mL) cooked.

Serves 4 or 5

1. In a nonstick saucepan sprayed with vegetable spray, heat oil over medium heat; add garlic, onions and carrots and cook, stirring occasionally, for 4 minutes or until the onion is softened.
2. Add beans, stock and cumin; bring to a boil. Cover, reduce heat to medium low and simmer for 20 minutes or until carrots are softened. Transfer to food processor and purée until smooth.
3. Ladle into bowls; sprinkle with coriander.

Make Ahead
✦ Prepare and refrigerate up to a day ahead and reheat gently before serving, adding more stock if too thick.

Nutritional Analysis (Per Serving)
✦ Calories: 147   ✦ Protein: 8 g   ✦ Cholesterol: 0 mg
✦ Sodium: 741 mg   ✦ Fat, total: 3 g   ✦ Carbohydrates: 25 g
✦ Fiber: 8 g   ✦ Fat, saturated: 0.3 g

Black Bean Soup with Wild Rice and Corn

1 cup	chopped onions	250 mL
1 cup	canned corn or frozen corn, thawed	250 mL
1/2 cup	finely chopped carrots	125 mL
1 1/2 tsp	minced garlic	7 mL
3 1/2 cups	vegetable or chicken stock	875 mL
1	can (19 oz/540 mL) tomatoes, with juice	1
1 cup	canned cooked black beans, rinsed and drained	250 mL
1/3 cup	wild rice	75 mL
1 tbsp	packed brown sugar	15 mL
1 1/2 tsp	ground cumin	7 mL
1 1/2 tsp	dried basil	7 mL
	Freshly ground black pepper	
3 tbsp	chopped fresh coriander or parsley	45 mL

Serves 6

1. In a large nonstick saucepan sprayed with vegetable spray, cook onions, corn, carrots and garlic over medium-high heat for 5 minutes or until starting to brown. Add stock, tomatoes, black beans, wild rice, brown sugar, cumin and basil; bring to a boil, breaking tomatoes with back of a spoon. Reduce heat to medium-low; cook, covered, for 30 minutes or until rice is tender.

2. Ladle soup into bowls. Season to taste with pepper; garnish with chopped coriander. Serve.

Tip

✦ A small dollop of low-fat sour cream or yogurt followed by a sprinkling of the coriander gives this soup an elegant look.

Nutritional Analysis (Per Serving)
- ✦ Calories: 130
- ✦ Protein: 6 g
- ✦ Cholesterol: 0 mg
- ✦ Sodium: 63 mg
- ✦ Fat, total: 1 g
- ✦ Carbohydrates: 30 g
- ✦ Fiber: 5 g
- ✦ Fat, saturated: 0.3 g

Cauliflower and White Bean Soup

1 tsp	vegetable oil	5 mL
1 tsp	minced garlic	5 mL
1 cup	chopped onions	250 mL
3 2/3 cups	chicken stock	900 mL
3 cups	cauliflower florets	750 mL
1 1/2 cups	canned white kidney beans, drained	375 mL
1 cup	peeled diced potatoes	250 mL
1/4 tsp	ground black pepper	1 mL
1/4 cup	chopped fresh dill (or 1 tsp/5mL dried dillweed)	50 mL
2 tbsp	chopped chives or green onions	25 mL

Parsley or basil can be substituted for dill.

Serves 6

1. In nonstick saucepan sprayed with vegetable spray, heat oil over medium heat. Add garlic and onions; cook for 4 minutes or until softened. Add stock, cauliflower, kidney beans, potatoes, pepper and dried dillweed, if using; bring to a boil. Cover, reduce heat to low and simmer for 20 to 25 minutes or until vegetables are tender.

2. Transfer soup to food processor or blender; purée. Serve garnished with fresh dill, if using, and chives.

Make Ahead

✦ Prepare and refrigerate up to a day ahead and reheat gently before serving, adding more stock if too thick.

Nutritional Analysis (Per Serving)
- ✦ Calories: 116
- ✦ Protein: 6 g
- ✦ Cholesterol: 0 mg
- ✦ Sodium: 731 mg
- ✦ Fat, total: 1 g
- ✦ Carbohydrates: 22 g
- ✦ Fiber: 5 g
- ✦ Fat, saturated: 0.2 g

Three-Bean Soup

2 tsp	vegetable oil	10 mL
2 tsp	minced garlic	10 mL
3/4 cup	chopped onions	175 mL
3/4 cup	chopped carrots	175 mL
4 cups	chicken or vegetable stock	1 L
1 1/4 cups	canned chickpeas, drained	300 mL
1 1/4 cups	canned red kidney beans, drained	300 mL
1 1/4 cups	canned white kidney beans, drained	300 mL
1 tsp	dried basil	5 mL
1/4 cup	chopped fresh parsley	50 mL

Fiber-up with beans: *Want to boost your fiber intake? Try chickpeas — they're a great alternative to meat or chicken in soups, pasta sauces and salads. One cup (250 mL) of cooked chickpeas packs 12.5 g fiber. That's one-half the recommended daily intake. Like other legumes (such as kidney beans, black beans and lentils), chickpeas contain mostly soluble fiber, which delays stomach emptying and keeps you feeling full longer. It also keeps your blood sugar stable and can help to lower elevated blood cholesterol.*

Serves 6

1. In saucepan sprayed with vegetable spray, heat oil over medium heat; add garlic, onions and carrots and cook for 5 minutes or until onion is softened. Add chicken stock and 1 cup (250 mL) each of the chickpeas and red and white kidney beans; add basil. Bring to a boil. Cover, reduce heat to low and let simmer for 15 minutes or until carrots are tender.

2. Transfer soup to blender or food processor and purée. Return puréed soup to saucepan and stir in remaining 1/4 cup (50 mL) each chickpeas, red and white kidney beans. Cook gently for 5 minutes or until heated through. Serve garnished with parsley.

Tips

✦ Any combination of cooked beans will work well.

✦ If cooking your own beans, use 1 cup (250 mL) of dry to make 3 cups (750 mL) cooked.

Make Ahead

✦ Prepare and refrigerate up to a day ahead and reheat gently before serving, adding more stock if too thick.

Nutritional Analysis (Per Serving)

✦ Calories: 187   ✦ Protein: 10 g   ✦ Cholesterol: 0 mg
✦ Sodium: 974 mg   ✦ Fat, total: 3 g   ✦ Carbohydrates: 31 g
✦ Fiber: 9 g   ✦ Fat, saturated: 0.3 g

White, Red and Black Bean Soup

2 tsp	vegetable oil	10 mL
2 tsp	minced garlic	10 mL
2/3 cup	chopped onions	150 mL
3/4 cup	chopped carrots	175 mL
1/3 cup	chopped celery	75 mL
3 3/4 cups	chicken or vegetable stock	925 mL
1 1/4 cups	canned black beans, drained	300 mL
1 1/4 cups	canned red kidney beans, drained	300 mL
1 1/4 cups	canned white kidney beans, drained	300 mL
1 1/4 tsp	dried basil	6 mL
1/2 tsp	dried oregano	2 mL
1/4 cup	chopped fresh basil or parsley	50 mL

Serves 6

1. In saucepan sprayed with vegetable spray, heat oil over medium heat; add garlic, onions, carrots and celery and cook for 5 minutes or until onions are softened. Add chicken stock and 1 cup (250 mL) each of the black, red and white kidney beans; add basil and oregano. Bring to a boil. Cover, reduce heat to low and let simmer for 15 minutes or until carrots are tender.

2. Transfer soup to blender or food processor and purée. Return puréed soup to saucepan and stir in remaining 1/4 cup (50 mL) each black, red and white kidney beans. Cook gently for 5 minutes or until heated through. Serve garnished with basil.

Tips

✦ Any other combination of cooked beans will work well.

✦ If cooking your own beans, use 1 cup (250 mL) of dry to make 3 cups (750 mL) cooked.

✦ Other dried herbs can replace basil and oregano. Try bay leaves and rosemary.

Make Ahead

✦ Prepare and refrigerate up to a day ahead. Reheat gently before serving, adding more stock if too thick.

Nutritional Analysis (Per Serving)
✦ Calories: 187 ✦ Protein: 10 g ✦ Cholesterol: 0 mg
✦ Sodium: 974 mg ✦ Fat: 3 g ✦ Carbohydrates: 31 g
✦ Fiber: 9 g

Pumpkin and White Bean Soup

2 tsp	vegetable oil	10 mL
2 tsp	minced garlic	10 mL
1 cup	chopped onions	250 mL
1/2 cup	chopped carrots	125 mL
1/2 cup	chopped celery	125 mL
3 1/2 cups	Basic Vegetable Stock (see recipe page 52)	875 mL
1	can (14 oz/398 mL) pumpkin (not pie filling)	1
1	can (19 oz/540 mL) white kidney beans, rinsed and drained	1
1	bay leaf	1
1 tsp	ground ginger	5 mL
1/4 cup	maple syrup	50 mL

In season, use fresh pumpkin. Bake for approximately 1 hour at 375°F (190°C) or until tender.

Serves 4 to 6

1. In a nonstick saucepan sprayed with vegetable spray, heat oil over medium-high heat. Add garlic, onions, carrots and celery; cook 4 minutes or until onions and celery are softened.
2. Stir in stock, pumpkin, beans, bay leaf and ginger. Bring to a boil; reduce heat, cover, and cook 15 to 20 minutes or until vegetables are tender.
3. Stir in maple syrup. Serve immediately.

Make Ahead
✦ Prepare up to 2 days in advance. Add more stock if too thick.
✦ Freeze for up to 4 weeks.

Nutritional Analysis (Per Serving)
✦ Calories: 175   ✦ Protein: 7 g   ✦ Cholesterol: 0 mg
✦ Sodium: 172 mg   ✦ Fat, total: 2 g   ✦ Carbohydrates: 34 g
✦ Fiber: 6 g   ✦ Fat, saturated: 0.3 g

Split-Pea Barley Vegetable Soup

1 tsp	vegetable oil	5 mL
1 1/2 tsp	minced garlic	7 mL
3/4 cup	chopped onions	175 mL
6 cups	Basic Vegetable Stock (see recipe, page 52)	1.5 L
1 1/2 cups	diced potatoes	375 mL
1 cup	diced carrots	250 mL
1/2 cup	dried yellow split peas	125 mL
1/3 cup	barley	75 mL
2	bay leaves	2
2 tsp	dried basil	10 mL
1 1/2 cups	green beans cut in 1-inch (2.5 cm) pieces	375 mL
1 cup	diced plum tomatoes	250 mL
1/4 tsp	freshly ground black pepper	1 mL

Serves 6 to 8

1. In a nonstick saucepan sprayed with vegetable spray, heat oil over medium heat. Add garlic and onions; cook 4 minutes or until softened.
2. Stir in stock, potatoes, carrots, split peas, barley, bay leaves and basil. Bring to a boil; reduce heat to medium-low, cover and cook 40 minutes or until peas and barley are tender.
3. Stir in green beans, tomatoes and pepper; cook, covered, 10 minutes or until green beans are tender-crisp.

Make Ahead
✦ Prepare Steps 1 and 2 up to 1 day in advance. Add beans and tomatoes when reheating and ready to serve.

Nutritional Analysis (Per Serving)
✦ Calories: 129   ✦ Protein: 6 g   ✦ Cholesterol: 0 mg
✦ Sodium: 20 mg   ✦ Fat, total: 1 g   ✦ Carbohydrates: 26 g
✦ Fiber: 4 g   ✦ Fat, saturated: 0.1 g

Yellow Split-Pea Soup

2 tsp	vegetable oil	10 mL
2 tsp	minced garlic	10 mL
1 cup	chopped onions	250 mL
1 cup	chopped carrots	250 mL
1 cup	chopped celery	250 mL
7 cups	basic vegetable stock	1.75 L
1 cup	diced potatoes	250 mL
1 cup	dried yellow split peas	250 mL

Garnish

¼ cup	2% plain yogurt (optional)	50 mL
¼ cup	chopped green onions	50 mL

The yellow split peas puréed in this soup give it a rich and creamy texture.

Serves 6 to 8

1. In a nonstick saucepan, heat oil over medium-high heat. Add garlic, onions, carrots and celery; cook 5 minutes or until vegetables are softened and starting to brown.
2. Stir in stock, potatoes and split peas. Bring to a boil; reduce heat to medium-low, cover and cook 40 minutes or until split peas are tender.
3. In a food processor or blender, purée soup. Serve hot with a dollop of yogurt, if desired, and sprinkled with green onions.

Make Ahead

✦ Prepare up to 2 days in advance, adding more stock if too thick.
✦ Freeze up to 4 weeks.

Nutritional Analysis (Per Serving)
✦ Calories: 136   ✦ Protein: 8 g   ✦ Cholesterol: 0 mg
✦ Sodium: 32 mg   ✦ Fat, total: 2 g   ✦ Carbohydrates: 24 g
✦ Fiber: 2 g   ✦ Fat, saturated: 0.2 g

Creamy Bean and Clam Chowder

1 tbsp	vegetable oil	15 mL
1½ cups	chopped onion	375 mL
2 tsp	crushed garlic	10 mL
1	can (5 oz/142 g) clams	1
2 cups	chicken stock	500 mL
1	medium potato, peeled and diced	1
1½ cups	drained canned white kidney beans	375 mL
2 tbsp	chopped fresh dill (or 1 tsp/5 mL dried dillweed)	25 mL
2 tbsp	chopped fresh chives or green onions	25 mL
1 tbsp	chopped fresh parsley (or 2 tsp/10 mL dried)	15 mL

Try other canned white beans such as navy beans or white pea beans.

Serves 4 to 6

1. In nonstick saucepan, heat oil; sauté onion and garlic until softened, approximately 5 minutes.
2. Drain clams, reserving juice; set clams aside. To saucepan, add clam juice, stock and potato; cover and simmer for 20 minutes or until potato is tender.
3. Add beans; cover and cook for 10 minutes. Purée in food processor until smooth. Return to saucepan; stir in reserved clams, dill, chives and parsley.

Make Ahead

✦ Prepare and refrigerate early in day and reheat gently before serving, adding more stock if too thick.

Nutritional Analysis (Per Serving)
✦ Calories: 159   ✦ Protein: 12 g   ✦ Cholesterol: 15 mg
✦ Sodium: 288 mg   ✦ Fat: 3 g   ✦ Carbohydrates: 19 g
✦ Fiber: 5 g

Clam and Scallop Chowder

2	cans (5 oz/142 g) baby clams	2
1 tsp	vegetable oil	5 mL
1 tsp	minced garlic	5 mL
1 cup	chopped onions	250 mL
3/4 cup	chopped celery	175 mL
3/4 cup	chopped carrots	175 mL
2 cups	chicken or fish stock	500 mL
1	can (19 oz/540 mL) tomatoes, puréed	1
1 1/2 cups	peeled, diced potatoes	375 mL
1 tsp	dried basil	5 mL
1 tsp	dried oregano	5 mL
1	bay leaf	1
8 oz	scallops, sliced	250 g

Canned tomatoes are available whole (with juice), crushed or puréed. If a recipe calls for puréed tomatoes but you only have whole, just purée them in a food processor.

Serves 6

1. Drain clams, reserving liquid; measure out 1 1/2 cups (375 mL) of clams for chowder and reserve the rest for another use.
2. In a nonstick saucepan sprayed with vegetable spray, heat oil over medium heat. Add garlic, onions, celery and carrots; cook for 4 minutes or until onion is softened. Add the reserved clam liquid, stock, tomatoes, potato, basil, oregano and bay leaf; bring to a boil. Cover, reduce heat to low and simmer for 35 minutes or until potatoes are tender. Stir in scallops and clams; cook for 5 minutes longer or until scallops are just done at center.

Tips

+ Shrimp or squid or any firm white fish can be used instead of scallops.
+ If using frozen scallops, defrost and drain excess liquid.

Make Ahead

+ Prepare up to a day ahead, but do not add scallops and clams until just ready to serve.

Nutritional Analysis (Per Serving)
+ Calories: 188   + Protein: 20 g   + Cholesterol: 46 mg
+ Sodium: 690 mg   + Fat, total: 2 g   + Carbohydrates: 20 g
+ Fiber: 3 g   + Fat, saturated: 0.3 g

Creamy Salmon Dill Bisque

6 oz	salmon fillet	150 g
2 tsp	margarine or butter	10 mL
1 tsp	minced garlic	5 mL
1 cup	chopped onions	250 mL
1 cup	chopped carrots	250 mL
1/2 cup	chopped celery	125 mL
1 tbsp	tomato paste	15 mL
2 1/4 cups	chicken stock	550 mL
1 1/2 cups	peeled, chopped potatoes	375 mL
1/2 cup	2% milk	125 mL
1/4 cup	chopped fresh dill	50 mL

Carrots contain beta carotene, which your body converts to vitamin A — an essential nutrient for normal vision, cell division and growth, and building immune compounds that fight infections, as well as healthy skin, bones and teeth. Beta carotene also acts as an antioxidant, protecting cells from damage caused by unstable free radical molecules, which scientists believe to play a role in the development of some cancers. Another good source of beta carotene is sweet potatoes.

When using margarine, choose a soft (non-hydrogenated) version to limit consumption of trans fats.

Serves 4

1. In nonstick pan sprayed with vegetable spray, cook salmon over high heat for 3 minutes, then turn and cook 2 minutes longer, or until just barely done at center. Set aside.

2. Melt margarine in nonstick saucepan sprayed with vegetable spray over medium heat. Add garlic, onions, carrots, and celery; cook for 5 minutes or until onion is softened. Add tomato paste, stock and potatoes; bring to a boil. Cover, reduce heat to low and simmer for 20 minutes or until carrots and potatoes are tender.

3. Transfer soup to food processor or blender and purée. Return to saucepan and stir in milk and dill. Flake the cooked salmon. Add to soup and serve.

Tips

✦ Canned, drained salmon can be used if fresh is unavailable.

✦ Leftover cooked salmon can also be used.

✦ Fresh basil can replace dill. If using dried herbs, use 1 tsp (5 mL) and add during cooking.

Make Ahead

✦ Prepare up to a day ahead, but do not add salmon until just ready to serve. Add more stock if soup is too thick.

Nutritional Analysis (Per Serving)

✦ Calories: 179 ✦ Protein: 12 g ✦ Cholesterol: 23 mg
✦ Sodium: 617 mg ✦ Fat, total: 5 g ✦ Carbohydrates: 23 g
✦ Fiber: 3 g ✦ Fat, saturated: 1 g

Gazpacho with Baby Shrimp

2¹/₂ cups	tomato juice	625 mL
4 tsp	red wine vinegar	20 mL
1 tsp	crushed garlic	5 mL
1 cup	diced sweet green pepper	250 mL
1 cup	diced sweet red or yellow pepper	250 mL
1¹/₄ cups	diced tomatoes	300 mL
1 cup	diced cucumber	250 mL
1 cup	chopped green onions	250 mL
1 cup	diced celery	250 mL
¹/₄ cup	chopped fresh parsley (or 1 tbsp/15 mL dried)	50 mL
2 tbsp	chopped fresh basil (or 2 tsp/10 mL dried)	25 mL
1 tbsp	lemon juice	15 mL
2 oz	cooked baby shrimp	50 g
Dash	Tabasco	Dash
	Pepper	
	Chopped fresh chives	

Serves 4 to 6

1. In large bowl, combine tomato juice, vinegar and garlic.
2. Mix together green and red peppers, tomatoes, cucumber, green onions and celery; add half to bowl. Place remaining half in food processor; purée until smooth. Add to bowl.
3. Add parsley, basil, lemon juice, shrimp, Tabasco, and pepper to taste; stir gently to combine well. Refrigerate until chilled. To serve, garnish each bowl with sprinkle of chives.

Tip

✦ Serve with a spoonful of yogurt on each serving.

Make Ahead

✦ Prepare and refrigerate up to a day before to allow flavors to blend and develop.

Nutritional Analysis (Per Serving)
✦ Calories: 58 ✦ Protein: 4 g ✦ Cholesterol: 18 mg
✦ Sodium: 413 mg ✦ Fat: 0.5 g ✦ Carbohydrates: 11 g
✦ Fiber: 3 g

Sweet Potato Soup with Split Peas and Ham

³/₄ cup	chopped onions	175 mL
³/₄ cup	chopped carrots	175 mL
1¹/₂ tsp	minced garlic	7 mL
6¹/₂ cups	chicken or beef stock	1.625 L
1¹/₂ cups	diced sweet potatoes	375 mL
³/₄ cup	dried yellow split peas	175 mL
¹/₃ cup	small soup pasta (such as orzo or ditali)	75 mL
1 cup	diced cooked ham	250 mL

When buying ham, make sure it's "fully cooked" or "ready-to-eat." Most store-bought cooked ham has been smoked to give it a rich and juicy flavor, yet it takes on other flavors when added to soup — or any other recipe.

Serves 6

1. In a nonstick saucepan sprayed with vegetable spray, cook onions, carrots and garlic over medium-high heat for 3 minutes or until softened. Add stock, sweet potatoes and split peas; bring to a boil. Reduce heat to medium-low; cook, covered, for 40 minutes or until split peas are tender.
2. Transfer mixture to a food processor; purée until smooth. Return soup to saucepan. Add pasta and ham; cook over medium heat, covered, for 8 minutes or until pasta is tender.

Nutritional Analysis (Per Serving)
✦ Calories: 289 ✦ Protein: 17 g ✦ Cholesterol: 28 mg
✦ Sodium: 200 mg ✦ Fat: 2 g ✦ Carbohydrates: 41 g
✦ Fiber: 2 g

Lentil Soup with Sausage and Tiny Pasta

6 oz	medium-spicy Italian sausage, casings removed	175 g
1 cup	chopped onions	250 mL
1½ tsp	minced garlic	7 mL
½ cup	finely chopped carrots	125 mL
5 cups	beef or chicken stock	1.25 L
1	can (19 oz/540 mL) tomatoes, crushed	1
½ cup	green lentils	125 mL
1½ tsp	packed brown sugar	7 mL
1 tsp	Italian seasoning	5 mL
1	bay leaf	1
⅓ cup	small pasta (orzo, ditali, stelline or tubetti)	75 mL

Lentils are an excellent source of folic acid and potassium and a good source of iron.

Serves 6

1. In a nonstick frying pan set over medium heat, cook sausage, stirring to break up meat, for 5 minutes or until no longer pink. Drain excess fat; set aside.

2. In a large nonstick saucepan sprayed with vegetable spray, cook onions and garlic over medium-high heat for 2 minutes or until softened. Add carrots; cook for 2 minutes. Add stock, tomatoes, lentils, brown sugar, Italian seasoning, bay leaf and sausage; bring to a boil. Reduce heat to medium-low; cook, covered, for 35 minutes.

3. Add pasta; cook, covered and stirring occasionally, for 10 minutes or until pasta and lentils are tender.

Nutritional Analysis (Per Serving)
- Calories: 223
- Protein: 10 g
- Cholesterol: 12 mg
- Sodium: 150 mg
- Fat, total: 8 g
- Carbohydrates: 29 g
- Fiber: 4 g
- Fat, saturated: 2 g

Tomato Rice Soup with Mushrooms and Beef

8 oz	boneless top sirloin beef steak, cut into ½-inch (1 cm) cubes	250 g
3 cups	chopped mushrooms	750 mL
¾ cup	chopped onions	175 mL
1½ tsp	minced garlic	7 mL
1	can (19 oz/540 mL) tomatoes, with juice	1
3½ cups	beef or chicken stock	875 mL
1 tbsp	packed brown sugar	15 mL
1 tsp	dried basil	5 mL
1 tsp	chili powder	5 mL
½ cup	long-grain white rice	125 mL

The long-grain white rice provides a nice light texture. Be careful not to overcook it, though; if you do, all those delicious grains will turn into a sticky mess!

Serves 6

1. In a nonstick saucepan sprayed with vegetable spray, cook beef over medium-high heat, stirring occasionally, for 3 minutes or until browned on all sides. Remove from pan; set aside.

2. Respray pan; add mushrooms, onions and garlic. Cook for approximately 5 minutes or until browned and tender; add tomatoes, stock, brown sugar, basil and chili powder. Bring to a boil; stir, breaking up tomatoes with back of a spoon. Add browned beef and rice; reduce heat to low. Cook, covered, for 20 minutes or until rice is tender.

Nutritional Analysis (Per Serving)
- Calories: 170
- Protein: 13 g
- Cholesterol: 29 mg
- Sodium: 187 mg
- Fat, total: 3 g
- Carbohydrates: 23 g
- Fiber: 2 g
- Fat, saturated: 1.3 g

Hearty Beef Soup with Lentils and Barley

6 oz	boneless round steak, cut into 1/2-inch (1 cm) cubes	175 g
2 tbsp	all-purpose flour	25 mL
1/2 cup	chopped onions	125 mL
1 tsp	minced garlic	5 mL
1/2 cup	chopped carrots	125 mL
1/2 cup	chopped green bell peppers	125 mL
1/2 cup	green lentils	125 mL
1	can (19 oz/540 mL) tomatoes, with juice	1
4 1/2 cups	beef or chicken stock	1.125 L
1/3 cup	pearl barley	75 mL
2 tsp	packed brown sugar	10 mL
1 1/2 tsp	dried basil	7 mL
2	bay leaves	2
1/4 tsp	freshly ground black pepper	1 mL

Lentils come in a wide variety of colors — including the common brown lentil, as well as black, yellow, red and orange. On their own, lentils are pretty b-o-o-o-r-ing. But when tossed into salads, soups or mixed with other grain dishes, they're sensational! What's more, lentils are high in fiber and are also as excellent source of folic acid and potassium. This recipe uses green lentils — not only do they cook faster, but they hold their shape better than red and yellow varieties (which have a tendency to dissolve as they cook).

Serves 4

1. In a bowl coat beef with flour; shake off excess. In a nonstick saucepan sprayed with vegetable spray, cook beef over medium-high heat for 5 minutes or until browned on all sides. Remove meat to a plate; respray pan. Add onions and garlic; cook for 2 minutes. Add carrots and green peppers; cook, stirring occasionally, for 4 minutes or until vegetables are softened.

2. Add browned beef, lentils, tomatoes, stock, barley, brown sugar, basil, bay leaves and pepper; bring to a boil, breaking up tomatoes with back of a spoon. Reduce heat to medium-low; cook, covered, for 45 minutes or until lentils and barley are tender. Ladle soup into bowls. Serve.

Tips

✦ Stewing beef is often used in a soup like this, but it takes a lot of cooking time before it becomes tender. To speed things up, try using more tender cuts of beef: either round or loin. Remember, too, that the smaller the cubes, the faster the meat tenderizes.

✦ *Pumping iron:* This soup is a great source of iron. At 5 mg per serving, it goes a long way toward meeting your daily iron requirements (women need 18 mg each day; men require 8 mg). Iron is used by your red blood cells to form hemoglobin, the molecule that transports oxygen from your lungs to your cells. If your body is deficient in iron, you'll feel lethargic, weak and you'll tire easily during exercise. This soup gets its iron boost from stewing beef, lentils and barley. For more on iron, see pages 175 and 191.

Nutritional Analysis (Per Serving)
✦ Calories: 300 ✦ Protein: 26 g ✦ Cholesterol: 41 mg
✦ Sodium: 300 mg ✦ Fat, total: 6 g ✦ Carbohydrates: 42 g
✦ Fiber: 9 g ✦ Fat, saturated: 2.3 g

Salads

◆ ◆

Tomato, Potato and Artichoke Salad with Oriental Dressing

1 lb	red potatoes (about 3)	500 g
3	plum tomatoes, seeded	3
1	can (14 oz/398 mL) artichoke hearts, drained and quartered	1
3/4 cup	chopped red onions	175 mL
1/2 cup	chopped fresh coriander	125 mL
1/3 cup	chopped green onions	75 mL

Dressing

2 tbsp	rice wine vinegar	25 mL
2 tbsp	soya sauce	25 mL
1 tbsp	sesame oil	15 mL
1 tbsp	vegetable oil	15 mL
1 tbsp	honey	15 mL
1 tsp	minced garlic	5 mL
1 tsp	minced gingerroot	5 mL

While commercially prepared artichoke hearts are convenient, it's really not very difficult to make your own. Just buy 6 fresh artichokes and rinse them well; with scissors, trim off the thorny tough tops of the outside layers. Rub these surfaces with lemon. Place the artichokes right-side up in boiling water with a squeeze of lemon juice; reduce to a simmer and cook, uncovered, for 20 minutes or until a leaf pulls away easily. Remove leaves and, with a spoon, scrape off the "fuzz" to reveal the tender, delicious artichoke heart.

Serves 4 to 6

1. Scrub but do not peel potatoes; cut into 1 1/2-inch (4 cm) pieces and put in a saucepan. Add cold water to cover; bring to a boil, reduce heat to simmer and cook until tender, about 15 minutes. Rinse under cold water and drain.

2. Cut tomatoes into 1 1/2-inch (4 cm) pieces. In a serving bowl, combine potatoes, tomatoes, artichokes, red onions, coriander and green onions.

3. *Make the dressing:* In a small bowl, whisk together vinegar, soya sauce, sesame oil, vegetable oil, honey, garlic and ginger. Just before serving, pour over salad; toss to coat.

Tips

✦ This salad makes a great side dish or main course.

✦ If eaten the next day, this salad will appear wilted but will have a more pronounced marinated flavor.

✦ When buying artichoke hearts for this recipe, be sure that they're packed in water, not oil. The oil-packed variety has double the calories and triple the fat — a huge difference!

Make Ahead

✦ Prepare salad and dressing up to 1 day in advance. Best if tossed just before serving.

Nutritional Analysis (Per Serving)
✦ Calories: 165 ✦ Protein: 4 g ✦ Cholesterol: 0 mg
✦ Sodium: 394 mg ✦ Fat, total: 5 g ✦ Carbohydrates: 29 g
✦ Fiber: 5 g ✦ Fat, saturated: 1 g

Three-Tomato Salad with Goat Cheese Dressing

Dressing

3 oz	goat cheese	75 g
1/4 cup	light sour cream	50 mL
3 tbsp	light mayonnaise	45 mL
1 1/2 tsp	dried basil	7 mL
1 tsp	minced garlic	5 mL

Salad

3 cups	chopped tomatoes (about 1 lb/500 g)	750 mL
3 cups	quartered plum tomatoes (about 1 lb/500 g)	750 mL
1 cup	chopped softened sun-dried tomatoes (see tip, at right)	250 mL

Serves 4 to 6

1. In a food processor, purée goat cheese, sour cream, mayonnaise, basil and garlic until smooth, scraping down sides of bowl once or twice.
2. In a serving bowl, combine tomatoes, plum tomatoes and sun-dried tomatoes.
3. Pour dressing over salad; toss to coat.

Tips

+ To soften sun-dried tomatoes, cover with boiling water and let soak 15 minutes; drain and chop.
+ Tomatoes and goat cheese are a great combination.
+ If yellow tomatoes are available, use them instead of regular tomatoes.

Make Ahead

+ Prepare salad and dressing early in the day. Toss just before serving.

Nutritional Analysis (Per Serving)

+ Calories: 114
+ Protein: 5 g
+ Cholesterol: 0 mg
+ Sodium: 298 mg
+ Fat, total: 5 g
+ Carbohydrates: 15 g
+ Fiber: 3 g
+ Fat, saturated: 0.3 g

Tomato, Avocado and Snow Pea Salad with Blue Cheese Dressing

4 oz	snow peas, cut in half	125 g
	Lettuce leaves	
Half	medium red or sweet onion, sliced	Half
Half	avocado, sliced thinly	Half
1	large tomato, sliced	1

Dressing

1/4 cup	crumbled blue cheese	50 mL
1/3 cup	2% yogurt	75 mL
1/4 tsp	crushed garlic	1 mL
	Salt and pepper	

Since avocado discolors quickly when sliced, assemble the salad just before serving.

Puréeing dressing gives it a smooth thin texture. Processing on and off allows pieces of blue cheese to remain.

Serves 4

1. Steam or microwave snow peas just until tender-crisp. Drain and rinse with cold water; drain well and pat dry.
2. Line serving platter with lettuce leaves. Decoratively arrange onion, avocado, tomato and snow peas over lettuce.
3. *Dressing:* In food processor, combine blue cheese, yogurt and garlic; process until just combined. Season with salt and pepper to taste. Drizzle over salad.

Make Ahead

✦ Prepare and refrigerate dressing up to a day before. Prepare salad just prior to serving.

Nutritional Analysis (Per Serving)
- ✦ Calories: 105
- ✦ Protein: 5 g
- ✦ Cholesterol: 7 mg
- ✦ Sodium: 140 mg
- ✦ Fat: 6 g
- ✦ Carbohydrates: 8 g
- ✦ Fiber: 2 g

Sweet Pepper Salad with Red Pepper Dressing

2 cups	chopped sweet red, green or yellow pepper	500 mL
1 cup	chopped cucumber	250 mL
1 cup	cherry tomatoes, cut into quarters	250 mL
1/2 cup	chopped red onion	125 mL
1/2 cup	chopped celery	125 mL

Dressing

2 tbsp	diced red onion	25 mL
1/4 cup	diced sweet red pepper	50 mL
1 tbsp	lemon juice	15 mL
2 tsp	red wine vinegar	10 mL
1 tbsp	water	15 mL
2 tbsp	olive oil	25 mL
1/2 tsp	crushed garlic	2 mL
1/2 tsp	Dijon mustard	2 mL
2 tbsp	chopped fresh parsley	25 mL
	Salt and pepper	

Serves 4

1. In salad bowl, combine red pepper, cucumber, tomatoes, onion and celery.
2. *Dressing:* In food processor, combine onion, red pepper, lemon juice, vinegar, water, oil, garlic, mustard, parsley, and salt and pepper to taste; process until combined. Pour over salad and toss to combine.

Tip

✦ Double the recipe for red pepper dressing and save half to serve as a wonderful side sauce for fish or chicken.

Make Ahead

✦ Prepare dressing up to a day before. Stir well and pour over salad just prior to serving.

Nutritional Analysis (Per Serving)
- ✦ Calories: 102
- ✦ Protein: 1 g
- ✦ Cholesterol: 0 mg
- ✦ Sodium: 37 mg
- ✦ Fat: 7 g
- ✦ Carbohydrates: 10 g
- ✦ Fiber: 2 g

Vegetable Salad with Feta Dressing

Salad

2 cups	chopped celery	500 mL
2 cups	chopped English cucumbers	500 mL
2 cups	chopped red bell peppers	500 mL
2 cups	chopped plum tomatoes	500 mL
1 cup	chopped red onions	250 mL
1/3 cup	sliced black olives	75 mL

Dressing

2 oz	feta cheese, crumbled	50 g
1/3 cup	light sour cream	75 mL
2 tbsp	2% plain yogurt	25 mL
1 tbsp	freshly squeezed lemon juice	15 mL
1 1/2 tsp	minced garlic	7 mL
1 1/4 tsp	dried oregano	6 mL

Serves 4 to 6

1. In a serving bowl, combine celery, cucumbers, red peppers, tomatoes, red onions and olives.
2. *Make the dressing:* In a food processor or blender, combine feta, sour cream, yogurt, lemon juice, garlic and oregano; process until smooth.
3. Pour dressing over salad; toss to coat.

Tip
✦ Try goat cheese instead of feta for a change.

Make Ahead
✦ Prepare salad and dressing early in the day. Toss just before serving.

Nutritional Analysis (Per Serving)
✦ Calories: 86   ✦ Protein: 4 g   ✦ Cholesterol: 9 mg
✦ Sodium: 213 mg   ✦ Fat, total: 3 g   ✦ Carbohydrates: 13 g
✦ Fiber: 3 g   ✦ Fat, saturated: 2 g

Warm Spinach and Mushroom Salad

Dressing

3 tbsp	balsamic vinegar	45 mL
4 tsp	olive oil	20 mL
1 tsp	minced garlic	5 mL

Salad

6 cups	washed, dried and torn spinach leaves	1.5 L
1/2 cup	chopped, softened sun-dried tomatoes (see tip, page 93)	125 mL
1/4 cup	toasted chopped walnuts	50 mL
2 tsp	vegetable oil	10 mL
1 tsp	minced garlic	5 mL
2 cups	sliced oyster mushrooms	500 mL
3/4 cup	sliced red onions	175 mL

Try this recipe with different mushrooms, such as cremini or, for a decadent evening, shiitake or chanterelles. Common mushrooms will also work well with this recipe.

Serves 4 to 6

1. In a small bowl, whisk together vinegar, olive oil and garlic. Set aside.
2. Put spinach, sun-dried tomatoes and walnuts in a large serving bowl.
3. In a large nonstick frying pan, heat oil over high heat. Add garlic, mushrooms and red onions; cook 6 minutes, or until mushrooms are browned and any excess liquid is absorbed. Quickly add hot vegetables and dressing to spinach and toss. Serve immediately.

Make Ahead
✦ Prepare dressing and sauté mushroom mixture early in the day. Do not mix with salad. When ready to serve, reheat mushroom mixture and toss with dressing and salad.

Nutritional Analysis (Per Serving)
✦ Calories: 108   ✦ Protein: 4 g   ✦ Cholesterol: 0 mg
✦ Sodium: 143 mg   ✦ Fat, total: 8 g   ✦ Carbohydrates: 9 g
✦ Fiber: 3 g   ✦ Fat, saturated: 1 g

Spinach Salad with Oranges and Mushrooms

8 cups	packed fresh spinach leaves, washed, dried and torn into bite-sized pieces	2 L
1½ cups	sliced mushrooms	375 mL
¾ cup	sliced water chestnuts	175 mL
½ cup	sliced red onions	125 mL
¼ cup	raisins	50 mL
2 tbsp	sliced or chopped almonds, toasted	25 mL
1	orange, peeled and sections cut into pieces	1

Dressing

3 tbsp	olive oil	45 mL
3 tbsp	balsamic vinegar	45 mL
2 tbsp	orange juice concentrate, thawed	25 mL
1 tbsp	honey	15 mL
1 tsp	grated orange zest	5 mL
1 tsp	minced garlic	5 mL

Serves 6

1. In large serving bowl, combine spinach, mushrooms, water chestnuts, red onions, raisins, almonds and orange pieces; toss well.

2. In small bowl whisk together olive oil, balsamic vinegar, orange juice concentrate, honey, orange zest and garlic; pour over salad and toss.

Tips

✦ Use 1½ cups (375 mL) canned, drained mandarins to replace the orange.

✦ Oyster mushrooms or other wild mushrooms are exceptionally tasty.

Make Ahead

✦ Prepare salad early in the day, keeping refrigerated. Prepare dressing up to 2 days ahead. Pour over salad just before serving.

Nutritional Analysis (Per Serving)
✦ Calories: 177 ✦ Protein: 5 g ✦ Cholesterol: 0 mg
✦ Sodium: 88 mg ✦ Fat, total: 10 g ✦ Carbohydrates: 21 g
✦ Fiber: 5 g ✦ Fat, saturated: 1 g

Creamy Coleslaw with Apples and Raisins

1	medium carrot, diced	1
⅓ cup	finely chopped red onion	75 mL
½ cup	finely chopped sweet red or green pepper	125 mL
2	green onions, diced	2
3 cups	thinly sliced white or red cabbage	750 mL
⅓ cup	diced (unpeeled) apple	75 mL
⅓ cup	raisins	75 mL

Dressing

¼ cup	light mayonnaise	50 mL
2 tbsp	2% yogurt	25 mL
2 tbsp	lemon juice	25 mL
1½ tsp	honey	7 mL
	Salt and pepper	

Serves 4

1. In serving bowl, combine carrot, red onion, red pepper, green onions, cabbage, apple and raisins.

2. *Dressing:* In small bowl, stir together mayonnaise, yogurt, lemon juice, honey, and salt and pepper to taste, mixing well. Pour over salad and toss gently to combine.

Tip

✦ For curry lovers, 1 tsp (5 mL) curry powder can be added to the dressing.

Make Ahead

✦ Prepare and refrigerate early in day and stir well before serving.

Nutritional Analysis (Per Serving)
✦ Calories: 137 ✦ Protein: 2 g ✦ Cholesterol: 4 mg
✦ Sodium: 119 mg ✦ Fat: 5 g ✦ Carbohydrates: 24 g
✦ Fiber: 3 g

Oriental Coleslaw

³/₄ cup	chopped snow peas	175 mL
3 cups	shredded green cabbage	750 mL
3 cups	shredded red cabbage	750 mL
1 cup	sliced water chestnuts	250 mL
1 cup	sliced red peppers	250 mL
³/₄ cup	canned mandarin oranges, drained	175 mL
2	medium green onions, chopped	2

Dressing

3 tbsp	brown sugar	45 mL
2 tbsp	rice wine vinegar	25 mL
2 tbsp	vegetable oil	25 mL
1 tbsp	soya sauce	15 mL
1 tbsp	sesame oil	15 mL
1 tsp	minced garlic	5 mL
1 tsp	minced gingerroot	5 mL

Get moving — being active every day is a sure way to achieve and maintain a healthy body weight. Regular physical activity will help you look and feel your best.

Serves 8 to 10

1. In saucepan of boiling water or microwave, blanch snow peas just until tender-crisp, approximately 1 to 2 minutes; refresh in cold water and drain. Place in serving bowl with shredded cabbage, water chestnuts, red peppers, mandarin oranges and green onions; toss well to combine.

2. In small bowl whisk together brown sugar, vinegar, vegetable oil, soya sauce, sesame oil, garlic and ginger; pour over salad and toss well.

Tips

✦ Other vegetables such as green beans or broccoli can replace snow peas.

✦ This is a great variation on the usual coleslaw.

Make Ahead

✦ Prepare salad and dressing early in the day. Best if tossed just before serving.

Nutritional Analysis (Per Serving)
✦ Calories: 81 ✦ Protein: 1 g ✦ Cholesterol: 0 mg
✦ Sodium: 116 mg ✦ Fat, total: 4 g ✦ Carbohydrates: 12 g
✦ Fiber: 2 g ✦ Fat, saturated: 0.4 g

Potato Salad with Crispy Fresh Vegetables

½ cup	chopped broccoli florets	125 mL
½ cup	snow peas, sliced	125 mL
4	medium potatoes, peeled, cooked and cubed	4
2	green onions, sliced	2
½ cup	chopped sweet red, yellow or green pepper	125 mL
1	celery stalk, diced	1
½ cup	finely chopped onions	125 mL
1	medium carrot, sliced	1
3 tbsp	finely chopped fresh dill (or 1 tsp/5 mL dried dillweed)	45 mL
¼ tsp	paprika	1 mL
2 tbsp	chopped fresh parsley	25 mL

Dressing

4 tsp	red wine vinegar	20 mL
2 tbsp	2% yogurt	25 mL
3 tbsp	light mayonnaise	45 mL
3 tbsp	lemon juice	45 mL
1½ tsp	Dijon mustard	7 mL
1 tsp	crushed garlic	5 mL
1 tbsp	vegetable oil	15 mL

Lighten up those high-fat recipes: *Got an old recipe you don't use now because it's high in fat? Try replacing some of the ingredients to make a low-fat version. Here are some examples (and the amount of fat and calories you'll save for each 1 cup/250 mL: for whipping (35%) cream, use evaporated 2% milk (save 57 g fat, 336 cal) or evaporated skim milk (save 88 g fat, 612 cal); for regular sour cream, use light (5%) sour cream (save 34 g fat, 203 cal) or non-fat plain yogurt (save 31 g fat, 260 cal); for regular mayonnaise, use light mayonnaise (save 33 g fat, 926 cal).*

Serves 4 to 6

1. In saucepan, blanch broccoli and snow peas in boiling water for 1 minute or just until color brightens. Drain and rinse with cold water; drain well and place in large salad bowl.
2. Add potatoes, green onions, red pepper, celery, chopped onions, carrot and dill.
3. *Dressing:* In small bowl, mix together vinegar, yogurt, mayonnaise, lemon juice, mustard, garlic and oil; pour over salad and mix gently. Garnish with paprika and parsley.

Tips

+ Vary the vegetables accompanying the potatoes in this unusual salad.
+ All the vegetables must be fresh, colorful and crisp looking.
+ For a sweeter salad, try balsamic vinegar.

Make Ahead

+ Toss salad with dressing early in day and refrigerate. Stir just before serving.

Nutritional Analysis (Per Serving)
+ Calories: 128 + Protein: 3 g + Cholesterol: 2 mg
+ Sodium: 85 mg + Fat: 5 g + Carbohydrates: 19 g
+ Fiber: 2 g

Vegetable and Bean Minestroni (page 77) ➤

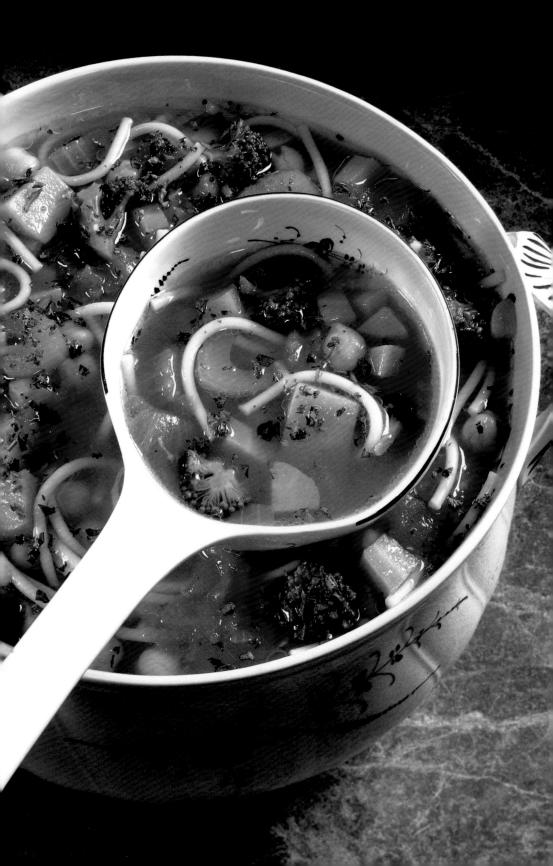

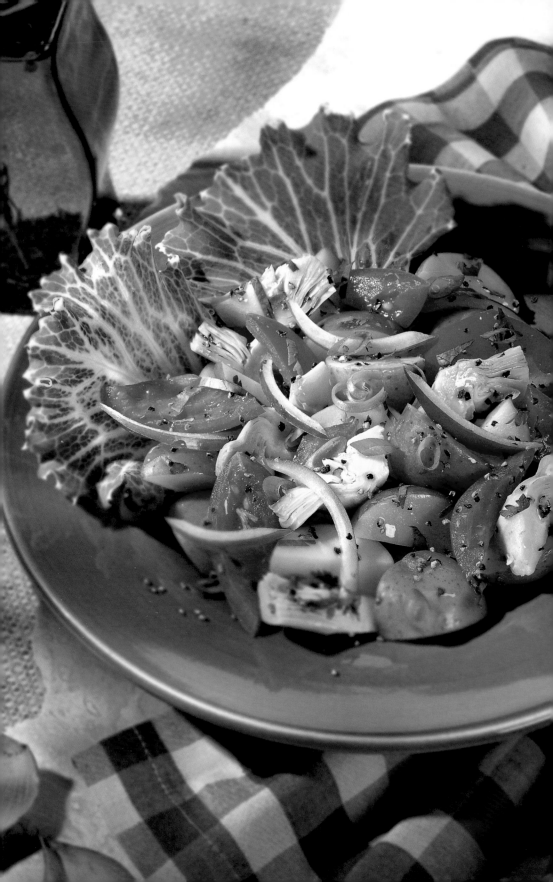

Pesto Potato Salad

2 lb	scrubbed whole red potatoes with skins on	1 kg
Pesto		
1¼ cups	packed fresh basil leaves	300 mL
3 tbsp	olive oil	45 mL
2 tbsp	toasted pine nuts	25 mL
2 tbsp	grated Parmesan cheese	25 mL
1 tsp	minced garlic	5 mL
¼ tsp	salt	1 mL
¼ cup	chicken stock or water	50 mL
1 cup	halved snow peas	250 mL
¾ cup	chopped red onions	175 mL
¾ cup	chopped red peppers	175 mL
¾ cup	chopped green peppers	175 mL
½ cup	corn kernels	125 mL
2	medium green onions, chopped	2
2 tbsp	toasted pine nuts	25 mL
2 tbsp	lemon juice	25 mL

Serves 8 to 10

1. Put potatoes in saucepan with cold water to cover; bring to a boil and cook for 20 to 25 minutes, or until easily pierced with a sharp knife. Drain and set aside.
2. Meanwhile, put basil, olive oil, pine nuts, Parmesan, garlic and salt in food processor; process until finely chopped. With the processor running, gradually add stock through the feed tube; process until smooth.
3. In saucepan of boiling water or microwave, blanch snow peas for 1 or 2 minutes, or until tender-crisp; refresh in cold water and drain. Place in large serving bowl, along with pesto, red onions, red and green peppers, corn, green onions, pine nuts and lemon juice. When potatoes are cool enough to handle, cut into wedges and add to serving bowl; toss well to combine.

Tips

✦ Use ¾ cup (175 mL) storebought pesto instead of making your own. Keep in mind that calories and fat will be higher.

✦ If basil is unavailable, try spinach or parsley leaves.

✦ Roasted corn kernels (1 cob) make a delicious replacement for canned kernels. Broil or barbecue corn for 15 minutes or until charred.

Make Ahead

✦ Prepare potatoes, pesto and vegetables up to a day ahead. Toss before serving.

✦ Tastes great the next day.

Nutritional Analysis (Per Serving)
✦ Calories: 154 ✦ Protein: 4 g ✦ Cholesterol: 1 mg
✦ Sodium: 124 mg ✦ Fat, total: 6 g ✦ Carbohydrates: 22 g
✦ Fiber: 3 g ✦ Fat, saturated: 1 g

◄ Tomato, Potato and Artichoke Salad with Oriental Dressing (page 90)

Broccoli, Apricot and Red Pepper Salad in a Creamy Dressing

4 cups	broccoli florets	1 L
1 cup	chopped carrots	250 mL
1 cup	sliced red bell peppers	250 mL
¾ cup	sliced water chestnuts	175 mL
½ cup	chopped red onions	125 mL
½ cup	chopped dried apricots or dates	125 mL
⅓ cup	raisins	75 mL
2 oz	feta cheese, crumbled	50 g

Dressing

¼ cup	chopped fresh dill	50 mL
¼ cup	light mayonnaise	50 mL
¼ cup	light sour cream	50 mL
2 tbsp	freshly squeezed lemon juice	25 mL
1½ tsp	minced garlic	7 mL
	Freshly ground black pepper, to taste	

Serves 4 to 6

1. Boil or steam broccoli 3 minutes or until tender-crisp; drain. Rinse under cold water; drain well.

2. In a large serving bowl, combine broccoli, carrots, red peppers, water chestnuts, red onions, apricots, raisins and feta cheese.

3. In a small bowl, whisk together dill, mayonnaise, sour cream, lemon juice and garlic. Pour over salad; toss to coat. Season to taste with pepper.

Make Ahead

✦ Prepare early in the day. Best served chilled.

Nutritional Analysis (Per Serving)
- ✦ Calories: 156
- ✦ Protein: 5 g
- ✦ Cholesterol: 8 mg
- ✦ Sodium: 184 mg
- ✦ Fat, total: 5 g
- ✦ Carbohydrates: 27 g
- ✦ Fiber: 4 g
- ✦ Fat, saturated: 2 g

Oriental Vegetable Salad

2½ cups	trimmed green beans	625 mL
2 cups	asparagus cut into 1-inch (2.5 cm) pieces	500 mL
1½ cups	halved snow peas	375 mL
1¾ cups	bean sprouts	425 mL
1½ cups	sliced red bell peppers	375 mL
1 cup	chopped baby corn cobs	250 mL
¾ cup	canned sliced water chestnuts, drained	175 mL
¾ cup	canned mandarin oranges, drained	175 mL

Dressing

4 tsp	soya sauce	20 mL
4 tsp	rice wine vinegar	20 mL
1 tbsp	olive oil	15 mL
1 tbsp	honey	15 mL
2 tsp	sesame oil	10 mL
2 tsp	toasted sesame seeds	10 mL
1½ tsp	minced garlic	7 mL
1 tsp	minced gingerroot	5 mL

Serves 4 to 6

1. Boil or steam green beans and asparagus for 2 to 3 minutes or until tender-crisp; drain. Rinse under cold water and drain; transfer to a large serving bowl.

2. Boil or steam snow peas 45 seconds or until tender-crisp; drain. Rinse under cold water and drain; add to serving bowl along with bean sprouts, red peppers, corn cobs, water chestnuts and mandarin oranges. Toss to combine.

3. In a small bowl, whisk together soya sauce, vinegar, olive oil, honey, sesame oil, sesame seeds, garlic and ginger. Pour over salad; toss to coat.

Nutritional Analysis (Per Serving)
- ✦ Calories: 139
- ✦ Protein: 6 g
- ✦ Cholesterol: 0 mg
- ✦ Sodium: 486 mg
- ✦ Fat, total: 5 g
- ✦ Carbohydrates: 22 g
- ✦ Fiber: 5 g
- ✦ Fat, saturated: 1 g

Broccoli, Snow Pea and Baby Corn Salad with Orange Dressing

2 cups	chopped broccoli florets	500 mL
1 cup	snow peas, cut into pieces	250 mL
1/2 cup	sliced onion	125 mL
Half	medium sweet red pepper, sliced	Half
3 cups	torn romaine lettuce	750 mL
3/4 cup	drained mandarin orange sections	175 mL
1/2 cup	sliced water chestnuts	125 mL
8	drained canned baby corn cobs	8
1 tbsp	raisins	15 mL
1 tbsp	chopped walnuts	15 mL

Dressing

3 tbsp	olive oil	45 mL
3 tbsp	frozen orange juice concentrate, thawed	45 mL
1 1/2 tsp	red wine vinegar	7 mL
1/2 tsp	crushed garlic	2 mL
4 tsp	lemon juice	20 mL
1 tsp	granulated sugar	5 mL

Serves 4 to 6

1. Steam or microwave broccoli and snow peas just until tender-crisp. Drain and rinse with cold water; drain again and pat dry. Place in serving bowl.

2. Add onion, red pepper, lettuce, oranges, water chestnuts, corn, raisins and walnuts.

3. *Dressing:* In small bowl, mix oil, orange juice concentrate, vinegar, garlic, lemon juice and sugar; pour over salad and toss well.

Tips

✦ Substitute other vegetables for those listed. Try asparagus instead of snow peas, yellow or green pepper instead of red pepper, or choose other lettuces.

✦ Orange juice concentrate provides the intense flavor — if you substitute orange juice, flavor will be less pronounced. Refreeze the remainder of thawed concentrate for making juice later.

Make Ahead

✦ Prepare dressing up to a day before. Toss with salad just before serving.

Nutritional Analysis (Per Serving)
✦ Calories: 150   ✦ Protein: 3 g   ✦ Cholesterol: 0 mg
✦ Sodium: 16 mg   ✦ Fat: 8 g   ✦ Carbohydrates: 19 g
✦ Fiber: 3 g

Baby Corn, Broccoli and Cauliflower Salad in a Creamy Citrus Dressing

2 cups	broccoli florets	500 mL
2 cups	cauliflower florets	500 mL
2 cups	chopped baby corn cobs	500 mL
2 cups	chopped red bell peppers	500 mL
1 cup	chopped water chestnuts	250 mL
¾ cup	chopped green onions	175 mL

Dressing

⅓ cup	chopped fresh coriander	75 mL
3 tbsp	olive oil	45 mL
3 tbsp	light sour cream	45 mL
2 tbsp	freshly squeezed lemon juice	25 mL
2 tbsp	freshly squeezed lime juice	25 mL
2 tbsp	light mayonnaise	25 mL
2 tsp	honey	10 mL
1½ tsp	minced garlic	7 mL
1 to 2 tsp	minced fresh jalapeño peppers	5 to 10 mL

> *To reduce the fat in recipes, use lower fat versions of sour cream and cottage, ricotta and cream cheeses.*

Serves 6 to 8

1. Boil or steam broccoli and cauliflower 5 minutes or until tender-crisp. Rinse under cold water and drain. Put in a serving bowl.
2. Stir baby corn, red peppers, water chestnuts and green onions into broccoli-cauliflower mixture.
3. *Make the dressing:* In a small bowl, whisk together coriander, olive oil, sour cream, lemon juice, lime juice, mayonnaise, honey, garlic and jalapeño peppers. Pour over salad; toss to coat. Chill and serve.

Tips

✦ For the best flavor, be sure to use fresh citrus juices. Bottled juice concentrates tend to be more acidic.

✦ 1 tsp (5 mL) chili powder can replace jalapeño peppers.

✦ Replace coriander with fresh dill or basil.

Make Ahead

✦ Prepare salad up to 1 day in advance. The salad will marinate.

Nutritional Analysis (Per Serving)
✦ Calories: 102   ✦ Protein: 3 g   ✦ Cholesterol: 0 mg
✦ Sodium: 460 mg   ✦ Fat, total: 6 g   ✦ Carbohydrates: 11 g
✦ Fiber: 2 g   ✦ Fat, saturated: 1 g

Grilled Vegetable Salad

1	medium zucchini	1
1	medium sweet red pepper	1
Half	large red onion	Half
12	small mushrooms	12
3 cups	mixed lettuce leaves (Boston, romaine, radicchio)	750 mL

Dressing

2 tbsp	lemon juice	25 mL
2 tbsp	water	25 mL
1 tbsp	brown sugar	15 mL
4 tsp	balsamic vinegar	20 mL
1 tsp	crushed garlic	5 mL
2 tbsp	olive oil	25 mL
	Salt and pepper	

If using wooden skewers, soak them in water for at least 30 minutes before using to prevent scorching.

Serves 4

1. Cut zucchini, red pepper and onion into 2-inch (5 cm) chunks. Alternately thread along with mushrooms onto barbecue skewers.
2. *Dressing:* In small bowl, combine lemon juice, water, sugar, vinegar and garlic; gradually whisk in oil. Season with salt and pepper to taste. Pour into dish large enough to hold skewers.
3. Add skewers to dressing; marinate for 20 minutes, turning often.
4. Grill vegetables until tender, basting with dressing and rotating often, approximately 15 minutes.
5. Remove vegetables from skewers and place on lettuce-lined serving platter. Pour any remaining dressing over vegetables.

Nutritional Analysis (Per Serving)
- Calories: 107
- Protein: 2 g
- Cholesterol: 0 mg
- Sodium: 8 mg
- Fat: 7 g
- Carbohydrates: 10 g
- Fiber: 2 g

Pear, Lettuce and Feta Cheese Salad

Dressing

2 tbsp	raspberry vinegar	25 mL
2½ tbsp	olive oil	35 mL
1 tsp	minced garlic	5 mL
1½ tsp	honey	7 mL
1 tsp	sesame oil	5 mL

Salad

4 cups	red or green leaf lettuce, washed, dried and torn into pieces	1 L
1½ cups	curly endive or escarole, washed, dried and torn into pieces	375 mL
1½ cups	radicchio, washed, dried and torn into pieces	375 mL
1 cup	diced pears (about 1 pear)	250 mL
2 oz	feta cheese, crumbled	50 g
⅓ cup	sliced black olives	75 mL

Serves 4 to 6

1. *Prepare the dressing:* In a small bowl, whisk together vinegar, olive oil, garlic, honey and sesame oil; set aside.
2. *Make the salad:* In a serving bowl, combine leaf lettuce, curly endive, radicchio, pears, feta and olives. Pour dressing over; toss gently to coat. Serve immediately.

Tip
- If you don't want the salad to wilt, use a larger amount of romaine lettuce.

Make Ahead
- Prepare salad and dressing early in the day. Toss just before serving

Nutritional Analysis (Per Serving)
- Calories: 108
- Protein: 2 g
- Cholesterol: 8 mg
- Sodium: 165 mg
- Fat, total: 8 g
- Carbohydrates: 8 g
- Fiber: 2 g
- Fat, saturated: 2 g

Sweet Cinnamon Waldorf Salad

2½ cups	diced apples	625 mL
¾ cup	diced celery	175 mL
1 cup	red or green seedless grapes, quartered	250 mL
1 cup	chopped red or green peppers	250 mL
⅓ cup	raisins	75 mL
½ cup	canned mandarin oranges, drained	125 mL
2 tbsp	finely chopped pecans	25 mL
Dressing		
¼ cup	light mayonnaise	50 mL
¼ cup	light (1%) sour cream	50 mL
2 tbsp	honey	25 mL
1 tbsp	lemon juice	15 mL
½ tsp	cinnamon	2 mL

Serves 6 to 8

1. In serving bowl, combine apples, celery, grapes, sweet peppers, raisins, mandarin oranges and pecans.
2. In small bowl, combine mayonnaise, sour cream, honey, lemon juice and cinnamon; mix thoroughly. Pour over salad and toss.

Tips

✦ For a nice change, use a combination of peas and apples to total 2½ cups (625 mL).
✦ Children like this salad as a dessert.

Make Ahead

✦ Prepare salad early in the day. Refrigerate and toss well just before serving. Keeps well for 2 days in refrigerator.

Nutritional Analysis (Per Serving)
✦ Calories: 116   ✦ Protein: 1 g   ✦ Cholesterol: 2 mg
✦ Sodium: 116 mg   ✦ Fat, total: 3 g   ✦ Carbohydrates: 24 g
✦ Fiber: 2 g   ✦ Fat, saturated: 0.4 g

Tortilla Bean Salad with Creamy Salsa Dressing

3 cups	romaine lettuce, washed, dried and torn into pieces	750 mL
1 cup	canned chickpeas, rinsed and drained	250 mL
1 cup	canned red kidney beans rinsed and drained	250 mL
1 cup	shredded carrots	250 mL
1 cup	chopped red bell peppers	250 mL
¾ cup	chopped red onions	175 mL
⅓ cup	chopped fresh coriander	75 mL
Dressing		
3 tbsp	salsa	45 mL
3 tbsp	light sour cream	45 mL
2 tbsp	light mayonnaise	25 mL
1 tsp	minced garlic	5 mL
¾ to 1 tsp	chili powder	4 to 5 mL
1 oz	tortilla chips, crushed (about 12)	25 g

Serves 4

1. In a large bowl, combine lettuce, chickpeas, kidney beans, carrots, red peppers, red onions and coriander.
2. *Make the dressing:* In a small bowl, whisk together salsa, sour cream, mayonnaise, garlic and chili powder.
3. Just before serving, pour dressing over salad. Toss to coat. Sprinkle with tortilla chips. Serve immediately.

Tips

✦ Use a mild or hot salsa, whichever you prefer.
✦ Vary beans and vegetables to your taste.

Make Ahead

✦ Prepare salad and dressing early in the day. Toss just before serving.

Nutritional Analysis (Per Serving)
✦ Calories: 263   ✦ Protein: 11 g   ✦ Cholesterol: 1 mg
✦ Sodium: 443 mg   ✦ Fat, total: 7 g   ✦ Carbohydrates: 42 g
✦ Fiber: 10 g   ✦ Fat, saturated: 1 g

Corn and Three-Bean Salad

8 oz	pasta wheels or small shell pasta	250 g
1 cup	canned black beans or chickpeas, drained	250 mL
3/4 cup	canned red kidney beans, drained	175 mL
3/4 cup	canned white kidney beans, drained	175 mL
3/4 cup	canned corn niblets, drained	175 mL
1 1/4 cups	diced sweet red peppers	300 mL
3/4 cup	diced carrots	175 mL
1/2 cup	diced red onions	125 mL
Dressing		
1/4 cup	lemon juice	50 mL
3 tbsp	vegetable oil	45 mL
3 tbsp	red wine or cider vinegar	45 mL
2 tsp	crushed garlic	10 mL
1/2 cup	chopped coriander or parsley	125 mL

Serves 6 to 8

1. Cook pasta in boiling water according to package instructions or until firm to the bite. Rinse with cold water. Drain and place in serving bowl.
2. Add all three beans, corn niblets, red peppers, carrots and onions.
3. *Make the dressing:* In small bowl combine lemon juice, oil, vinegar, garlic and coriander. Pour over dressing, and toss.

Make Ahead

✦ Prepare salad and dressing separately up to a day ahead. Pour dressing over top just before serving.

Nutritional Analysis (Per Serving)
- ✦ Calories: 277
- ✦ Protein: 10 g
- ✦ Cholesterol: 0 mg
- ✦ Sodium: 293 mg
- ✦ Fat, total: 7 g
- ✦ Carbohydrates: 46 g
- ✦ Fiber: 7 g
- ✦ Fat, saturated: 0.6 g

Bean Salad with Fresh Vegetables and Feta Cheese

3/4 cup	drained cooked white or red kidney beans	175 mL
3/4 cup	drained cooked chickpeas	175 mL
1 cup	chopped tomato	250 mL
1/2 cup	chopped onion	125 mL
1/2 cup	chopped celery	125 mL
1/2 cup	chopped sweet green or red pepper	125 mL
1 oz	feta cheese, crumbled	25 g
	Lettuce leaves	
Dressing		
3 tbsp	lemon juice	45 mL
1 tsp	crushed garlic	5 mL
1 tsp	dried basil (or 2 tbsp/25 mL chopped fresh)	5 mL
1/2 tsp	dried oregano (or 1 tbsp/15 mL chopped fresh)	2 mL
2 tbsp	vegetable oil	25 mL

Serves 4

1. In bowl, combine beans, chickpeas, tomato, onion, celery, green pepper and feta cheese.
2. *Dressing:* In small bowl, combine lemon juice, garlic, basil and oregano; whisk in oil. Pour over salad and stir gently to mix well.
3. Line serving bowl with lettuce leaves; top with salad.

Tip

✦ Other crisp vegetables such as broccoli, corn or cucumbers can be substituted.

Make Ahead

✦ Combine with dressing a few hours before eating and let marinate. Stir before arranging in lettuce-lined bowl.

Nutritional Analysis (Per Serving)
- ✦ Calories: 201
- ✦ Protein: 8 g
- ✦ Cholesterol: 6 mg
- ✦ Sodium: 103 mg
- ✦ Fat: 9 g
- ✦ Carbohydrates: 23 g
- ✦ Fiber: 6 g

Pasta and Bean Salad with Creamy Basil Dressing

Dressing

1½ cups	tightly packed fresh basil leaves	375 mL
3 tbsp	grated low-fat Parmesan cheese	45 mL
2 tbsp	toasted pine nuts	25 mL
1½ tsp	minced garlic	7 mL
⅓ cup	low-fat yogurt	75 mL
3 tbsp	fresh lemon juice	45 mL
3 tbsp	light mayonnaise	45 mL
3 tbsp	water	45 mL
1 tbsp	olive oil	15 mL
¼ tsp	freshly ground black pepper	1 mL

Salad

12 oz	medium shell pasta	375 g
¾ cup	canned black beans, rinsed and drained	175 mL
¾ cup	canned chickpeas, rinsed and drained	175 mL
¾ cup	canned red kidney beans, rinsed and drained	175 mL
¾ cup	diced red onions	175 mL
½ cup	shredded carrots	125 mL
2 cups	diced ripe plum tomatoes	500 mL

The lowdown on deli pasta salads: *With only 2 tsp (10 mL) fat per serving, this pasta salad is a great source of low-fat nutrition. But that's not the case with all pasta salads. In fact, the kind typically sold at your local deli can pack as much as 7 tsp (35 mL) of hidden fat (from mayonnaise, cheese and olives) per 1½-cup serving. So stay at home and make this recipe. And if you want to cut even more fat, use fat-free mayonnaise and sour cream.*

Serves 8

1. In a food processor or blender, combine basil, Parmesan cheese, pine nuts and garlic; process until finely chopped. Add yogurt, lemon juice, mayonnaise, water, olive oil and pepper; purée until smooth. Set aside.

2. In a large pot of boiling water, cook pasta for 8 to 10 minutes or until tender but firm; drain. Rinse under cold running water; drain.

3. In a serving bowl, combine pasta, black beans, chickpeas, kidney beans, red onions, carrots and plum tomatoes. Pour dressing over salad; toss to coat well. Serve immediately.

Tips

✦ For those times when you run out of fresh garlic, keep a jar of commercially prepared crushed garlic in the fridge. The garlic is preserved in oil, but the amount of fat added is negligible. Keep in mind that since the garlic has already been crushed, its flavor is less intense. So always add a little more to recipes than you would for fresh garlic.

✦ Canned beans are quick and convenient (you can keep a wide variety on hand in your pantry) and, if you rinse them well, are good for most recipes. Of course, freshly prepared beans are still the best. But time may be a problem. If so, instead of soaking beans overnight, use the quick-soak method: Cover beans with cold water in a saucepan and bring to a boil; cook for 2 minutes. Remove from heat and let them sit for 1 hour. Drain, replace the water and cook over medium-low heat until beans are tender.

Nutritional Analysis (Per Serving)
- ✦ Calories: 456
- ✦ Protein: 18 g
- ✦ Cholesterol: 3 mg
- ✦ Sodium: 178 mg
- ✦ Fat, total: 10 g
- ✦ Carbohydrates: 75 g
- ✦ Fiber: 7 g
- ✦ Fat, saturated: 2.1 g

Italian Bean Pasta Salad

12 oz	medium shell pasta	375 g
2¹⁄₂ cups	chopped tomatoes	625 mL
³⁄₄ cup	diced sweet green peppers	175 mL
³⁄₄ cup	diced red onions	175 mL
²⁄₃ cup	canned red kidney beans, drained	150 mL
²⁄₃ cup	canned white kidney beans, drained	150 mL
²⁄₃ cup	canned chickpeas, drained	150 mL
3 oz	feta cheese, crumbled	75 g
Dressing		
¹⁄₄ cup	lemon juice	50 mL
3 tbsp	olive oil	45 mL
1 tbsp	red wine vinegar	15 mL
2 tsp	crushed garlic	10 mL
2¹⁄₂ tsp	dried basil	12 mL
1¹⁄₂ tsp	dried oregano	7 mL

Serves 6 to 8 as an appetizer

1. Cook pasta in boiling water according to package instructions or until firm to the bite. Rinse with cold water. Drain and place in serving bowl.
2. Add tomatoes, green peppers, onions, three beans and feta cheese.
3. *Make the dressing:* In small bowl add lemon juice, oil, vinegar, garlic, basil and oregano. Mix well. Pour over pasta, and toss.

Make Ahead

✦ Prepare salad and dressing early in the day. Toss up to 2 hours ahead.

Nutritional Analysis (Per Serving)

✦ Calories: 333   ✦ Protein: 11 g   ✦ Cholesterol: 8 mg
✦ Sodium: 266 mg   ✦ Fat, total: 9 g   ✦ Carbohydrates: 53 g
✦ Fiber: 7 g   ✦ Fat, saturated: 2 g

Cold Oriental Noodles with Sesame Dressing

Dressing		
¹⁄₄ cup	Basic Vegetable Stock (see page 52)	50 mL
3 tbsp	honey	45 mL
2 tbsp	tahini	25 mL
1 tbsp	rice wine vinegar	15 mL
1 tbsp	sesame oil	15 mL
1 tbsp	soya sauce	15 mL
1¹⁄₂ tsp	toasted sesame seeds	7 mL
1 tsp	minced garlic	5 mL
1 tsp	minced gingerroot	5 mL
Salad		
8 oz	medium-size rice noodles	250 g
1 cup	asparagus cut in ¹⁄₂-inch (1 cm) pieces	250 mL
1 cup	chopped broccoli	250 mL
1 cup	chopped red bell peppers	250 mL
¹⁄₂ cup	chopped green onions	125 mL
¹⁄₃ cup	chopped fresh coriander	75 mL

Serves 4 to 6

1. In a food processor or blender, purée stock, honey, tahini, vinegar, sesame oil, soya sauce, sesame seeds, garlic and ginger. Set aside.
2. Pour boiling water over noodles to cover; soak 15 minutes or until soft. Drain; rinse with cold water and put in serving bowl.
3. Boil or steam asparagus and broccoli, about 1 minute or until tender-crisp. Rinse under cold water, drain and add to noodles. Add red peppers, green onions and coriander.
4. Pour dressing over noodles and vegetables; toss to coat.

Make Ahead

✦ Prepare salad early in the day. Keep salad and dressing separate. Toss just before serving.

Nutritional Analysis (Per Serving)

✦ Calories: 240   ✦ Protein: 3 g   ✦ Cholesterol: 0 mg
✦ Sodium: 156 mg   ✦ Fat, total: 6 g   ✦ Carbohydrates: 47 g
✦ Fiber: 2 g   ✦ Fat, saturated: 1 g

Penne with Brie Cheese, Tomatoes and Basil

12 oz	penne	375 g
1½ lb	chopped tomatoes	750 g
2 tsp	crushed garlic	10 mL
1 cup	chopped red onions	250 mL
3 oz	diced Brie cheese	75 g
⅓ cup	sliced black olives	75 mL
⅔ cup	chopped fresh basil (or 2 tsp/10 mL dried)	150 mL
3 tbsp	olive oil	45 mL
2 tbsp	lemon juice	25 mL
1 tbsp	red wine vinegar	15 mL
	Pepper	

Sweet Vidalia onions are great to use in season.

Serves 6 to 8 as an appetizer

1. Cook pasta in boiling water according to package instructions or until firm to the bite. Rinse with cold water. Drain and place in serving bowl.
2. Add tomatoes, garlic, onions, cheese, olives, basil, oil, lemon juice, vinegar and pepper. Mix well.

Tips
✦ This recipe needs little oil because the tomatoes give it the necessary liquid. Use ripe juicy tomatoes.

Make Ahead
✦ Prepare tomato dressing early in day and let marinate. Do not toss until ready to serve.

Nutritional Analysis (Per Serving)
- ✦ Calories: 299
- ✦ Protein: 9 g
- ✦ Cholesterol: 9 mg
- ✦ Sodium: 155 mg
- ✦ Fat, total: 10 g
- ✦ Carbohydrates: 43 g
- ✦ Fiber: 4 g
- ✦ Fat, saturated: 3 g

Cold Penne with Fresh Tomato, Sweet Peppers and Coriander

12 oz	penne	375 g
Vegetable Dressing		
2 cups	thinly sliced sweet red and/or yellow peppers	500 mL
2 cups	chopped tomatoes	500 mL
¾ cup	diced cucumbers	175 mL
¾ cup	sliced red onions	175 mL
¼ cup	chopped green onions	50 mL
½ cup	chopped coriander or dill	125 mL
3 tbsp	olive oil	45 mL
3 tbsp	lime or lemon juice	45 mL
2 tsp	crushed garlic	10 mL

Use juicy ripe tomatoes for extra liquid in salad.

Serves 6

1. Cook pasta in boiling water according to package instructions or until firm to the bite. Rinse with cold water. Drain and place in serving bowl.
2. *Make the dressing:* Add sweet peppers, tomatoes, cucumbers, red and green onions, coriander, oil, lime juice and garlic. Toss and serve cold.

Make Ahead
✦ Prepare vegetable dressing early in day and allow to marinate. Toss just before serving.

Nutritional Analysis (Per Serving)
- ✦ Calories: 350
- ✦ Protein: 10 g
- ✦ Cholesterol: 0 mg
- ✦ Sodium: 15 mg
- ✦ Fat, total: 8 g
- ✦ Carbohydrates: 60 g
- ✦ Fiber: 4 g
- ✦ Fat, saturated: 1 g

Chilled Penne Salad with Fresh Tomatoes, Yellow Pepper and Basil

8 oz	penne noodles	250 g
2½ cups	chopped tomatoes	625 mL
1 cup	thinly sliced sweet yellow or green pepper	250 mL
½ cup	chopped fresh basil (or 1½ tsp/7 mL dried)	125 mL
⅓ cup	shredded mozzarella cheese	75 mL
1 tsp	crushed garlic	5 mL
2 tbsp	olive oil	25 mL
1 tbsp	lemon juice	15 mL
2	green onions, sliced	2

Serves 4 to 6

1. Cook penne according to package directions or until firm to the bite. Drain and place in serving bowl.
2. Add tomatoes, yellow pepper, basil, cheese, garlic, oil and lemon juice; toss well. Sprinkle with green onions. Chill for at least 2 hours before serving.

Tip

✦ Substitute rotini or medium shell pasta for the noodles.

Make Ahead

✦ Make early in day. Toss well just before serving.

Nutritional Analysis (Per Serving)
✦ Calories: 228   ✦ Protein: 7 g   ✦ Cholesterol: 3 mg
✦ Sodium: 189 mg ✦ Fat: 6 g   ✦ Carbohydrates: 35 g
✦ Fiber: 2 g

Penne Salad with Tomatoes, Goat Cheese and Basil

12 oz	penne	375 g
3 cups	chopped tomatoes	750 mL
2 tsp	crushed garlic	10 mL
2 tbsp	olive oil	25 mL
2 tbsp	balsamic vinegar	25 mL
3 oz	goat cheese, crumbled	75 g
¾ cup	chopped fresh basil (or 2 tsp/10 mL dried)	175 mL
⅓ cup	sliced black olives	75 mL
	Pepper	

Try feta cheese instead of goat cheese.

Serves 6

1. Cook pasta in boiling water according to package instructions or until firm to the bite. Rinse with cold water. Drain and place in serving bowl.
2. Add tomatoes, garlic, oil, vinegar, cheese, basil, olives and pepper. Toss until cheese begins to melt.

Tip

✦ Apple cider vinegar can replace balsamic vinegar.

Make Ahead

✦ Prepare tomato dressing early in day to marinate. Do not toss until ready to serve.

Nutritional Analysis (Per Serving)
✦ Calories: 333   ✦ Protein: 11 g   ✦ Cholesterol: 4 mg
✦ Sodium: 167 mg ✦ Fat, total: 8 g   ✦ Carbohydrates: 54 g
✦ Fiber: 4 g   ✦ Fat, saturated: 2 g

Penne and Mushroom Salad with Creamy Balsamic Dressing

Dressing

1/3 cup	low-fat sour cream	75 mL
2 tbsp	light mayonnaise	25 mL
2 tbsp	balsamic vinegar	25 mL
2 tbsp	fresh lemon juice	25 mL
1 1/2 tbsp	honey	20 mL
1 tsp	minced garlic	5 mL
1 tsp	hot Asian chili sauce (optional)	5 mL

Salad

1 lb	mushrooms, cleaned and quartered	500 g
3/4 cup	chopped red bell peppers	175 mL
1/2 cup	chopped fresh coriander	125 mL
1/2 cup	chopped red onions	125 mL
1/3 cup	sliced black olives	75 mL
2 oz	light feta cheese, crumbled	50 g
12 oz	penne	375 g

Serves 6

1. In a bowl combine sour cream, mayonnaise, balsamic vinegar, lemon juice, honey, garlic and chili sauce; whisk well. Set aside.

2. In a large nonstick frying pan sprayed with vegetable spray, cook mushrooms over medium-high heat for 5 minutes or until softened and releasing moisture. Drain, discarding liquid. In a serving bowl, combine mushrooms, red peppers, coriander, red onions, black olives and feta cheese. Pour dressing over; toss to coat well.

3. In a large pot of boiling water, cook penne for 8 to 10 minutes or until tender but firm; drain. Rinse under cold running water; drain well. Add to salad; toss well. Serve.

Nutritional Analysis (Per Serving)
- Calories: 364
- Protein: 12 g
- Cholesterol: 18 mg
- Sodium: 252 mg
- Fat, total: 8.3 g
- Carbohydrates: 62 g
- Fiber: 4 g
- Fat, saturated: 3.6 g

Tex-Mex Rotini Salad

8 oz	rotini	250 g
1 1/2 cups	diced ripe plum tomatoes	375 mL
1 cup	canned red kidney beans, rinsed and drained	250 mL
1 cup	canned corn kernels, rinsed and drained	250 mL
1/2 cup	chopped fresh coriander	125 mL
1/2 cup	chopped green onions	125 mL

Dressing

1/3 cup	barbecue sauce	75 mL
2 1/2 tbsp	cider vinegar	35 mL
2 tsp	molasses	10 mL
1 tsp	minced jalapeño pepper (optional)	5 mL
1 oz	baked tortilla chips (about 12)	25 g

Serves 4

1. In a large pot of boiling water, cook rotini for 8 to 10 minutes or until tender but firm; drain. Rinse under cold running water; drain. In a serving bowl combine pasta, tomatoes, kidney beans, corn, coriander and green onions.

2. In a bowl combine barbecue sauce, cider vinegar, molasses and jalapeño pepper; whisk well. Pour dressing over salad; toss to coat well. Garnish with crumbled tortilla chips. Serve.

Nutritional Analysis (Per Serving)
- Calories: 393
- Protein: 16 g
- Cholesterol: 0 mg
- Sodium: 196 mg
- Fat, total: 2 g
- Carbohydrates: 80 g
- Fiber: 2 g
- Fat, saturated: 0.3 g

Pasta Salad with Apricots, Dates and Orange Dressing

12 oz	medium shell pasta	375 g
1½ cups	diced sweet red or green peppers	375 mL
¾ cup	diced dried apricots	175 mL
¾ cup	diced dried dates	175 mL
½ cup	chopped green onions	125 mL
Dressing		
3 tbsp	balsamic vinegar	45 mL
3 tbsp	frozen orange juice concentrate, thawed	45 mL
3 tbsp	olive oil	45 mL
2 tbsp	lemon juice	25 mL
2 tbsp	water	25 mL
1½ tsp	crushed garlic	7 mL
½ cup	chopped parsley	125 mL

This pasta salad goes well with a grilled fish or chicken entrée.

Serves 6 to 8

1. Cook pasta in boiling water according to package instructions or until firm to the bite. Rinse with cold water. Drain and place in serving bowl.
2. Add sweet peppers, apricots, dates and green onions.
3. *Make the dressing:* In small bowl combine vinegar, orange juice concentrate, oil, lemon juice, water, garlic and parsley. Pour over salad, and toss. Toss just before serving.

Make Ahead

✦ Prepare salad and dressing early in day.

Nutritional Analysis (Per Serving)

✦ Calories: 307   ✦ Protein: 7 g   ✦ Cholesterol: 0 mg
✦ Sodium: 8 mg   ✦ Fat, total: 6 g   ✦ Carbohydrates: 58 g
✦ Fiber: 4 g   ✦ Fat, saturated: 0.8 g

Rotini Salad with Oriental Vegetable Sauce

12 oz	rotini	375 g
Sauce		
1 cup	diced cucumbers	250 mL
1 cup	diced carrots	250 mL
1 cup	diced sweet red peppers	250 mL
⅓ cup	chopped green onions	75 mL
¼ cup	chopped coriander or parsley	50 mL
3 tbsp	vegetable oil	45 mL
2 tsp	sesame oil	10 mL
3 tbsp	rice wine vinegar	45 mL
¼ cup	chicken stock	50 mL
1 tbsp	soya sauce	15 mL
2 tsp	minced gingerroot	10 mL
2 tsp	crushed garlic	10 mL

Use ginger marinated in oil, available in the vegetable section of the grocery store. It's easy to use and keeps indefinitely in the refrigerator.

Serves 6 to 8 as an appetizer

1. Cook pasta in boiling water according to package instructions or until firm to the bite. Rinse with cold water. Drain and place in serving bowl.
2. Make the sauce: In food processor, combine cucumbers, carrots, red peppers, onions, coriander, both oils, vinegar, stock, soya sauce, ginger and garlic. Process on and off for 30 seconds until finely diced. Pour over pasta, and toss.

Tip

✦ Zucchini can replace the cucumber.

Make Ahead

✦ Prepare pasta and sauce early in day. Toss up to 2 hours earlier. Toss again just before serving.

Nutritional Analysis (Per Serving)

✦ Calories: 256   ✦ Protein: 7 g   ✦ Cholesterol: 0 mg
✦ Sodium: 167 mg   ✦ Fat, total: 7 g   ✦ Carbohydrates: 41 g
✦ Fiber: 2 g   ✦ Fat, saturated: 0.6 g

Creamy Seafood Pasta Salad

12 oz	medium shell pasta	375 g
1 lb	mixed seafood (combination of scallops, shrimp, squid and/or firm white fish fillets) cut into 2-inch (5 cm) pieces	500 g
1½ cups	diced sweet red peppers	375 mL
1 cup	diced sweet green peppers	250 mL
¾ cup	diced red onions	175 mL
¾ cup	thinly sliced carrots	175 mL
½ cup	chopped green onions	125 mL
Dressing		
1 cup	2% yogurt	250 mL
⅓ cup	light mayonnaise	75 mL
½ cup	chopped fresh dill (or 1½ tbsp/20 mL dried)	125 mL
2 tbsp	lemon juice	25 mL
2 tsp	crushed garlic	10 mL
1 tsp	Dijon mustard	5 mL

Serves 6 to 8 as an appetizer

1. Cook pasta in boiling water according to package instructions or until firm to the bite. Rinse with cold water. Drain and place in serving bowl.
2. In medium nonstick skillet sprayed with vegetable spray, sauté seafood just until cooked, approximately 3 minutes. Set aside.
3. Add red and green peppers, onions, carrots and green onions to pasta. Add seafood.
4. *Make the dressing:* In small bowl combine yogurt, mayonnaise, dill, lemon juice, garlic and mustard. Pour over pasta. Toss and chill.

Make Ahead

✦ Pasta salad and dressing can be prepared early in day. Do not toss until ready to serve.

Nutritional Analysis (Per Serving)
✦ Calories: 374   ✦ Protein: 23 g   ✦ Cholesterol: 89 mg
✦ Sodium: 191 mg   ✦ Fat, total: 6 g ✦ Carbohydrates: 59 g
✦ Fiber: 7 g   ✦ Fat, saturated: 0.9 g

Creamy Crabmeat Salad over Macaroni

8 oz	macaroni or small shell pasta	250 g
12 oz	crabmeat, chopped	375 g
Sauce		
1 cup	tomato juice	250 mL
¼ cup	chili sauce	50 mL
1 tsp	crushed garlic	5 mL
¾ cup	chopped cucumbers	175 mL
½ cup	chopped celery	125 mL
½ cup	chopped sweet green peppers	125 mL
⅓ cup	chopped red onions	75 mL
½ cup	chopped parsley	125 mL
¼ cup	light mayonnaise	50 mL

Serves 6 to 8 as an appetizer

1. Cook pasta in boiling water according to package instructions or until firm to the bite. Rinse with cold water. Drain and place in serving bowl. Add chopped crabmeat.
2. *Make the sauce:* In food processor combine tomato juice, chili sauce, garlic, cucumbers, celery, green peppers, onions, parsley and mayonnaise. Process on and off just until vegetables are finely chopped. Pour over pasta; toss and chill for at least 1 hour.

Make Ahead

✦ Prepare sauce up to a day ahead. Do not toss until ready to serve.

Cooked shrimp, scallops or squid, or a combination, are delicious as a replacement for crabmeat.

Nutritional Analysis (Per Serving)
✦ Calories: 205   ✦ Protein: 14 g   ✦ Cholesterol: 26 mg
✦ Sodium: 510 mg   ✦ Fat, total: 3 g ✦ Carbohydrates: 30 g
✦ Fiber: 2 g   ✦ Fat, saturated: 0.3 g

Wild Rice with Feta Cheese Dressing

3 cups	chicken stock or water	750 mL
½ cup	wild rice	125 mL
½ cup	white rice	125 mL
3	medium asparagus, chopped	3
½ cup	chopped broccoli	125 mL
1	stalk celery, chopped	1
⅓ cup	chopped carrot	75 mL
2	green onions, chopped	2
½ cup	chopped sweet red or green pepper	125 mL
¾ cup	chopped tomato	175 mL

Dressing

½ tsp	crushed garlic	2 mL
1 tbsp	lemon juice	15 mL
1½ tsp	red wine vinegar	7 mL
3 tbsp	crumbled feta cheese	45 mL
¾ tsp	dried oregano (or 1 tbsp/15 mL chopped fresh)	4 mL
3 tbsp	olive oil	45 mL

> *Did you know that wild rice isn't really a rice at all? It's a long-grain marsh grass, characterized by a distinctively nutty flavor and chewy texture. It takes longer to cook than white rice — approximately 45 minutes. Avoid overcooking or it will become starchy.*

Serves 4 to 6

1. In saucepan, bring stock to boil; add wild and white rice and reduce heat. Cover and simmer for 25 to 30 minutes or until just tender. Drain, rinse with cold water and place in serving bowl.

2. Blanch asparagus and broccoli in boiling water until still crisp. Drain and rinse with cold water. Add to bowl along with celery, carrot, green onions, red pepper and tomato; mix well.

3. *Dressing:* In small bowl, whisk together garlic, lemon juice, vinegar, cheese, oregano and oil until well combined. Pour over rice mixture and mix well. Serve at room temperature or chilled.

Tips

✦ You can use 1 cup (250 mL) wild rice and omit the white rice to make a very sophisticated salad.

✦ Goat cheese instead of feta would also suit this salad.

Make Ahead

✦ Make early in the day and stir well before serving.

Nutritional Analysis (Per Serving)
✦ Calories: 224   ✦ Protein: 7 g   ✦ Cholesterol: 4 mg
✦ Sodium: 809 mg   ✦ Fat: 9 g   ✦ Carbohydrates: 29 g
✦ Fiber: 2 g

Polynesian Wild Rice Salad

2 cups	chicken stock	500 mL
1/2 cup	white rice	125 mL
1/2 cup	wild rice	125 mL
1 cup	halved snow peas	250 mL
1 cup	chopped red peppers	250 mL
3/4 cup	chopped celery	175 mL
2/3 cup	sliced water chestnuts	150 mL
1/2 cup	canned mandarin oranges, drained	125 mL
2	medium green onions, chopped	2

Dressing

2 tsp	orange juice concentrate, thawed	10 mL
2 tsp	honey	10 mL
1 tsp	soya sauce	5 mL
1 tsp	vegetable oil	5 mL
1/2 tsp	sesame oil	2 mL
1/2 tsp	lemon juice	2 mL
1/2 tsp	minced garlic	2 mL
1/4 tsp	minced gingerroot	1 mL

Serves 4 to 6

1. Bring stock to boil in medium saucepan; add wild rice and white rice. Cover, reduce heat to medium-low and simmer for 15 to 20 minutes, or until rice is tender and liquid is absorbed. Rinse with cold water. Put rice in serving bowl.

2. In a saucepan of boiling water or microwave, blanch snow peas for 1 or 2 minutes or until tender-crisp; refresh in cold water and drain. Add to serving bowl along with red peppers, celery, water chestnuts, mandarin oranges and green onions; toss well.

3. In small bowl, whisk together orange juice concentrate, honey, soya sauce, vegetable oil, sesame oil, lemon juice, garlic and ginger; pour over salad and toss well.

Nutritional Analysis (Per Serving)
- Calories: 169
- Protein: 5 g
- Cholesterol: 0 mg
- Sodium: 388 mg
- Fat, total: 2 g
- Carbohydrates: 36 g
- Fiber: 2 g
- Fat, saturated: 0.2 g

Rice, Black Bean and Red Pepper Salad

2 cups	chicken stock or water	500 mL
1/2 cup	wild rice	125 mL
1/2 cup	white rice	125 mL
1 cup	chopped red peppers	250 mL
1 cup	chopped snow peas	250 mL
1 cup	canned black beans, drained	250 mL
1/2 cup	corn kernels	125 mL
1/3 cup	chopped red onions	75 mL
1/3 cup	chopped fresh coriander or parsley	75 mL
1	medium green onion, chopped	1

Dressing

3 tbsp	olive oil	45 mL
2 tbsp	lemon juice	25 mL
1 tbsp	red wine vinegar	15 mL
1 tsp	minced garlic	5 mL

Serves 6

1. Bring stock or water to boil in a saucepan; add wild rice and white rice. Cover, reduce heat to medium-low and simmer for 20 minutes or until rice is tender. Remove from heat and let stand for 5 minutes, or until all liquid is absorbed. Rinse with cold water and put in large serving bowl.

2. Add red peppers, snow peas, black beans, corn, red onions, coriander and green onion to rice and toss to combine.

3. In small bowl whisk together olive oil, lemon juice, red wine vinegar and garlic; pour over salad and toss well.

Nutritional Analysis (Per Serving)
- Calories: 251
- Protein: 8 g
- Cholesterol: 0 mg
- Sodium: 437 mg
- Fat, total: 8 g
- Carbohydrates: 40 g
- Fiber: 5 g
- Fat, saturated: 1 g

Southwest Barley Salad

Salad

3 cups	vegetable or chicken stock	750 mL
¾ cup	pearl barley	175 mL
1 cup	canned corn kernels, drained	250 mL
1 cup	canned black beans, rinsed and drained	250 mL
¾ cup	chopped red bell peppers	175 mL
½ cup	chopped green bell peppers	125 mL
½ cup	chopped green onions	125 mL

Dressing

½ cup	medium salsa	125 mL
3 tbsp	low-fat sour cream	45 mL
2 tbsp	fresh lime or lemon juice	25 mL
½ cup	chopped fresh coriander	125 mL
1 tsp	minced garlic	5 mL

Slow-burning carbs keep you going: *Carbohydrates provide energy, but not all in the same way. The "glycemic index" (GI) measures how quickly a food will raise your blood sugar. High-GI foods raise blood sugar quickly, giving you a burst of energy; but this also causes your pancreas to release a large amount of insulin, which lowers your blood sugar, so your quick energy boost is followed by a "crash." Low-GI foods take longer to digest; blood sugar rises slowly, without creating a surge of insulin, so the energy lasts longer. Low-GI carbs include oatmeal, bran cereals, rye bread, barley, citrus fruit, yogurt and milk. For more on GI see pages 6 and 7.*

Serves 6

1. In a saucepan over high heat, bring stock to a boil. Add barley; reduce heat to medium-low. Simmer, covered, for 40 minutes or until barley is tender and liquid is absorbed. Transfer to a serving bowl; cool to room temperature. Add corn, black beans, red peppers, green peppers and green onions.

2. In a bowl combine salsa, sour cream, lime juice, coriander and garlic. Pour dressing over salad; toss to coat well.

Tip

♦ This colorful salad looks great if served in a shaped tortilla shell. Mexican restaurants often use this type of presentation, but because they typically deep-fry the tortilla shell, it adds a lot of fat and calories. Here's a low-fat version: Place a 10-inch (25 cm) flour tortilla (these are available a variety of flavors and colors) in an 8- to 10-inch (20 to 25 cm) fluted baking tin. Bake at 400°F (200°C) for 5 minutes or until slightly browned and the tortilla is holding its shape. Fill with salad and enjoy!

Nutritional Analysis (Per Serving)

- ♦ Calories: 230
- ♦ Protein: 10 g
- ♦ Cholesterol: 4 mg
- ♦ Sodium: 200 mg
- ♦ Fat, total: 2.5 g
- ♦ Carbohydrates: 41 g
- ♦ Fiber: 9 g
- ♦ Fat, saturated: 1.3 g

Kasha with Beans and Salsa Dressing

Dressing		
½ cup	chopped fresh coriander	125 mL
⅓ cup	medium salsa	75 mL
¼ cup	low-fat sour cream	50 mL
3 tbsp	light mayonnaise	45 mL
2 tbsp	water	25 mL
1 tsp	minced garlic	5 mL
Salad		
1½ cups	vegetable or chicken stock	375 mL
¾ cup	whole grain kasha	175 mL
½ cup	canned red kidney beans, rinsed and drained	125 mL
½ cup	canned chickpeas, rinsed and drained	125 mL
½ cup	chopped red onions	125 mL

Serves 4

1. In a bowl combine coriander, salsa, sour cream, mayonnaise, water and garlic. Set aside.
2. In a saucepan over high heat, bring stock to boil. Meanwhile, in a nonstick saucepan set over medium-high heat, toast kasha for 1 minute. Add hot stock; return to a boil, stirring. Reduce heat to medium-low; cook, covered, for 10 minutes or until kasha is tender and liquid is absorbed. Set aside to cool.
3. In a serving bowl, combine cooled kasha, red kidney beans, chickpeas and red onions. Pour dressing over; toss to coat well. Serve at room temperature or heat in microwave to serve warm.

Nutritional Analysis (Per Serving)
- Calories: 167
- Protein: 7 g
- Cholesterol: 5 mg
- Sodium: 200 mg
- Fat, total: 6 g
- Carbohydrates: 23 g
- Fiber: 3 g
- Fat, saturated: 1.3 g

Millet Salad with Dried Fruit in an Oriental Lime Dressing

1 cup	millet	250 mL
2 cups	vegetable or chicken stock	500 mL
1 tsp	grated lime zest	5 mL
2 tbsp	fresh lime juice	25 mL
1 tbsp	honey	15 mL
1 tbsp	sesame oil	15 mL
1 tbsp	light soya sauce	15 mL
1 tsp	minced garlic	5 mL
⅓ cup	diced dried apples	75 mL
⅓ cup	diced dried apricots	75 mL
⅓ cup	dried cherries or raisins	75 mL
⅓ cup	chopped fresh coriander	75 mL
⅓ cup	chopped green onions	75 mL
⅓ cup	diced prunes	75 mL

Serves 4

1. In a nonstick skillet over medium-high heat, toast millet for 1 minute.
2. In a saucepan over high heat, bring stock to a boil. Add millet; reduce heat to low. Cook, covered, for 25 minutes or until grain is tender. Drain if any excess liquid. Set aside to cool.
3. In a bowl combine lime zest, lime juice, honey, sesame oil, soya sauce and garlic; whisk well.
4. In a serving bowl, combine millet, apples, apricots, cherries, coriander, green onions and prunes. Pour dressing over salad; toss to coat well. Serve.

Nutritional Analysis (Per Serving)
- Calories: 375
- Protein: 8 g
- Cholesterol: 0 mg
- Sodium: 40 mg
- Fat, total: 6 g
- Carbohydrates: 73 g
- Fiber: 8 g
- Fat, saturated: 0.9 g

Asian Tabbouleh Salad with Soya Orange Dressing

Salad

2 cups	Basic Vegetable Stock (see recipe, page 52) or water	500 mL
1½ cups	bulgur wheat	375 mL
1 cup	finely chopped red bell peppers	250 mL
1 cup	finely chopped water chestnuts	250 mL
½ cup	finely chopped green onions	125 mL
⅓ cup	chopped fresh coriander	75 mL
1 cup	broccoli florets	250 mL
1 cup	chopped snow peas	250 mL

Dressing

4 tsp	orange juice concentrate	20 mL
4 tsp	honey	20 mL
2½ tsp	sesame oil	12 mL
2½ tsp	soya sauce	12 mL
1 tsp	minced garlic	5 mL
1 tsp	freshly squeezed lemon juice	5 mL
¾ tsp	minced gingerroot	4 mL

Be sure not to buy orange juice concentrate with added sugar; these are often labelled orange juice "punch" or "cocktail." A great substitute for orange juice concentrate is unsweetened pineapple juice concentrate.

Serves 4 to 6

1. In a saucepan bring stock or water to a boil. Stir in bulgur, cover and turn heat off. Let stand 15 minutes; drain, rinse with cold water and place in a serving bowl. Stir in red peppers, water chestnuts, green onions and coriander.

2. Boil or steam broccoli florets and snow peas 2 minutes or until tender-crisp. Rinse under cold water, drain and add to bulgur mixture.

3. *Make the dressing:* In a small bowl, whisk together orange juice concentrate, honey, sesame oil, soya sauce, garlic, lemon juice and ginger. Pour over bulgur mixture and toss to coat. Serve chilled or at room temperature.

Tips

✦ Bulgur wheat can often be found in grocery stores next to the rice and other grains. If not, health food stores always carry it.

✦ Bulgur can be replaced with couscous or quinoa.

✦ Coriander can be replaced with basil, parsley or dill.

✦ This salad is a great source of fiber.

Make Ahead

✦ Prepare early in the day. Dressing can be poured over early, allowing salad to marinate.

Nutritional Analysis (Per Serving)

✦ Calories: 200 ✦ Protein: 7 g ✦ Cholesterol: 0 mg
✦ Sodium: 131 mg ✦ Fat, total: 3 g ✦ Carbohydrates: 41 g
✦ Fiber: 9 g ✦ Fat, saturated: 0.4 g

Tabbouleh Greek Style

¾ cup	bulgur	175 mL
½ cup	finely chopped red onion	125 mL
1 cup	diced cucumber	250 mL
1½ cups	diced tomatoes	375 mL
2	green onions, sliced thinly	2
¼ cup	sliced pitted black olives	50 mL
2 oz	feta cheese, crumbled	50 g

Dressing

⅓ cup	chopped fresh parsley	75 mL
⅓ cup	chopped fresh mint	75 mL
2 tbsp	lemon juice	25 mL
2 tbsp	vegetable oil	25 mL
1 tsp	crushed garlic	5 mL
¾ tsp	dried basil (or 2 tbsp/25 mL chopped fresh)	4 mL
½ tsp	dried oregano (or 1 tbsp/15 mL chopped fresh)	2 mL

Herbs for health: *Can adding herbs to meals reduce your cancer risk? Evidence is sketchy, but it may not hurt to try. Herbs contain a number of phytochemicals that interact in the body. Some examples: coriander leaves (cilantro) and parsley, related to the carrot family, have polyacetylenes (immune enhancers) and phthalides (antioxidants); rosemary, mint, oregano, sage and thyme contain quinones (antioxidants); and chives, a cousin of garlic, are full of the same allyl sulfur compounds (immune enhancers, antioxidants).*

Serves 4 to 6

1. Cover bulgur with 2 cups (500 mL) boiling water; soak for 20 minutes. Drain well and place in large serving bowl.
2. Add onion, cucumber, tomatoes, green onions, olives and feta; mix well.
3. *Dressing:* In small bowl, combine parsley, mint, lemon juice, oil, garlic, basil and oregano; pour over tabbouleh. Mix well. Refrigerate until chilled.

Tips

✦ After salad is mixed, it may be chopped in food processor using off/on motion until desired consistency is reached.

✦ Fresh herbs can be preserved by standing them in a glass with water covering the stems. Place plastic wrap over the glass and refrigerate.

Make Ahead

✦ Prepare early in day and stir just before serving.

Nutritional Analysis (Per Serving)

✦ Calories: 152   ✦ Protein: 4 g   ✦ Cholesterol: 8 mg
✦ Sodium: 164 mg   ✦ Fat: 7 g   ✦ Carbohydrates: 18 g
✦ Fiber: 4 g

Quinoa Salad with Fennel, Red Pepper and Apricots in an Orange Dressing

2 cups	vegetable or chicken stock	500 mL
1 cup	quinoa, rinsed	250 mL
1 cup	diced fennel	250 mL
1 cup	diced red bell peppers	250 mL
1 cup	diced snow peas	250 mL
1/2 cup	diced dried apricots	125 mL
1/4 cup	dried cranberries or dried cherries or raisins	50 mL

Dressing

2 tbsp	raspberry vinegar	25 mL
2 tbsp	orange juice concentrate	25 mL
1 tbsp	honey	15 mL
1 tbsp	olive oil	15 mL
1 tsp	minced garlic	5 mL

Serves 4

1. In a saucepan over high heat, bring stock to a boil. Meanwhile, in a nonstick skillet over medium-high heat, lightly toast quinoa for 1 minute. Add quinoa to stock; reduce heat to medium-low. Cook, covered, for 15 minutes or until tender and liquid is absorbed. Transfer to a serving bowl.

2. When quinoa has cooled, add fennel, red peppers, snow peas, apricots and dried cranberries.

3. In a bowl combine vinegar, orange juice concentrate, honey, olive oil and garlic; whisk well. Pour dressing over salad; toss to coat well. Serve.

Nutritional Analysis (Per Serving)
- Calories: 339
- Protein: 9 g
- Cholesterol: 0 mg
- Sodium: 188 mg
- Fat, total: 7 g
- Carbohydrates: 64 g
- Fiber: 7 g
- Fat, saturated: 0.9 g

Shrimp and Macaroni Salad with Creamy Russian Dressing

8 oz	macaroni or any small shell pasta	250 g
6 oz	raw shrimp, shelled	175 g
1/3 cup	light mayonnaise	75 mL
1/3 cup	low-fat sour cream	75 mL
1/4 cup	sweet tomato chili sauce	50 mL
1/2 cup	minced green bell peppers	125 mL
1/2 cup	minced red bell peppers	125 mL
1/2 cup	minced red onions	125 mL

Be sure that you don't mistakenly use hot chili sauce instead of the sweet tomato chili sauce called for in the recipe. (That is, unless you like your salad really lively!)

Serves 4

1. In a pot of boiling water, cook macaroni for 8 to 10 minutes or until tender but firm; drain. Rinse under cold running water; drain.

2. If using large or jumbo shrimp, cut into halves. In a nonstick frying pan sprayed with vegetable spray, cook shrimp over medium-high heat for 2 minutes or until pink. In a bowl combine mayonnaise, sour cream and chili sauce.

3. In a serving bowl, combine green peppers, red peppers, red onions, pasta, shrimp and sauce; toss to coat well. Best served chilled.

Nutritional Analysis (Per Serving)
- Calories: 374
- Protein: 17 g
- Cholesterol: 69 mg
- Sodium: 233 mg
- Fat, total: 9 g
- Carbohydrates: 54 g
- Fiber: 3 g
- Fat, saturated: 2.8 g

Salmon Penne Salad

Dressing

²/₃ cup	buttermilk	150 mL
3 tbsp	light mayonnaise	45 mL
1¹/₂ tbsp	fresh lemon juice	20 mL
2 tsp	honey	10 mL
1¹/₂ tsp	Dijon mustard	7 mL
1¹/₂ tsp	minced garlic	7 mL
¹/₄ tsp	freshly ground black pepper	1 mL
¹/₄ tsp	salt	1 mL

Salad

8	stalks asparagus, trimmed and cut into 1¹/₂-inch (4 cm) lengths	8
8 oz	penne	250 g
³/₄ cup	chopped red bell peppers	175 mL
¹/₂ cup	chopped green onions	125 mL
¹/₃ cup	chopped fresh dill (or 1 tsp/5 mL dried)	75 mL
6 oz	salmon fillet	175 g

To cut back on fat and calories, use reduced fat mayonnaise, spreads and salad dressings and soft non-hydrogenated margarine.

Serves 4
Preheat broiler or set grill to medium-high

1. In a bowl combine buttermilk, mayonnaise, lemon juice, honey, Dijon mustard, garlic, pepper and salt. Set aside.

2. In a pot of boiling water, cook asparagus for 1 minute or until tender-crisp. Drain; rinse with cold water until cool.

3. In a large pot of boiling water, cook penne for 8 to 10 minutes or until tender but firm; drain. Rinse under cold running water; drain. In a serving bowl, combine pasta, asparagus, red peppers, green onions and dill; toss to combine well.

4. Broil or grill salmon, turning once, for 10 minutes per 1-inch (2.5 cm) thickness or until cooked through; flake with a fork. Add salmon to salad. Pour dressing over; toss to coat well.

Tips

✦ Most varieties of salmon come from the Pacific coast. The best is the highly flavored Chinook or King salmon. Although higher in fat, these varieties are also rich in omega-3 fatty acids, which help lower blood cholesterol. For this recipe, use salmon fillets or steaks, whichever you prefer.

✦ *Butterless buttermilk:* Despite its rich-sounding name, buttermilk has only 2 g fat for every 1 cup (250 mL). That's the same amount of fat as in 1% milk. Buttermilk gets its thick consistency from bacterial cultures added during processing, which convert the sugar in the milk into lactic acid. The result is milk that tastes rich, tart and buttery. It's great in pancakes and muffins, and makes wonderfully creamy salad dressings — without the cream!

Nutritional Analysis (Per Serving)

✦ Calories: 389 ✦ Protein: 19 g ✦ Cholesterol: 29 mg
✦ Sodium: 318 mg ✦ Fat, total: 9 g ✦ Carbohydrates: 58 g
✦ Fiber: 3 g ✦ Fat, saturated: 1.8 g

Salmon Salad with Peanut Lime Dressing

8 oz	skinless salmon, cut into ½-inch (1 cm) cubes	250 g
2 cups	halved snow peas	500 mL
6 cups	well-packed romaine lettuce, washed, dried and torn into bite-size pieces	1.5 L
2 cups	sliced red peppers	500 mL
1 cup	sliced baby corn cobs	250 mL
½ cup	chopped fresh coriander or parsley	125 mL

Dressing

3 tbsp	lime juice	45 mL
2 tbsp	peanut butter	25 mL
2 tbsp	water	25 mL
2 tbsp	honey	25 mL
1 tbsp	soya sauce	15 mL
1 tbsp	vegetable oil	15 mL
2 tsp	sesame oil	10 mL
1½ tsp	minced garlic	7 mL
1 tsp	minced ginger	5 mL

Serves 8

1. Heat nonstick skillet sprayed with vegetable spray over high heat; add salmon cubes and cook for 2½ minutes, turning frequently, or until just done at center. Set aside.

2. Blanch snow peas in boiling water or microwave for 1 minute or until tender-crisp; refresh in cold water and drain. Place in serving bowl with salmon, romaine, red peppers, baby corn and coriander; toss gently.

3. In small bowl whisk together lime juice, peanut butter, water, honey, soya sauce, vegetable oil, sesame oil, garlic and ginger; pour over salad and toss gently.

Tips

✦ Dressing is great as a marinade or for stir-fry. Keeps well for days in refrigerator.

✦ Great with tuna, swordfish or other tasty fish.

✦ If you wish, use canned salmon or tuna.

Make Ahead

✦ Prepare salad and dressing early in the day. Keep separate until ready to serve.

Nutritional Analysis (Per Serving)

✦ Calories: 141   ✦ Protein: 9 g   ✦ Cholesterol: 16 mg
✦ Sodium: 324 mg   ✦ Fat, total: 7 g   ✦ Carbohydrates: 13 g
✦ Fiber: 3 g   ✦ Fat, saturated: 0.9 g

Chicken and Asparagus Salad with Lemon Dill Vinaigrette

12	baby red potatoes (or 4 small white)	12
8 oz	boneless skinless chicken breasts, cubed	250 g
¼ cup	water	50 mL
¼ cup	white wine	50 mL
8 oz	asparagus, trimmed and cut into small pieces	250 g
2	small heads Boston lettuce, torn into pieces	2

Lemon Dill Vinaigrette

3 tbsp	balsamic vinegar	45 mL
2 tbsp	lemon juice	25 mL
1 tbsp	water	15 mL
1	large green onion, minced	1
¾ tsp	garlic	4 mL
2 tbsp	chopped fresh dill (or 1 tsp/5 mL dried dillweed)	25 mL
3 tbsp	olive oil	45 mL

What makes balsamic vinegar so sensational — and expensive? Well, it's made from one type of grape (Trebbiano), and aged for years (often 12 or more) in special casks, which give the vinegar its characteristic sweetness and purplish-brown color. In fact, the oldest balsamic vinegars are often more highly prized (and costly) than vintage wines! Such vinegars should be treated with respect and used sparingly to highlight simple foods — a plate of mixed greens or strawberries, for example.

Serves 4 to 6

1. In saucepan of boiling water, cook potatoes until just tender. Peel and cut into cubes. Place in salad bowl and set aside.

2. In saucepan, bring chicken, water and wine to boil; reduce heat, cover and simmer for approximately 2 minutes or until chicken is no longer pink. Drain and add to potatoes in bowl.

3. Steam or microwave asparagus until just tender-crisp; drain and add to bowl. Add lettuce.

4. *Lemon Dill Vinaigrette:* In bowl, whisk together vinegar, lemon juice, water, onion, garlic and dill; whisk in oil until combined. Pour over chicken mixture; toss to coat well.

Tips

✦ Containing both protein and carbohydrates, this salad is a complete meal.

✦ Substitute broccoli or fresh green beans for the asparagus.

Nutritional Analysis (Per Serving)
- ✦ Calories: 199
- ✦ Protein: 11 g
- ✦ Cholesterol: 20 mg
- ✦ Sodium: 33 mg
- ✦ Fat: 8 g
- ✦ Carbohydrates: 19 g
- ✦ Fiber: 3 g

Pesto Potato Salad (page 97) ➤
Overleaf: Linguine with Caramelized Onions, Tomatoes and Basil (page 135)

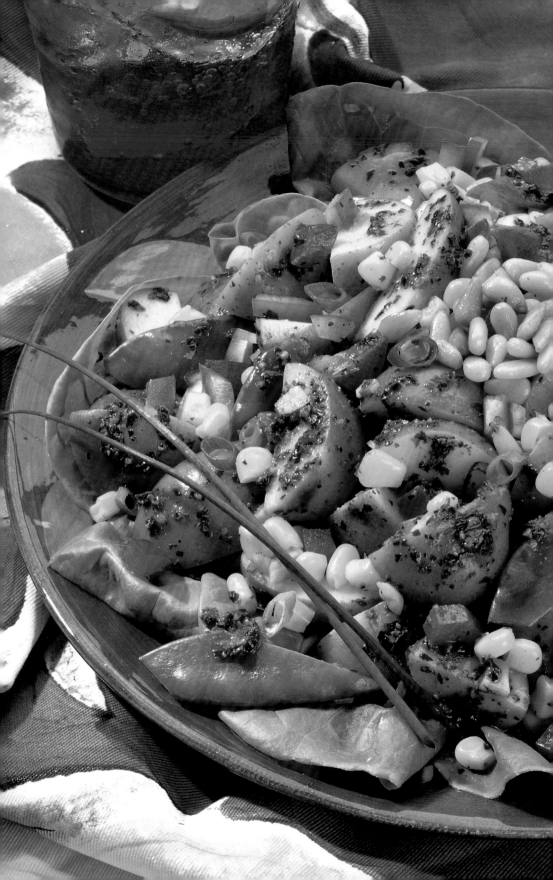

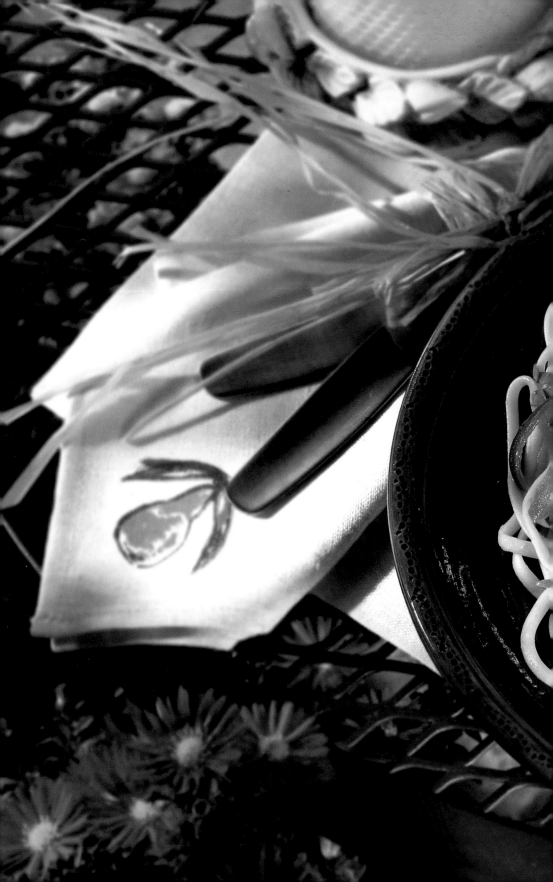

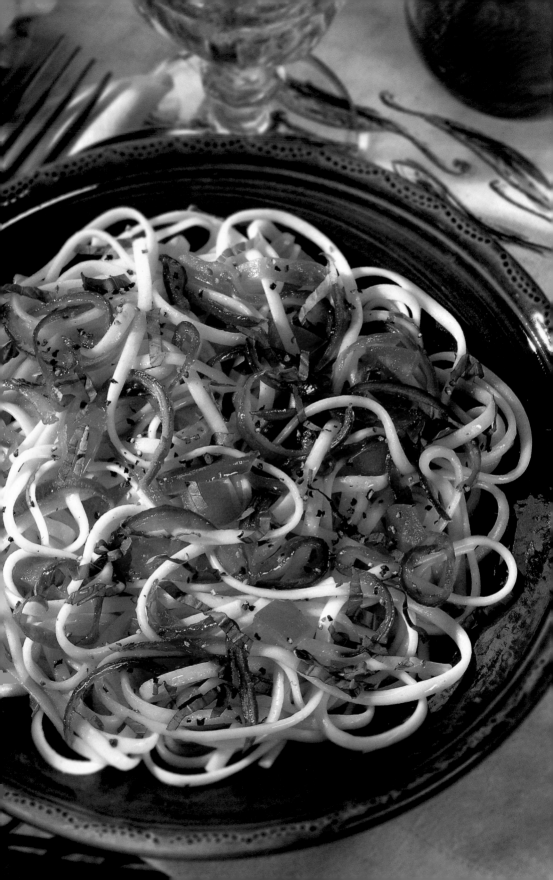

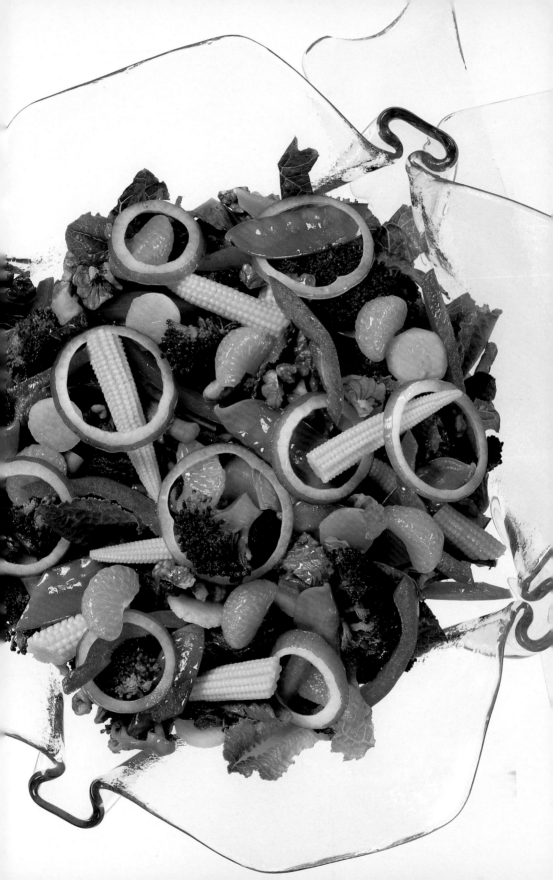

Chicken Salad with Tarragon and Pecans

10 oz	boneless skinless chicken breast, cubed	300 g
¾ cup	chopped sweet red or green pepper	175 mL
¾ cup	chopped carrot	175 mL
¾ cup	chopped broccoli florets	175 mL
¾ cup	chopped snow peas	175 mL
¾ cup	chopped red onion	175 mL
1 tbsp	chopped pecans, toasted	15 mL

Dressing

½ cup	2% yogurt	125 mL
2 tbsp	lemon juice	25 mL
2 tbsp	light mayonnaise	25 mL
1 tsp	crushed garlic	5 mL
1 tsp	Dijon mustard	5 mL
¼ cup	chopped fresh parsley	50 mL
2 tsp	dried tarragon (or 3 tbsp/45 mL chopped fresh)	10 mL
	Salt and pepper	

Serves 4

1. In small saucepan, bring 2 cups (500 mL) water to boil; reduce heat to simmer. Add chicken; cover and cook just until no longer pink inside, 2 to 4 minutes. Drain and place in serving bowl.

2. Add red pepper, carrot, broccoli, snow peas and onion; toss well.

3. *Dressing:* In small bowl, combine yogurt, lemon juice, mayonnaise, garlic, mustard, parsley, tarragon, and salt and pepper to taste; pour over chicken and mix well. Taste and adjust seasoning. Sprinkle with pecans.

Tips

✦ If tarragon is unavailable, substitute ¼ cup (50 mL) chopped fresh dill.

✦ Fresh tuna or swordfish are delicious substitutes for chicken.

✦ Toast pecans in small skillet on medium heat until browned, 2 to 3 minutes.

Make Ahead

✦ Prepare and refrigerate salad and dressing separately early in day, but do not mix until ready to serve.

Nutritional Analysis (Per Serving)
✦ Calories: 187 ✦ Protein: 20 g ✦ Cholesterol: 42 mg
✦ Sodium: 151 mg ✦ Fat: 6 g ✦ Carbohydrates: 13 g
✦ Fiber: 3 g

Chicken Tarragon Pasta Salad

12 oz	rotini or fusilli	375 g
12 oz	skinless, boneless chicken breast, cut into 1-inch (2.5 cm) cubes	375 g
1½ cups	chopped broccoli	375 mL
½ cup	diced carrots	125 mL
1½ cups	diced red peppers	375 mL
¾ cup	diced green peppers	175 mL
½ cup	diced red onions	125 mL

Dressing

½ cup	2% yogurt	125 mL
⅓ cup	light mayonnaise	75 mL
3 tbsp	lemon juice	45 mL
⅓ cup	chopped fresh tarragon or dill (or 3 tsp/15 mL dried)	75 mL
2½ tbsp	honey	35 mL
2 tsp	crushed garlic	10 mL
1½ tsp	Dijon mustard	7 mL

To cut back on fat, try buttermilk, skim milk and 1% milk; yogurt and cottage cheese containing less than 1% milk fat; puddings made with skim milk; and reduced-fat ice cream and sherbet.

Serves 6 to 8 as an appetizer

1. Cook pasta in boiling water according to package instructions or until firm to the bite. Rinse with cold water. Drain and place in serving bowl.

2. In nonstick skillet sprayed with vegetable spray, sauté chicken until no longer pink, approximately 3 minutes. Cool. Add to pasta.

3. Blanch broccoli and carrots in boiling water just until tender, approximately 3 minutes. Drain and refresh with cold water; add to pasta. Add red and green peppers and onions.

4. *Make the dressing:* In small bowl combine yogurt, mayonnaise, lemon juice, tarragon, honey, garlic and mustard until mixed. Pour over pasta, and toss.

Tips

✦ Other vegetables can be used as long as the total amount is not exceeded.

✦ Try coriander or parsley as an herb.

Make Ahead

✦ Salad and dressing can be made up to a day ahead. Do not toss until ready to serve.

Nutritional Analysis (Per Serving)
✦ Calories: 331   ✦ Protein: 19 g   ✦ Cholesterol: 34 mg
✦ Sodium: 131 mg ✦ Fat, total: 6 g ✦ Carbohydrates: 51 g
✦ Fiber: 4 g   ✦ Fat, saturated: 0.9 g

Oriental Chicken Salad with Mandarin Oranges, Snow Peas and Asparagus

12 oz	skinless, boneless chicken breasts	375 g
1 cup	asparagus cut into 1-inch (2.5 cm) pieces	250 mL
1¼ cups	halved snow peas	300 mL
1 cup	sliced baby corn cobs	250 mL
1 cup	bean sprouts	250 mL
1 cup	canned mandarin oranges, drained	250 mL
1½ cups	sliced red or green peppers	375 mL
¾ cup	sliced water chestnuts	175 mL
2	medium green onions, chopped	2

Dressing

2 tbsp	orange juice concentrate, thawed	25 mL
1 tbsp	rice wine vinegar	15 mL
1 tbsp	soya sauce	15 mL
2 tsp	honey	10 mL
2 tsp	vegetable oil	10 mL
1 tsp	sesame oil	5 mL
1 tsp	minced gingerroot	5 mL
1 tsp	minced garlic	5 mL

Serves 6

1. In nonstick skillet sprayed with vegetable spray, sauté chicken breasts and cook approximately 7 minutes, or until browned on both sides and just done at center. Let chicken cool, then cut into ½ inch (1 cm) cubes and place in large serving bowl.

2. In boiling water or microwave, blanch asparagus for 2 minutes or until tender-crisp; refresh in cold water and drain. As well, cook snow peas for 45 seconds or until tender-crisp; refresh in cold water and drain. Place in serving bowl with chicken. Add baby corn, bean sprouts, mandarin oranges, red peppers, water chestnuts and green onions to bowl and toss.

3. In small bowl, whisk together orange juice concentrate, vinegar, soya sauce, honey, vegetable oil, sesame oil, ginger and garlic; pour over salad and toss.

Tips

+ Replace chicken with shrimp, pork or steak.
+ Broccoli or green beans can replace asparagus.
+ Thinly sliced carrots (julienned) can replace bean sprouts.

Make Ahead

+ Prepare salad and dressing early in the day, keeping separate until ready to serve.
+ Dressing can keep for days.

Nutritional Analysis (Per Serving)
+ Calories: 155 + Protein: 17 g + Cholesterol: 33 mg
+ Sodium: 434 mg + Fat, total: 3 g + Carbohydrates: 17 g
+ Fiber: 2 g + Fat, saturated: 0.5 g

Thai Beef Salad

8 oz	boneless steak, sliced thinly	250 g
1¾ cups	halved snow peas	425 mL
5 cups	well-packed romaine lettuce, washed, dried and torn into bite-size pieces	1.25 L
1 cup	chopped cucumber	250 mL
¾ cup	sliced red onions	175 mL
¾ cup	sliced water chestnuts	175 mL
¾ cup	canned mandarin oranges, drained	175 mL
1	medium red pepper, sliced	1

Dressing

1½ tbsp	orange juice concentrate, thawed	20 mL
4 tsp	honey	20 mL
1 tbsp	rice wine vinegar	15 mL
1 tbsp	soya sauce	15 mL
2 tsp	vegetable oil	10 mL
2 tsp	sesame oil	10 mL
1 tsp	minced garlic	5 mL
¾ tsp	minced gingerroot	4 mL
½ tsp	grated orange zest	2 mL

Serves 6

1. In nonstick skillet sprayed with vegetable spray, cook beef over high heat for 90 seconds or until just done at center. Drain any excess liquid. Put in large serving bowl.

2. In a saucepan of boiling water or microwave, blanch snow peas for 1 or 2 minutes, or until tender-crisp; refresh in cold water and drain. Place in serving bowl, along with lettuce, cucumber, red onions, water chestnuts, mandarin oranges and red pepper.

3. In small bowl whisk together orange juice concentrate, honey, vinegar, soya sauce, vegetable oil, sesame oil, garlic, ginger and orange zest; pour over salad and toss well.

Tips

+ Use a good-quality steak such as rib eye, sirloin or porterhouse.

+ You can use leftover roast beef or cooked steak.

+ Chicken or pork can replace steak.

+ Dressing is great for other salads.

Make Ahead

+ Prepare dressing up to 2 days in advance. Toss just before serving.

Nutritional Analysis (Per Serving)
+ Calories: 156   + Protein: 11 g   + Cholesterol: 18 mg
+ Sodium: 207 mg   + Fat, total: 5 g + Carbohydrates: 18 g
+ Fiber: 3 g   + Fat, saturated: 1 g

Pasta, Pizza and Wraps

continued on next page

✦ ✦

Pizza

Wraps

Cheddar Cheese and Parmesan Sauce

1 tbsp	margarine or butter	15 mL
1 tbsp	all-purpose flour	15 mL
½ cup	2% milk	125 mL
½ cup	chicken stock	125 mL
½ cup	grated cheddar cheese	125 mL
2 tbsp	grated Parmesan cheese	25 mL
½ tsp	Dijon mustard (optional)	2 mL

Great over cooked vegetables or fish.

For a more intense flavor, try Swiss or blue cheese instead of cheddar.

When using margarine, choose a soft (non-hydrogenated) version to limit consumption of trans fats.

Makes 1⅓ cups (325 mL)

1. In small nonstick saucepan, melt margarine over medium heat. Add flour and mix until smooth.
2. Gradually add milk and stock and whisk constantly until mixture begins to thicken slightly, approximately 3 to 4 minutes. Add cheeses and mustard and whisk just until cheese melts.

Tip
+ For a basic white sauce, just delete the cheese, mustard and chicken stock, and use 1 cup (250 mL) milk.

Make Ahead
+ Prepare up to a day ahead. Gently reheat, adding more liquid if too thick.

Nutritional Analysis (Per Tablespoon/15 mL)
+ Calories: 30   + Protein: 1 g   + Cholesterol: 7 mg
+ Sodium: 65 mg   + Fat: 1 g   + Carbohydrates: 1 g
+ Fiber: 0 g

Mushroom Sauce

1½ cups	sliced mushrooms	375 mL
1 tbsp	margarine or butter	15 mL
1 tbsp	all-purpose flour	15 mL
½ cup	chicken or beef stock	125 mL
½ cup	2% milk	125 mL
⅛ tsp	pepper	0.5 mL

If available, use wild mushrooms, such as oyster or chanterelle.

When using margarine, choose a soft (non-hydrogenated) version to limit consumption of trans fats.

Makes 1½ cups (375 mL)

1. In nonstick skillet sprayed with vegetable spray, sauté mushrooms on high heat until browned, approximately 4 minutes. Set aside.
2. In small nonstick saucepan, melt margarine; add flour and stir until combined.
3. Add stock and milk; cook on low heat, stirring constantly, until thickened, 4 to 5 minutes. Add pepper and mushrooms.

Tip
+ Serve over cooked beef, veal, chicken or pork.

Make Ahead
+ Prepare and refrigerate up to a day ahead, then gently reheat. Add more stock or milk if too thick.

Nutritional Analysis (Per Tablespoon/15 mL)
+ Calories: 43   + Protein: 2 g   + Cholesterol: 1 mg
+ Sodium: 101 mg   + Fat: 2 g   + Carbohydrates: 3 g
+ Fiber: 0 g

Pesto Sauce

½ cup	well-packed chopped fresh parsley	125 mL
½ cup	well-packed chopped fresh basil	125 mL
¼ cup	water or chicken stock	50 mL
1 tbsp	toasted pine nuts	15 mL
2 tbsp	grated Parmesan cheese	25 mL
3 tbsp	olive oil	45 mL
¾ tsp	crushed garlic	4 mL

Makes ¾ cup (175 mL)

1. In food processor, combine parsley, basil, water, pine nuts, Parmesan, oil and garlic; process until smooth.

Tips
✦ You can be creative with pesto sauces by substituting different leaves, such as spinach or coriander, or using a combination of different leaves.

✦ Serve over ¾ lb (375 g) pasta.

✦ Serve over cooked fish or chicken.

Make Ahead
✦ Refrigerate for up to a week or freeze for up to 6 weeks.

Nutritional Analysis (Per Tablespoon/15 mL)
✦ Calories: 39   ✦ Protein: 1 g   ✦ Cholesterol: 1 mg
✦ Sodium: 17 mg   ✦ Fat: 4 g   ✦ Carbohydrates: 1 g
✦ Fiber: 0.3 g

Creamy Pesto Sauce

1 cup	packed fresh basil	250 mL
¼ cup	light sour cream	50 mL
2 tbsp	light mayonnaise	25 mL
1½ tbsp	grated Parmesan cheese	22 mL
1 tbsp	olive oil	15 mL
1 tbsp	toasted pine nuts	15 mL
1½ tsp	freshly squeezed lemon juice	7 mL
1 tsp	minced garlic	5 mL

Serves 6 to 8

1. In a food processor, combine basil, sour cream, mayonnaise, Parmesan, oil, pine nuts, lemon juice and garlic; process until smooth.

Tip
✦ Use this sauce in recipes that call for pesto. You can use the store-bought variety, but it is much higher in fat and calories.

Make Ahead
✦ Prepare up to 3 days in advance or freeze up to 3 weeks.

Nutritional Analysis (Per Tablespoon/15 mL)
✦ Calories: 33   ✦ Protein: 1 g   ✦ Cholesterol: 1 mg
✦ Sodium: 39 mg   ✦ Fat, total: 3 g   ✦ Carbohydrates: 1 g
✦ Fiber: 0 g   ✦ Fat, saturated: 1 g

Sun-Dried Tomato Pesto

4 oz	sun-dried tomatoes	125 g
1½ tsp	crushed garlic	7 mL
1 cup	water or chicken stock	250 mL
½ cup	chopped fresh parsley	125 mL
¼ cup	chopped fresh basil	50 mL
3 tbsp	olive oil	45 mL
2 tbsp	toasted pine nuts	25 mL
3 tbsp	grated Parmesan cheese	45 mL

Makes enough for 1½ lb (750 g) of pasta.

Great over bruschetta.

Makes 1⅓ cups (325 mL)

1. In bowl, pour enough boiling water over tomatoes to cover; let sit for 15 minutes or until soft enough to cut. Drain and cut into smaller pieces.
2. In food processor, combine tomatoes, garlic, water, parsley, basil, oil, pine nuts and Parmesan; process until well blended.

Tips

✦ Toss with pasta or rice, or serve over cooked fish or chicken.

✦ If sauce is too thick, add a little water to thin.

Make Ahead

✦ Prepare up to 2 days in advance or freeze for up to 3 months.

Nutritional Analysis (Per Tablespoon/15 mL)
✦ Calories: 35 ✦ Protein: 0 g ✦ Cholesterol: 0 mg
✦ Sodium: 46 mg ✦ Fat: 2 g ✦ Carbohydrates: 1 g
✦ Fiber: 0 g

Quick Basic Tomato Sauce

1 lb	pasta (any variety)	500 g
2 tsp	olive oil	10 mL
⅔ cup	finely chopped onions	150 mL
2 tsp	crushed garlic	10 mL
1	can (28 oz/796 mL) plum tomatoes, crushed	1
¼ cup	grated Parmesan cheese (optional)	50 mL

Other finely diced vegetables can be added, as well as basil and oregano to taste.

Serves 6 to 8

1. In large nonstick saucepan, heat oil; sauté onions and garlic for 3 minutes, stirring often.
2. Add tomatoes and cook on low heat for 15 to 20 minutes, stirring occasionally, or until reduced slightly. Pour over pasta. Add cheese if using, and toss.

Tip

✦ If a thicker sauce is desired, add 2 tbsp (25 mL) tomato paste during the cooking.

Make Ahead

✦ Refrigerate for up to 2 days, or freeze for up to 6 weeks. After defrosting, add 2 tbsp (25 mL) tomato paste to thicken. Heat for 15 minutes.

Nutritional Analysis (Per Serving)
✦ Calories: 270 ✦ Protein: 9 g ✦ Cholesterol: 0 mg
✦ Sodium: 167 mg ✦ Fat, total: 2 g ✦ Carbohydrates: 53 g
✦ Fiber: 3 g ✦ Fat, saturated: 0.4 g

Thick and Rich Tomato Sauce

1 lb	pasta (any variety)	500 g
1 tbsp	vegetable oil	15 mL
2 tsp	crushed garlic	10 mL
½ cup	chopped onions	125 mL
½ cup	chopped sweet green peppers	125 mL
½ cup	chopped carrots	125 mL
1	can (28 oz/796 mL) crushed tomatoes	1
¼ cup	red wine	50 mL
2 tbsp	tomato paste	25 mL
1	bay leaf	1
1 tsp	dried oregano	5 mL
1 tsp	dried basil	5 mL

Canned plum tomatoes are a good choice.

Serves 6 to 8

1. In large nonstick saucepan, heat oil; sauté garlic, onions, green peppers and carrots until softened, approximately 10 minutes.

2. Add tomatoes, wine, tomato paste, bay leaf, oregano and basil; cover and simmer for approximately 20 minutes, stirring occasionally. Discard bay leaf. Purée if desired.

Tip

✦ For a meat sauce, add 8 oz (250 g) ground beef, chicken, veal or pork after vegetables have been cooked. Sauté meat until no longer pink. Drain all fat. Then continue with recipe.

Make Ahead

✦ Refrigerate up to a day ahead or freeze for up to 6 weeks. When reheating add 2 tbsp (25 mL) tomato paste to thicken.

Nutritional Analysis (Per Serving)
- ✦ Calories: 303
- ✦ Protein: 10 g
- ✦ Cholesterol: 0 mg
- ✦ Sodium: 176 mg
- ✦ Fat, total: 3 g
- ✦ Carbohydrates: 58 g
- ✦ Fiber: 4 g
- ✦ Fat, saturated: 0.4 g

Tortellini with Creamy Tomato Sauce

1 lb	cheese tortellini	500 g
2 cups	tomato sauce	500 mL
2 tbsp	chopped fresh basil (or 1 tsp/5 mL dried)	25 mL
2 tbsp	chopped fresh parsley (or 2 tsp/10 mL dried)	25 mL
	Pepper	
½ cup	milk	125 mL
3 tbsp	grated Parmesan cheese	45 mL

Using milk or light cream instead of whipping cream provides just as much taste, with a significant reduction in fat.

Serves 4 to 6

1. Cook tortellini according to package directions or until firm to the bite. Drain and place in serving bowl.

2. Meanwhile, in medium saucepan, bring tomato sauce, basil, parsley, and pepper to taste to simmer. Add milk and 2 tbsp (25 mL) of the Parmesan; cook for 1 minute. Pour over pasta and mix well; sprinkle with remaining cheese.

Make Ahead

✦ Make sauce and refrigerate a day before, then gently rewarm before pouring over cooked pasta.

Nutritional Analysis (Per Serving)
- ✦ Calories: 218
- ✦ Protein: 14 g
- ✦ Cholesterol: 110 mg
- ✦ Sodium: 733 mg
- ✦ Fat: 6 g
- ✦ Carbohydrates: 25 g
- ✦ Fiber: 2 g

Rigatoni with Tomato Bean Sauce

1 tsp	vegetable oil	5 mL
2 tsp	minced garlic	10 mL
½ cup	chopped carrots	125 mL
1 cup	chopped zucchini	250 mL
1 cup	chopped onions	250 mL
8 oz	lean ground beef	250 g
1	can (19 oz/540 mL) tomatoes, crushed	1
1 cup	chicken stock	250 mL
1½ cups	canned white kidney beans, drained and mashed	375 mL
2 tsp	dried basil	10 mL
2 tsp	chili powder	10 mL
1 tsp	dried oregano	5 mL
1	bay leaf	1
1 lb	rigatoni	500 g
¼ cup	grated Parmesan cheese	50 mL

Serves 8

1. In large nonstick saucepan sprayed with vegetable spray, heat oil over medium-high heat. Add garlic, carrots, zucchini and onions; cook for 8 minutes or until softened and browned, stirring occasionally. Add a little water if vegetables begin to burn. Add beef and cook, stirring to break it up, for 2 minutes or until no longer pink. Add tomatoes, stock, beans, basil, chili powder, oregano and bay leaf; bring to a boil, reduce heat to medium-low and simmer for 30 minutes, covered, stirring occasionally, or until carrots are tender and sauce is thickened.

2. Meanwhile, in large pot of boiling water, cook pasta according to package directions or until tender but firm; drain and place on serving platter. Pour sauce over pasta and sprinkle with Parmesan.

Tips

✦ Red kidney beans or small white navy beans can replace white beans.

✦ Mashing the beans gives more texture to sauce.

✦ Great as leftovers the next day. Add more stock if too dry.

Make Ahead

✦ Sauce can be made up to 2 days ahead or frozen for up to 6 weeks.

Nutritional Analysis (Per Serving)

✦ Calories: 361   ✦ Protein: 18 g   ✦ Cholesterol: 18 mg
✦ Sodium: 452 mg   ✦ Fat, total: 7 g   ✦ Carbohydrates: 57 g
✦ Fiber: 7 g   ✦ Fat, saturated: 2 g

Rigatoni with Roasted Tomato Sauce

12 oz	rigatoni pasta	375 g
8 to 10	small tomatoes (plum or roma)	8 to 10
2 tsp	olive oil	10 mL
2 tsp	crushed garlic	10 mL
³/₄ cup	chopped onions	175 mL
1 cup	sliced mushrooms	250 mL
¹/₂ cup	frozen green peas, thawed	125 mL
¹/₂ cup	chopped fresh basil (or 2 tsp/10 mL dried)	125 mL
¹/₄ cup	grated Parmesan cheese	50 mL
	Pepper	

If you need to control your salt intake, cut back on anything smoked or pickled, dehydrated mixes and most canned foods — choose fresh or homemade without added salt, instead.

Serves 4 o 6
Preheat oven to broil

1. Cook pasta in boiling water according to package instructions or until firm to the bite. Drain and place in serving bowl.
2. Meanwhile, broil or grill tomatoes until black on the outside, approximately 15 minutes, turning once. Do not peel. Place in food processor and purée. Set aside.
3. In large nonstick skillet, heat oil; sauté garlic and onions until tender, approximately 4 minutes. Add mushrooms and sauté for 2 minutes. Add tomato purée, green peas and basil; cook for 3 minutes.
4. Pour over pasta. Sprinkle with cheese and pepper. Toss.

Tip

✦ For a sophisticated pasta, use wild mushrooms, such as oyster or cremini.

Make Ahead

✦ Prepare sauce early in day. Reheat gently, adding some water if sauce is too thick.

Nutritional Analysis (Per Serving)
✦ Calories: 318 ✦ Protein: 12 g ✦ Cholesterol: 3 mg
✦ Sodium: 94 mg ✦ Fat, total: 4 g ✦ Carbohydrates: 59 g
✦ Fiber: 6 g ✦ Fat, saturated: 1 g

Fettuccine with Black Olives
in a Spicy Tomato Sauce

12 oz	fettuccine	375 g
2 tsp	vegetable oil	10 mL
2 tsp	crushed garlic	10 mL
¾ cup	finely diced onions	175 mL
½ cup	finely diced celery	125 mL
½ cup	finely diced carrots	125 mL
⅓ cup	sliced black olives	75 mL
4	anchovies, minced	4
2 tsp	capers	10 mL
2½ cups	crushed tomatoes (canned or fresh)	625 mL
1 tbsp	tomato paste	15 mL
2 tsp	dried basil	10 mL
1 tsp	dried oregano	5 mL
¼ tsp	cayenne pepper	1 mL
3 tbsp	grated Parmesan cheese	45 mL

This sauce suits any type of pasta.

Serves 6

1. Cook pasta in boiling water according to package instructions or until firm to the bite. Drain and place in serving bowl.
2. In large nonstick skillet, heat oil; sauté garlic, onions, celery and carrots until soft, approximately 5 minutes. Add olives, anchovies, capers, tomatoes, tomato paste, basil, oregano and cayenne. Simmer 20 minutes on low heat, stirring occasionally. Pour over pasta. Sprinkle with cheese and toss.

Make Ahead

✦ Refrigerate up to 2 days ahead or freeze up to 1 week. When reheating, add more tomato paste if sauce is too thin.

Nutritional Analysis (Per Serving)
✦ Calories: 319 ✦ Protein: 12 g ✦ Cholesterol: 4 mg
✦ Sodium: 337 mg ✦ Fat, total: 5 g ✦ Carbohydrates: 58 g
✦ Fiber: 5 g ✦ Fat, saturated: 1 g

Penne Marinara

8 oz	penne	250 g
2 tsp	vegetable oil	10 mL
⅔ cup	diced onions	150 mL
2 tsp	crushed garlic	10 mL
2 tsp	chopped capers	10 mL
¼ cup	chopped fresh basil (or 1 tsp/5 mL dried)	50 mL
½ tsp	dried oregano	2 mL
1	bay leaf	1
1	can (19 oz/540 mL) crushed tomatoes	1
⅓ cup	pitted black olives, sliced	75 mL
1 tbsp	tomato paste	15 mL
3 tbsp	grated Parmesan cheese	45 mL
	Parsley	

Any type of pasta suits this dish.

Serves 4

1. Cook pasta in boiling water according to package instructions or until firm to the bite. Drain and place in serving bowl.
2. In nonstick skillet, heat oil; sauté onions and garlic until onions are soft, approximately 3 minutes. Add capers, basil, oregano, bay leaf, tomatoes, olives and tomato paste. Simmer for 15 minutes, stirring occasionally. Pour over pasta. Sprinkle with cheese and toss well. Garnish with parsley.

Make Ahead

✦ Refrigerate up to 2 days ahead or freeze up to 2 weeks. When reheating, add 1 tbsp (15 mL) of tomato paste if sauce is too watery.

Nutritional Analysis (Per Serving)
✦ Calories: 339 ✦ Protein: 12 g ✦ Cholesterol: 4 mg
✦ Sodium: 471 mg ✦ Fat, total: 7 g ✦ Carbohydrates: 58 g
✦ Fiber: 5 g ✦ Fat, saturated: 2 g

Pasta with Creole Sauce, Olives and Sweet Peppers

12 oz	penne	375 g
2 tsp	vegetable oil	10 mL
2 tsp	crushed garlic	10 mL
1 cup	chopped onions	250 mL
3/4 cup	chopped sweet green bell peppers	175 mL
3/4 cup	chopped sweet red bell peppers	175 mL
2 1/2 cups	canned or fresh crushed tomatoes	625 mL
16	large green olives, pitted and sliced	16
1 tbsp	chili powder	15 mL
1/4 tsp	cayenne	1 mL
	Parsley	

Substitute black olives for green if desired. Increase spiciness by adding more cayenne.

Serves 6

1. Cook pasta in boiling water according to package instructions or until firm to the bite. Drain and place in serving bowl.

2. In large nonstick skillet, heat oil; sauté garlic, onions and green and red peppers. Simmer until soft, approximately 5 minutes. Add tomatoes, olives, chili powder and cayenne. Simmer for 15 minutes, stirring occasionally until thickened. Pour over pasta. Sprinkle with parsley, and toss.

Make Ahead

✦ Prepare up to a day ahead. Reheat gently, adding a little water if sauce thickens.

Nutritional Analysis (Per Serving)
- ✦ Calories: 312
- ✦ Protein: 10 g
- ✦ Cholesterol: 0 mg
- ✦ Sodium: 210 mg
- ✦ Fat, total: 4 g
- ✦ Carbohydrates: 61 g
- ✦ Fiber: 6 g
- ✦ Fat, saturated: 0.3 g

Pasta with Spicy Mushroom Tomato Sauce

12 oz	bow-tie pasta or penne	375 g
2 tsp	vegetable oil	10 mL
2 tsp	crushed garlic	10 mL
1 cup	diced onions	250 mL
3 1/2 cups	chopped mushrooms	875 mL
1 cup	prepared tomato sauce or Quick Basic Tomato Sauce (see recipe, page 129)	250 mL
3/4 cup	2% milk	175 mL
1 1/2 tsp	dried basil	7 mL
1 tsp	dried oregano	5 mL
2 tsp	chili powder	10 mL
1/3 cup	grated Parmesan cheese	75 mL
	Parsley	

Use oyster mushrooms for a highlighted texture and flavor. For a spicier flavor, add 1/4 tsp (1 mL) cayenne pepper.

Serves 4 to 6

1. Cook pasta in boiling water according to package instructions or until firm to the bite. Drain and place in serving bowl.

2. In large nonstick skillet, heat oil; sauté garlic and onions until soft, approximately 5 minutes. Add mushrooms and sauté for another 5 minutes.

3. Add tomato sauce, milk, basil, oregano and chili. Simmer for 5 minutes, just until sauce begins to thicken. Pour over pasta. Sprinkle with cheese and toss. Garnish with parsley.

Make Ahead

✦ Prepare sauce early in day. Reheat, adding more milk if sauce thickens.

Nutritional Analysis (Per Serving)
- ✦ Calories: 362
- ✦ Protein: 16 g
- ✦ Cholesterol: 6 mg
- ✦ Sodium: 221 mg
- ✦ Fat, total: 7 g
- ✦ Carbohydrates: 62 g
- ✦ Fiber: 7 g
- ✦ Fat, saturated: 2 g

Linguine with Caramelized Onions, Tomatoes and Basil

2 tsp	vegetable oil	10 mL
2 tsp	minced garlic	10 mL
2 tbsp	packed brown sugar	25 mL
6 cups	thinly sliced red onions	1.5 L
2 cups	diced plum tomatoes	500 mL
3/4 cup	Basic Vegetable Stock (see recipe, page 52)	175 mL
1/2 cup	chopped fresh basil (or 1 1/2 tsp/7 mL dried)	125 mL
1/4 tsp	freshly ground black pepper	1 mL
12 oz	linguine	375 g

Try Vidalia onions when in season (usually in the spring).

Serves 4

1. In a large nonstick saucepan, heat oil over medium-low heat. Add garlic, sugar and red onions; cook, stirring often, 30 minutes or until browned and very soft.

2. Stir in tomatoes, stock, basil and pepper; cook 5 minutes longer or until heated through.

3. Meanwhile, in a pot of boiling water, cook linguine until tender but firm. Drain and toss with sauce.

Make Ahead
✦ Cook onions 1 day in advance. Reheat, then continue recipe.

Nutritional Analysis (Per Serving)
- ✦ Calories: 508
- ✦ Protein: 16 g
- ✦ Cholesterol: 0 mg
- ✦ Sodium: 28 mg
- ✦ Fat, total: 5 g
- ✦ Carbohydrates: 102 g
- ✦ Fiber: 7 g
- ✦ Fat, saturated: 0.4 g

Rotini with Fresh Tomatoes and Feta Cheese

8 oz	rotini noodles	250 g
1 1/2 tsp	vegetable oil	7 mL
2 tsp	crushed garlic	10 mL
1/2 cup	chopped onions	125 mL
2 cups	chopped ripe tomatoes	500 mL
1/2 cup	crumbled feta cheese	125 mL
1/4 cup	chopped fresh basil	50 mL
2 tbsp	grated Parmesan cheese	25 mL
1/4 cup	black olives, pitted and sliced	50 mL
	Pepper	

This dish is similar to a Greek pasta salad. Ripe tomatoes are a must.

Serves 4

1. Cook pasta according to package directions or until firm to the bite. Drain and place in serving bowl.

2. Meanwhile, in nonstick skillet, heat oil; sauté garlic and onions for 2 minutes. Add tomatoes and cook for 2 minutes, stirring constantly. Add to pasta.

3. Add feta, basil, Parmesan, olives, and pepper to taste; mix well.

Tip
✦ Serve either warm or cold.

Make Ahead
✦ If serving cold, prepare early in day and allow to marinate. Toss well before serving.

Nutritional Analysis (Per Serving)
- ✦ Calories: 333
- ✦ Protein: 12 g
- ✦ Cholesterol: 17 mg
- ✦ Sodium: 548 mg
- ✦ Fat: 8 g
- ✦ Carbohydrates: 52 g
- ✦ Fiber: 3 g

Rotini with Tomatoes, Black Olives and Goat Cheese

1 tbsp	vegetable oil	15 mL
1½ tsp	crushed garlic	7 mL
1 cup	chopped onions	250 mL
1	can (19 oz/540 mL) tomatoes, puréed	1
¼ cup	sliced pitted black olives	50 mL
1 tsp	dried basil (or 2 tbsp/25 mL chopped fresh)	5 mL
	Red pepper flakes	
2 oz	goat cheese	50 g
12 oz	penne noodles	375 g
1 tbsp	grated Parmesan cheese	15 mL
	Chopped fresh parsley	

Delicious served warm or cold.

Serves 4 to 6

1. In large nonstick saucepan, heat oil; sauté garlic and onions for 5 minutes. Add tomatoes, olives, basil, and red pepper flakes to taste; cover and simmer for 10 minutes, stirring often. Add goat cheese, stirring until melted.

2. Meanwhile, cook pasta according to package directions or until firm to the bite. Drain and place in serving bowl. Toss with sauce. Sprinkle with Parmesan cheese and garnish with parsley.

Make Ahead

✦ If serving cold, prepare and refrigerate early in day and toss again prior to serving.

Nutritional Analysis (Per Serving)
- ✦ Calories: 305
- ✦ Protein: 10 g
- ✦ Cholesterol: 9 mg
- ✦ Sodium: 539 mg
- ✦ Fat: 6 g
- ✦ Carbohydrates: 51 g
- ✦ Fiber: 3 g

Penne with Spicy Marinara Sauce

1½ tsp	vegetable oil	7 mL
½ cup	chopped onion	125 mL
1 tsp	crushed garlic	5 mL
1½ tsp	capers	7 mL
1	can (19 oz/540 mL) tomatoes, puréed	1
⅓ cup	sliced pitted black olives	75 mL
1 tbsp	tomato paste	15 mL
1½ tsp	dried basil (or 3 tbsp/45 mL chopped fresh)	7 mL
½ tsp	dried oregano	2 mL
1	bay leaf	1
	Red pepper flakes	
8 oz	penne noodles	250 g
4 tsp	grated Parmesan cheese	20 mL

For a spicier sauce, increase the red pepper flakes.

Serves 4

1. In large nonstick skillet, heat oil; sauté onion, garlic and capers for 3 minutes.

2. Add tomatoes, olives, tomato paste, basil, oregano, bay leaf and red pepper flakes to taste; cover and simmer for 10 to 15 minutes or until thickened slightly and flavors are blended. Discard bay leaf.

3. Meanwhile, cook penne according to package directions or until firm to the bite. Drain and place in serving bowl. Toss with sauce. Sprinkle with cheese.

Make Ahead

✦ Sauce can be prepared and refrigerated 2 days in advance, or frozen up to 1 month.

Nutritional Analysis (Per Serving)
- ✦ Calories: 296
- ✦ Protein: 10 g
- ✦ Cholesterol: 1 mg
- ✦ Sodium: 603 mg
- ✦ Fat: 5 g
- ✦ Carbohydrates: 54 g
- ✦ Fiber: 4 g

Pasta with Fresh Tomatoes, Basil and Cheese

12 oz	thin pasta (capellini or spaghettini)	375 g
1 tbsp	olive oil	15 mL
2 tsp	crushed garlic	10 mL
1¾ lb	chopped tomatoes	875 g
⅓ cup	chicken stock	75 mL
⅓ cup	sliced black olives	75 mL
½ cup	chopped fresh basil (or 2 tsp/10 mL dried)	125 mL
⅓ cup	grated Parmesan cheese	75 mL
	Pepper	

If using fresh basil, you'll get a more pronounced flavor if you add the basil after the pasta is tossed with the sauce. (Dried basil is added during the cooking.)

Serves 6

1. Cook pasta in boiling water according to package instructions or until firm to the bite. Drain and place in serving bowl.
2. In large nonstick skillet, heat oil; add garlic, tomatoes, stock and black olives; sauté for 2 minutes or just until hot. Pour over pasta. Add basil, cheese and pepper. Toss.

Tips

✦ Finely chop tomatoes when using thin pasta. Chop more coarsely if using wider pasta such as fettuccine.

✦ Romano cheese can replace Parmesan.

Make Ahead

✦ Prepare sauce up to a day ahead. Reheat gently, adding a little stock if too dense.

Nutritional Analysis (Per Serving)
✦ Calories: 318   ✦ Protein: 12 g   ✦ Cholesterol: 4 mg
✦ Sodium: 221 mg   ✦ Fat, total: 6 g   ✦ Carbohydrates: 55 g
✦ Fiber: 5 g   ✦ Fat, saturated: 2 g

Pasta with Ripe Tomato, Basil and Ricotta Cheese Sauce

12 oz	rotini	375 g
3 cups	chopped ripe tomatoes	750 mL
⅓ cup	green onions	75 mL
2 tbsp	olive oil	25 mL
⅔ cup	chopped fresh basil (or 1 tbsp/15 mL dried)	150 mL
1 cup	ricotta cheese	250 mL
2 tsp	crushed garlic	10 mL
⅓ cup	sliced black olives	75 mL

Serves 6

1. Cook pasta in boiling water according to package instructions or until firm to the bite. Drain and place in serving bowl.
2. Add tomatoes, onions, oil, basil, ricotta cheese, garlic and olives. Toss.

Tip

✦ Use juicy ripe tomatoes for extra moisture.

Make Ahead

✦ Combine all ingredients except pasta early in day. Toss just before serving.

Nutritional Analysis (Per Serving)
✦ Calories: 371   ✦ Protein: 15 g   ✦ Cholesterol: 13 mg
✦ Sodium: 226 mg   ✦ Fat, total: 10 g   ✦ Carbohydrates: 57 g
✦ Fiber: 5 g   ✦ Fat, saturated: 3 g

Roasted Garlic and Tomatoes with Ricotta Cheese over Rotini

1	head garlic, top ½ inch (1 cm) cut off, loosely wrapped in foil	1
5	large ripe plum tomatoes, cut in half crosswise	5
½ cup	5% ricotta cheese	125 mL
2 oz	feta cheese, crumbled	50 g
½ cup	chopped fresh basil (or 1 tsp/5 mL dried)	125 mL
1 tbsp	olive oil	15 mL
½ tsp	freshly ground black pepper	2 mL
12 oz	rotini	375 g

Serves 6
Preheat oven to 450°F (230°C)
Baking sheet lined with foil

1. Place garlic and tomatoes on prepared baking sheet. Roast in preheated oven for 30 minutes or until tomatoes are charred; let cool. Squeeze garlic out of skins.

2. In a food processor or blender, combine roasted tomatoes (with their juices) and garlic; pulse on and off several times until combined but still chunky. Transfer mixture to a bowl; add ricotta cheese, feta cheese, basil, olive oil and pepper. Set aside.

3. In a large pot of boiling water, cook rotini for 8 to 10 minutes or until tender but firm; drain. In a serving bowl combine pasta and sauce; toss well. Serve immediately.

Tip

✦ In the refrigerator, basil only keeps for a day or two. So try to buy basil no earlier than a day before you need it. And when you get home, don't wash the leaves; just put the basil in a paper bag (or perforated plastic bag). Basil also bruises easily — quickly turning from a beautiful green to an ugly brown-black color — so don't chop it until just before you're ready to add it to the recipe.

Lower-fat nut? If you're looking for a healthy snack, try roasted soynuts — a tasty source of soy protein with only 136 calories and 6 g fat per 1-oz (28 g) serving. That's a lot less fat than you'll find in the same amount of peanuts (14 g fat), macadamias (21 g), walnuts (18 g) or cashews (15 g). Soynuts also contain more protein, and they're the only nut that contains health-enhancing isoflavones. Try them plain, barbecued, onion-flavored or garlic-flavored.

Nutritional Analysis (Per Serving)
✦ Calories: 310 ✦ Protein: 12 g ✦ Cholesterol: 16 mg
✦ Sodium: 150 mg ✦ Fat, total: 7 g ✦ Carbohydrates: 49 g
✦ Fiber: 3 g ✦ Fat, saturated: 3.1 g

Spaghetti with Sun-Dried Tomatoes and Broccoli

8 oz	spaghetti	250 g
1/2 cup	sun-dried tomatoes	125 mL
2 cups	chopped broccoli	500 mL
2 1/2 cups	chopped tomatoes	625 mL
2 tbsp	olive oil	25 mL
1 1/2 tsp	crushed garlic	7 mL
Dash	crushed dried chilies	Dash
1/2 cup	chopped fresh basil (or 2 tsp/10 mL dried)	125 mL
3 tbsp	grated Parmesan cheese	45 mL

Instead of dried chilies, use 1/8 tsp (1 mL) cayenne pepper.

Buy dry sun-dried tomatoes, not those marinated in oil.

Serves 4

1. Cook pasta in boiling water according to package instructions or until firm to the bite. Drain and place in serving bowl.
2. Pour boiling water over sun-dried tomatoes. Let soak for 15 minutes. Drain, then chop. Add to pasta.
3. Blanch broccoli in boiling water just until barely tender. Rinse with cold water, drain and add to pasta. Add tomatoes, oil, garlic, chilies, basil and cheese. Toss.

Make Ahead

✦ Prepare pasta up to 2 hours earlier, leaving at room temperature. Toss before serving.

Nutritional Analysis (Per Serving)
- ✦ Calories: 366
- ✦ Protein: 14 g
- ✦ Cholesterol: 4 mg
- ✦ Sodium: 125 mg
- ✦ Fat, total: 9 g
- ✦ Carbohydrates: 60 g
- ✦ Fiber: 7 g
- ✦ Fat, saturated: 2 g

Linguine Alfredo

3/4 lb	linguine noodles	375 g
4 tsp	margarine	20 mL
2 tbsp	all-purpose flour	25 mL
2 cups	2% milk	500 mL
1/4 cup	grated Parmesan cheese	50 mL
1/4 tsp	nutmeg	1 mL
	Pepper	

You can dress up this dish with the simple addition of 1/2 cup (125 mL) diced steamed snow peas or red pepper, or 1/2 cup (125 mL) diced cooked ham.

When using margarine, choose a soft (non-hydrogenated) version to limit consumption of trans fats.

Serves 4

1. Cook linguine according to package directions or until firm to the bite. Drain and place in serving bowl.
2. Meanwhile, in small saucepan, melt margarine; add flour and cook, stirring, for 30 seconds. Add milk and cook on medium heat, stirring constantly, just until thickened, approximately 3 minutes. Add cheese, nutmeg, and pepper to taste; stir until combined. Pour over pasta and toss well.

Make Ahead

✦ Sauce can be made and refrigerated for up to 2 days ahead. Reheat gently, adding more milk to thin.

Nutritional Analysis (Per Serving)
- ✦ Calories: 470
- ✦ Protein: 18 g
- ✦ Cholesterol: 13 mg
- ✦ Sodium: 545 mg
- ✦ Fat: 9 g
- ✦ Carbohydrates: 77 g
- ✦ Fiber: 3 g

Fettuccine Alfredo
with Red Pepper and Snow Peas

8 oz	fettuccine noodles	250 g
1½ tsp	margarine	7 mL
½ cup	sliced sweet red pepper	125 mL
½ cup	snow peas	125 mL
2 tbsp	chopped fresh parsley	25 mL

Sauce

1 tbsp	margarine	15 mL
1 tbsp	all-purpose flour	15 mL
½ cup	2% milk	125 mL
¾ cup	chicken stock	175 mL
⅓ cup	grated Parmesan cheese	75 mL
	Pepper	

There are high-fat dishes — and then there's fettuccine Alfredo. Prepared in the traditional manner — with liberal amounts of whipping (35%) cream, butter, Parmesan cheese and sometimes even eggs — a plate of this pasta and sauce contains as much as 97 g fat (58% calories from fat). Yikes! That's a whole day's worth for a healthy male. So be kind to your arteries — try this skinny version of fettuccine Alfredo, which cuts the fat by a whopping 90%.

When using margarine, choose a soft (non-hydrogenated) version to limit consumption of trans fats.

Serves 4

1. Cook pasta according to package directions or until firm to the bite. Drain and place in serving bowl.

2. Meanwhile, in nonstick skillet, melt margarine; sauté red pepper and snow peas just until tender. Add to pasta.

3. *Sauce:* In small nonstick saucepan, melt margarine; add flour and cook, stirring, for 1 minute. Add milk and stock; simmer, stirring constantly, just until thickened, 3 to 5 minutes. Stir in cheese until melted. Season with pepper to taste. Pour over pasta mixture and combine well. Garnish with parsley.

Tip

✦ Try asparagus, broccoli or yellow pepper for a variation of this colorful dish.

Make Ahead

✦ Sauce can be made in advance and refrigerated; reheat gently, adding more milk to thin.

Nutritional Analysis (Per Serving)

✦ Calories: 306 ✦ Protein: 12 g ✦ Cholesterol: 56 mg
✦ Sodium: 587 mg ✦ Fat: 9 g ✦ Carbohydrates: 42 g
✦ Fiber: 3 g

Artichoke Cheese Dill Sauce over Rotini

12 oz	rotini	375 g
1	can (14 oz/398 mL) artichoke hearts, drained	1
2/3 cup	vegetable or chicken stock	150 mL
1/2 cup	chopped red onions	125 mL
1/2 cup	shredded low-fat mozzarella cheese	125 mL
1/3 cup	shredded low-fat Swiss cheese	75 mL
1/3 cup	chopped fresh dill (or 1 tsp/5 mL dried)	75 mL
1/3 cup	low-fat sour cream	75 mL
2 tbsp	light mayonnaise	25 mL
2 tbsp	fresh lemon juice	25 mL
1 tsp	minced garlic	5 mL
	Fresh chopped parsley	

Serves 6

1. In a large pot of boiling water, cook rotini for 8 to 10 minutes or until tender but firm; drain.
2. Meanwhile, in a food processor combine artichokes, stock, red onions, mozzarella cheese, Swiss cheese, dill, sour cream, mayonnaise, lemon juice and garlic; process until smooth. Transfer to a nonstick saucepan; cook over medium heat, stirring frequently, for 4 minutes or until heated through.
3. In a serving bowl, combine pasta and sauce; toss well. Garnish with fresh chopped parsley. Serve immediately.

Nutritional Analysis (Per Serving)
- Calories: 310
- Protein: 14 g
- Cholesterol: 15 mg
- Sodium: 193 mg
- Fat, total: 7 g
- Carbohydrates: 49 g
- Fiber: 6 g
- Fat, saturated: 3.2 g

Broccoli Pesto Fettuccine

2 cups	broccoli florets	500 mL
1/2 cup	chopped fresh basil or parsley	125 mL
3 tbsp	olive oil	45 mL
3 tbsp	grated Parmesan cheese	45 mL
3 tbsp	toasted pine nuts	45 mL
1 1/2 tsp	minced garlic	7 mL
1/2 cup	chicken stock	125 mL
12 oz	fettuccine	375 g

This is a great variation on pesto sauce. To make a complete meal, add 8 oz (250 g) sautéed chicken, fish or beef.

Serves 6

1. Cook broccoli in boiling water or in microwave for 4 minutes, or until tender. Drain and put in food processor along with basil, olive oil, Parmesan, pine nuts and garlic; process until finely chopped. With machine running, add stock through the feed tube; process until smooth.
2. In large pot of boiling water, cook pasta according to package directions, or until tender but firm; drain and place in serving bowl. Pour broccoli pesto over top and toss.

Tip
- Toast pine nuts on top of stove in a nonstick skillet for 2 minutes or until browned.

Make Ahead
- Prepare pesto early in the day, keeping covered. Pour over hot pasta just before serving.

Nutritional Analysis (Per Serving)
- Calories: 322
- Protein: 11 g
- Cholesterol: 2 mg
- Sodium: 149 mg
- Fat, total: 11 g
- Carbohydrates: 45 g
- Fiber: 3 g
- Fat, saturated: 2 g

Parsley and Basil Pesto Spaghettini

8 oz	spaghettini	250 g
1/2 cup	well-packed basil leaves	125 mL
1/2 cup	well-packed parsley leaves	125 mL
1/4 cup	water or chicken stock	50 mL
3/4 tsp	crushed garlic	4 mL
2 tbsp	olive oil	25 mL
2 tbsp	grated Parmesan cheese	25 mL
1 tsp	lemon juice	5 mL
1 tbsp	toasted pine nuts	15 mL

Try 1 cup (250 mL) basil and omit the parsley for a more intense flavor. Pesto can be made from other leaves such as fresh spinach and coriander.

Serves 4

1. Cook pasta according to package directions or until firm to the bite. Drain and place in serving bowl.
2. Meanwhile, in food processor, purée basil, parsley, water, garlic, oil, cheese, lemon juice and pine nuts until smooth. Pour over pasta; mix well.

Tip

✦ Toast nuts on top of stove in skillet or in 400°F (200°C) oven for 2 minutes.

Make Ahead

✦ Prepare pesto without cheese and freeze up to 6 months or refrigerate for 1 week. Bring pesto to room temperature and add cheese just before tossing with pasta.

Nutritional Analysis (Per Serving)
- ✦ Calories: 315 ✦ Protein: 9 g ✦ Cholesterol: 2 mg
- ✦ Sodium: 330 mg ✦ Fat: 10 g ✦ Carbohydrates: 46 g
- ✦ Fiber: 3 g

Pesto with Parsley, Dill and Basil Leaves

12 oz	spaghettini	375 g
2/3 cup	Italian parsley leaves, well packed down	150 mL
1 cup	basil leaves, well packed down	250 mL
1/3 cup	fresh dill, well packed down	75 mL
1/4 cup	olive oil	50 mL
1/3 cup	chicken stock	75 mL
3 tbsp	grated Parmesan cheese	45 mL
2 tsp	crushed garlic	10 mL
2 tbsp	toasted pine nuts	25 mL

For a different taste, try switching the given amounts of parsley, basil or dill.

Any nuts can replace pine nuts. Walnuts and pecans are delicious.

Serves 6 to 8

1. Cook pasta in boiling water according to package instructions or until firm to the bite. Drain and place in serving bowl.
2. In food processor, purée parsley, basil and dill leaves, oil, stock, cheese and garlic until well combined, approximately 30 seconds. Pour over pasta. Sprinkle with pine nuts, and toss.

Tips

✦ Dry leaves well after washing.
✦ Toast pine nuts on top of stove in skillet for 2 to 3 minutes, until brown.

Make Ahead

✦ Refrigerate up to 3 days or freeze up to 6 weeks.

Nutritional Analysis (Per Serving)
- ✦ Calories: 277 ✦ Protein: 10 g ✦ Cholesterol: 2 mg
- ✦ Sodium: 70 mg ✦ Fat, total: 9 g ✦ Carbohydrates: 41 g
- ✦ Fiber: 2 g ✦ Fat, saturated: 2 g

Pasta with Spinach Pesto

12 oz	pasta (any variety)	375 g
1½ cups	fresh spinach, washed and well packed down	375 mL
¼ cup	water or chicken stock	50 mL
3 tbsp	olive oil	45 mL
2 tbsp	toasted pine nuts	25 mL
3 tbsp	grated Parmesan cheese	45 mL
1½ tsp	crushed garlic	7 mL
	Pepper	

Dry spinach well after washing.

Serves 4 to 6

1. Cook pasta in boiling water according to package instructions or until firm to the bite. Drain and place in serving bowl.
2. Meanwhile, in food processor, purée spinach, water, oil, nuts, cheese, garlic and pepper until smooth. Pour over pasta.

Tips

✦ For variety, add to pasta 8 to 12 oz (250 to 375 g) of cooked meat, chicken or fish.

✦ Toast pine nuts on top of stove in skillet for 2 to 3 minutes, until brown.

Make Ahead

✦ Refrigerate sauce up to 3 days ahead or freeze for up to 6 weeks.

Nutritional Analysis (Per Serving)
✦ Calories: 325   ✦ Protein: 10 g   ✦ Cholesterol: 2 mg
✦ Sodium: 73 mg   ✦ Fat, total: 10 g   ✦ Carbohydrates: 48 g
✦ Fiber: 2 g   ✦ Fat, saturated: 2 g

Basil Pesto Sauce over Pasta

12 oz	linguine	375 g
1¼ cups	chopped fresh basil, well packed down	300 mL
⅓ cup	chicken stock or water	75 mL
2 tbsp	toasted pine nuts	25 mL
2 tbsp	grated Parmesan cheese	25 mL
3 tbsp	olive oil	45 mL
1 tsp	crushed garlic	5 mL

Dry basil well after washing.

Replace pine nuts with pecans or walnuts.

Serves 6

1. Cook pasta in boiling water according to package instructions or until firm to the bite. Drain and place in serving bowl.
2. In food processor, purée basil, stock, pine nuts, cheese, oil and garlic until smooth. Pour over pasta, and toss.

Tips

✦ Toast nuts on top of stove in skillet for 2 to 3 minutes, until brown.

✦ If the basil flavor is too strong, use half basil and half parsley.

Make Ahead

✦ Refrigerate up to 5 days ahead, or freeze up to 6 weeks.

Nutritional Analysis (Per Serving)
✦ Calories: 321   ✦ Protein: 10 g   ✦ Cholesterol: 1 mg
✦ Sodium: 66 mg   ✦ Fat, total: 10 g   ✦ Carbohydrates: 48 g
✦ Fiber: 2 g   ✦ Fat, saturated: 2 g

Fettuccine with Spring Vegetables in a Goat Cheese Sauce

1½ cups	halved snow peas or sugar snap peas	375 mL
1 cup	asparagus cut into 1-inch (2.5 cm) pieces	250 mL
1 cup	cherry tomatoes, cut in half	250 mL

Sauce

1 tbsp	margarine or butter	15 mL
2 tbsp	all-purpose flour	25 mL
1 cup	2% milk	250 mL
1 cup	chicken stock	250 mL
⅓ cup	sun-dried tomatoes	75 mL
3 tbsp	grated Parmesan cheese	45 mL
4 oz	goat cheese	125 g
¼ tsp	ground black pepper	1 mL
12 oz	fettuccine	375 g

Sugar snap peas are a cross between the common green pea and the snow pea. And as the name suggests, they are wonderfully sweet! Unfortunately, they are only available at certain times of the year (usually spring and fall), and when you do find them, they are almost always expensive. But they're worth it! Be sure you don't overcook these little treasures or they'll lose their crunch. If you can't find any sugar snap peas for this recipe, substitute snow peas.

When using margarine, choose a soft (non-hydrogenated) version to limit consumption of trans fats.

Serves 6

1. Pour boiling water over sun-dried tomatoes and allow to soften for 15 minutes. Drain and chop. Set aside.

2. In a saucepan of boiling water or in microwave, cook snow peas for 1 minute or until tender-crisp; refresh in cold water and drain. Repeat with asparagus for 2 minutes or until tender-crisp; refresh in cold water and drain. Put peas, asparagus and cherry tomatoes in large serving bowl.

3. In saucepan, melt margarine over medium heat; add flour and cook, stirring, for 1 minute. Gradually add milk and stock and cook, stirring, until sauce begins to thicken slightly, approximately 4 minutes. Reduce heat to low; add sun-dried tomatoes, Parmesan and goat cheeses and pepper. Stir until cheese melts. Remove from heat.

4. In large pot of boiling water, cook pasta according to package directions or until tender but firm; drain and add to serving bowl. Pour sauce over pasta and toss.

Tips

+ Broccoli can replace asparagus.

+ If cherry tomatoes are unavailable, use chopped plum tomatoes.

+ Use dry sun-dried tomatoes, not those soaked in oil. Buy them in bulk and keep them in freezer.

Make Ahead

+ Prepare cheese sauce up to a day ahead, adding more stock before serving if too thick.

Nutritional Analysis (Per Serving)

+ Calories: 351   + Protein: 15 g   + Cholesterol: 6 mg
+ Sodium: 394 mg   + Fat, total: 8 g   + Carbohydrates: 55 g
+ Fiber: 3 g   + Fat, saturated: 2 g

Corn and Three-Bean Salad (page 103) ➤

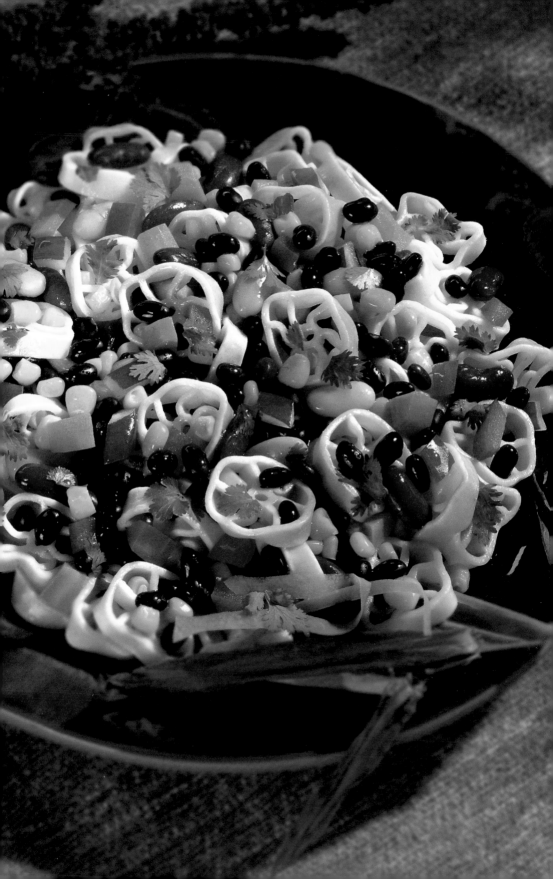

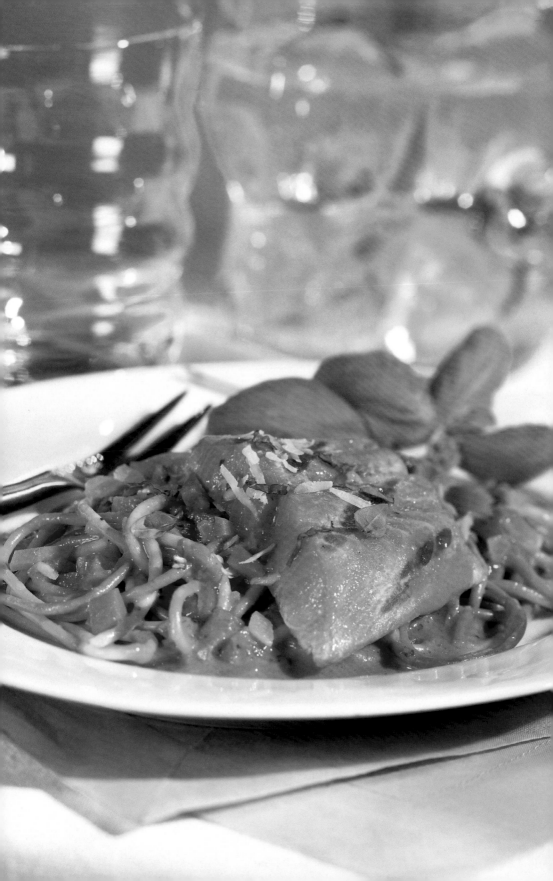

Pasta with Fresh Spring Vegetables and Mint

12 oz	angel hair pasta (fine strand)	375 g
1 tbsp	olive oil	15 mL
2 tsp	crushed garlic	10 mL
4 oz	chopped snow peas	125 g
1 cup	diced zucchini	250 mL
1	small carrot, finely diced	1
1 cup	finely diced sweet red peppers	250 mL
1 cup	frozen green peas	250 mL
2½ cups	cold chicken or vegetable stock	625 mL
2 tbsp + 2 tsp	all-purpose flour	35 mL
½ cup	chopped fresh mint (or 1½ tsp/7 mL dried)	125 mL

Serves 6

1. Cook pasta in boiling water according to package instructions or until firm to the bite. Drain and place in serving bowl.

2. In large nonstick skillet, heat oil; sauté garlic, snow peas, zucchini, carrot and red peppers until just tender, for 5 to 8 minutes. Add peas and sauté for 2 minutes.

3. Meanwhile, in small bowl, combine stock with flour until smooth. Add to vegetables and simmer just until slightly thickened, approximately 4 minutes, stirring constantly. Add mint and pour over pasta. Toss.

Tip

✦ Finely diced vegetables are best suited to the angel hair pasta. If vegetables are chopped in larger pieces, use linguine or fettuccine.

Make Ahead

✦ Sauté vegetables early in day until barely tender, approximately 4 minutes. Add frozen peas, but do not cook. Continue with recipe just before serving.

Nutritional Analysis (Per Serving)
✦ Calories: 319   ✦ Protein: 11 g   ✦ Cholesterol: 0 mg
✦ Sodium: 416 mg   ✦ Fat, total: 4 g   ✦ Carbohydrates: 60 g
✦ Fiber: 4 g   ✦ Fat, saturated: 0.5 g

◄ Grilled Salmon Fillet with Creamy Basil-Tomato Sauce (page 161)

Grilled Balsamic Vegetables over Penne

1	medium red onion, cut in half horizontally	1
1	medium zucchini, cut lengthwise into 4 strips	1
3	medium sweet peppers (green, red and/or yellow)	3
2	medium tomatoes, cut in half horizontally	2
1 lb	penne	500 g

Dressing

3 tbsp	lemon juice	45 mL
3 tbsp	balsamic vinegar	45 mL
1/4 cup	olive oil	50 mL
2 tsp	crushed garlic	10 mL

> *What's the difference between green and red bell peppers? Red peppers are left to ripen longer on the plant (which also makes them more expensive) and they are much higher in vitamins A and C. Today, bell peppers come in a variety of other shades — including yellow, orange, brown and purple. Use them interchangeably to add a rainbow of colors to your recipes!*

Serves 6 to 8
Preheat oven to broil or start barbecue

1. Place all vegetables on grill or barbecue. Grill onion for 25 minutes, turning until charred. Grill zucchini for 15 minutes until charred, turning as necessary. Grill sweet peppers for 15 minutes until charred. Grill tomatoes for 12 to 15 minutes until charred, rotating as necessary. Let vegetables cool for 10 minutes.

2. Remove top, skin and seeds of sweet peppers. Chop all vegetables into medium diced pieces, keeping juices. Set aside.

3. Meanwhile, cook pasta in boiling water according to package instructions or until firm to the bite. Drain and place in serving bowl. Add vegetables.

4. *Make the dressing:* Combine lemon juice, vinegar, oil and garlic. Pour over pasta, and toss.

Tips

+ Try alternating different vegetables such as eggplant, yellow zucchini or fennel.

+ If possible use one green, one red and one yellow or orange sweet pepper for brilliant color.

Make Ahead

+ Grill vegetables early in day. Chop before cooking pasta.

Nutritional Analysis (Per Serving)
+ Calories: 322
+ Protein: 10 g
+ Cholesterol: 0 mg
+ Sodium: 9 mg
+ Fat, total: 7 g
+ Carbohydrates: 55 g
+ Fiber: 4 g
+ Fat, saturated: 1 g

Spinach Cheese Tortellini in Puréed Vegetable Sauce

1 lb	cheese and/or spinach tortellini	500 g
Sauce		
1 tbsp	margarine or butter	15 mL
1 tsp	crushed garlic	5 mL
1 cup	finely diced carrots	250 mL
1 cup	finely diced zucchini	250 mL
1½ cups	chicken or vegetable stock	375 mL
⅓ cup	chopped fresh basil (or 1½ tsp/7 mL dried)	75 mL
2 tbsp	grated Parmesan cheese	25 mL

You can substitute sweet potatoes for carrots.

Serves 6

1. Cook pasta in boiling water according to package instructions or until firm to the bite. Drain and place in serving bowl.
2. *Make the sauce:* In small nonstick skillet, melt margarine; add garlic, carrots and zucchini. Cook until tender, approximately 8 minutes. Add stock and basil; simmer on medium heat for 5 minutes. Purée in food processor on and off for 30 seconds. Pour over pasta. Add cheese, and toss.

Make Ahead

✦ Prepare sauce early in day. Reheat gently, adding more stock if sauce becomes too dense.

Nutritional Analysis (Per Serving)
✦ Calories: 296   ✦ Protein: 12 g   ✦ Cholesterol: 4 mg
✦ Sodium: 510 mg   ✦ Fat, total: 9 g   ✦ Carbohydrates: 42 g
✦ Fiber: 3 g   ✦ Fat, saturated: 2 g

Teriyaki Rotini with Bell Peppers, Snow Peas and Sesame Sauce

¼ cup	packed brown sugar	50 mL
¼ cup	water	50 mL
¼ cup	light soya sauce	50 mL
3 tbsp	rice wine vinegar	45 mL
1 tbsp	all-purpose flour	15 mL
2 tsp	sesame seeds	10 mL
2 tsp	sesame oil	10 mL
2 tsp	minced garlic	10 mL
1½ tsp	minced gingerroot	7 mL
12 oz	rotini	375 g
1½ cups	julienned red or yellow bell peppers	375 mL
1 cup	julienned snow peas	250 mL
½ cup	chopped green onions	125 mL

Serves 6

1. In a bowl combine brown sugar, water, soya sauce, vinegar, flour, sesame seeds, sesame oil, garlic and ginger; whisk well. Set aside.
2. In a large pot of boiling water, cook rotini for 8 to 10 minutes or until tender but firm; drain. Meanwhile, in a nonstick wok or large nonstick saucepan sprayed with vegetable spray, cook peppers and snow peas over medium-high heat for 3 minutes or until tender-crisp. Add sauce; cook for 2 minutes or until thickened and hot.
3. In a serving bowl combine pasta and sauce; toss well. Sprinkle with green onions; serve.

Nutritional Analysis (Per Serving)
✦ Calories: 296   ✦ Protein: 9 g   ✦ Cholesterol: 0 mg
✦ Sodium: 359 mg   ✦ Fat, total: 3 g   ✦ Carbohydrates: 58 g
✦ Fiber: 3 g   ✦ Fat, saturated: 0.5 g

Asparagus Frittata with Roasted Red Peppers and Linguine

2 oz	linguine, broken	50 g
1/2 cup	chopped onions	125 mL
1 tsp	minced garlic	5 mL
1 cup	finely chopped asparagus	250 mL
2	large eggs	2
3	large egg whites	3
1/4 cup	low-fat evaporated milk	50 mL
1 tsp	Dijon mustard	5 mL
1/3 cup	chopped roasted red bell peppers	75 mL
3 tbsp	chopped fresh dill (or 1 tsp/5 mL dried)	45 mL
2 oz	Brie cheese, chopped or feta cheese, crumbled	50 g
2 tsp	vegetable oil	10 mL

Serves 6

1. In a pot of boiling water, cook linguine for 8 to 10 minutes or until tender but firm; drain. Rinse under cold running water; drain. Set aside.

2. In a 12-inch (30 cm) nonstick frying pan sprayed with vegetable spray, cook onions and garlic over medium-high heat for 5 minutes or until golden and tender. Add asparagus; cook, stirring often, for 2 minutes or until tender-crisp. Remove from pan; cool.

3. In a bowl combine eggs, egg whites, evaporated milk and Dijon mustard; whisk well. Add roasted peppers, dill, Brie cheese, pasta and cooled vegetable mixture.

4. Wipe out frying pan; heat oil over medium-low heat. Pour in frittata mixture; cook for 5 minutes. Gently lift sides of frittata, letting uncooked egg mixture flow beneath. Cook, covered, for 3 minutes or until frittata is set. Slip onto a serving platter; serve warm or at room temperature.

Tip

✦ Brie cheese is so rich and creamy, it just has to be packed with fat and calories, right? Not at all! In fact, 1 oz (25 g) has 100 calories and 9 g fat — about the same as (or slightly less than) other average-fat cheeses. The other good thing is that with a cheese as rich-tasting as Brie, you don't need to use much. In fact, this frittata, serving 6 people, has only 2 oz (50 g) Brie — a lot of flavor for only 3 g fat!

Nutritional Analysis (Per Serving)
✦ Calories: 131 ✦ Protein: 8 g ✦ Cholesterol: 83 mg
✦ Sodium: 162 mg ✦ Fat, total: 7 g ✦ Carbohydrates: 10 g
✦ Fiber: 1 g ✦ Fat, saturated: 2.5 g

Linguine with Bok Choy and Snow Peas in Oyster Sauce

Sauce

²/₃ cup	vegetable or chicken stock	150 mL
¼ cup	oyster sauce	50 mL
1 tbsp	rice wine vinegar	15 mL
1 tbsp	cornstarch	15 mL
2 tsp	sesame oil	10 mL
2 tsp	packed brown sugar	10 mL
1 tsp	hot Asian chili sauce (optional)	5 mL
8 oz	linguine (regular or whole wheat)	250 g
1 tsp	vegetable oil	5 mL
1½ tsp	minced garlic	7 mL
1 tsp	minced gingerroot	5 mL
3 cups	thinly sliced bok choy	750 mL
1 cup	thinly sliced red bell peppers	250 mL
1 cup	shredded carrots	250 mL
1 cup	halved snow peas	250 mL

The view on vitamin C: *American researchers have linked the daily use of vitamin C pills to a lower risk of cataracts in women. They found that women who supplemented their diet for 10 years or longer had more than a 70% lower risk for early cataract formation. While the study didn't measure how much vitamin C was taken, your best bet is to eat at least one vitamin C–rich food a day (e.g. citrus fruit, broccoli, bok choy, red pepper, tomato juice). This recipe provides a great start, at 123 mg per serving.*

Serves 4

1. In a bowl combine vegetable stock, oyster sauce, rice wine vinegar, cornstarch, sesame oil, brown sugar and Asian chili sauce. Set aside.

2. In a large pot of boiling water, cook linguine for 8 to 10 minutes or until tender but firm; drain. Meanwhile, in a nonstick wok or large skillet sprayed with vegetable spray, heat oil over medium-high heat. Add garlic and ginger; cook for 1 minute. Add bok choy, red peppers, carrots and snow peas; cook for 4 minutes or until vegetables are tender-crisp. Add sauce; cook for 1 minute or until thickened and bubbly.

3. In a serving bowl, combine sauce and pasta; toss well. Serve immediately.

Tip

✦ Bok choy is also known as pak choy or Chinese white cabbage — although it shouldn't be confused with Chinese cabbage, which is another name for napa cabbage. (I wish they'd get these names straightened out!) Anyway, it's a delicious vegetable — mild, with a nice crunch that makes it ideal for salads and stir-fries. Baby bok choy is, perhaps surprisingly, exactly what it sounds like: a more delicate (and sweeter) version of regular bok choy.

Nutritional Analysis (Per Serving)

✦ Calories: 266 ✦ Protein: 9 g ✦ Cholesterol: 0 mg
✦ Sodium: 222 mg ✦ Fat, total: 5 g ✦ Carbohydrates: 49 g
✦ Fiber: 6 g ✦ Fat, saturated: 0.5 g

Fettuccine with Creamy Wild Mushroom Sauce

12 oz	fettuccine	375 g
2 tsp	oil	10 mL
1½ tsp	crushed garlic	7 mL
⅔ cup	diced onions	150 mL
3½ cups	sliced wild or regular mushrooms (oyster, portobello or shiitake)	875 mL
6 tbsp	sweet wine (port or Madeira)	90 mL
6 tbsp	chicken stock	90 mL
1½ cups	2% milk	375 mL
5 tsp	all-purpose flour	25 mL
⅓ cup	finely chopped chives or green onions	75 mL

If you're trying to control your calorie intake, watch your portion sizes. Stick to the serving sizes suggested by the food guide.

Serves 4 to 6

1. Cook pasta in boiling water according to package instructions or until firm to the bite. Drain and place in serving bowl.
2. In large nonstick skillet, heat oil; sauté garlic and onions until soft, approximately 3 minutes. Add mushrooms and sauté until soft, approximately 5 minutes. Add wine and cook for 3 minutes.
3. Meanwhile, in small bowl, combine stock, milk and flour until dissolved. Add to mushroom mixture and simmer on medium heat for 5 minutes, stirring often. (Sauce may curdle initially; continue simmering.) Pour over pasta. Sprinkle with chives, and toss.

Tip
✦ If a sweet sauce is not desired, use dry white or red wine.

Make Ahead
✦ Prepare sauce early in day. Reheat gently, adding more milk if sauce thickens.

Nutritional Analysis (Per Serving)
✦ Calories: 364　✦ Protein: 14 g　✦ Cholesterol: 5 mg
✦ Sodium: 95 mg　✦ Fat, total: 5 g　✦ Carbohydrates: 64 g
✦ Fiber: 6 g　✦ Fat, saturated: 1 g

Oyster Mushrooms, Warm Spinach and Oranges over Rice Noodles

Sauce

6 tbsp	water	90 mL
1/4 cup	balsamic vinegar	50 mL
3 tbsp	orange juice concentrate	45 mL
3 tbsp	packed brown sugar	45 mL
1 1/2 tbsp	olive oil	20 mL
3 cups	sliced oyster mushrooms	750 mL
3/4 cup	chopped red onions	175 mL
1 tsp	minced garlic	5 mL
8 oz	broad rice noodles	250 g
4 cups	packed fresh spinach leaves, washed and torn	1 L
1/2 cup	drained canned mandarin oranges	125 mL

Serves 4

1. In a bowl combine water, balsamic vinegar, orange juice concentrate, brown sugar and olive oil; whisk well. Set aside.
2. In a large nonstick frying pan sprayed with vegetable spray, cook mushrooms, onions and garlic over medium-high heat, stirring occasionally, for 10 minutes or until browned. Add sauce; cook for 1 minute or until bubbly. Remove from heat; set aside.
3. In a large pot of boiling water, cook rice noodles for 5 minutes or until tender; drain. In a serving bowl combine pasta, sauce, spinach and mandarin oranges; toss well. Serve immediately.

Nutritional Analysis (Per Serving)
+ Calories: 293
+ Protein: 6 g
+ Cholesterol: 0 mg
+ Sodium: 60 mg
+ Fat, total: 6 g
+ Carbohydrates: 57 g
+ Fiber: 3 g
+ Fat, saturated: 0.8 g

Ravioli with Mushroom Sauce

1 lb	cheese ravioli	500 g
2 tsp	margarine or butter	10 mL
1 1/2 tsp	crushed garlic	7 mL
3 cups	sliced wild or regular mushrooms	750 mL
2 tbsp	all-purpose flour	25 mL
1/3 cup	dry white wine	75 mL
3/4 cup	chicken or vegetable stock	175 mL
3/4 cup	2% milk	175 mL
1/3 cup	finely chopped chives or green onions	75 mL
1/4 cup	grated Parmesan cheese	50 mL
	Pepper	

If using wild mushrooms, try oyster, which are less expensive and have great texture.

Serves 4 to 6

1. Cook pasta in boiling water according to package instructions or until firm to the bite. Drain and place in serving bowl.
2. In medium nonstick saucepan, melt margarine; sauté garlic and mushrooms for 5 minutes, just until mushrooms are cooked. Add flour and cook for 1 minute, stirring constantly. Add wine and cook for 1 minute. Slowly add stock and milk; simmer on medium heat for 5 minutes, or just until sauce slightly thickens, stirring constantly. Pour over pasta. Sprinkle with chives, Parmesan cheese and pepper. Toss.

Make Ahead
+ Prepare sauce early in day. Add more stock if sauce thickens.

Nutritional Analysis (Per Serving)
+ Calories: 322
+ Protein: 15 g
+ Cholesterol: 6 mg
+ Sodium: 373 mg
+ Fat, total: 9 g
+ Carbohydrates: 45 g
+ Fiber: 4 g
+ Fat, saturated: 2 g

Penne with Wild Mushrooms

12 oz	penne	375 g
1 tsp	margarine or butter	5 mL
3 cups	sliced wild mushrooms (oyster, cremini, portobello)	750 mL
2 tsp	olive oil	10 mL
2 tsp	crushed garlic	10 mL
1 cup	diced onions	250 mL
1 lb	chopped tomatoes (about 3 cups/750 mL)	500 g
2 cups	2% milk	500 mL
4 tsp	all-purpose flour	20 mL
1/2 cup	fresh chopped basil (or 2 tsp/10 mL dried)	125 mL
	Pepper	

> *When using margarine, choose a soft (non-hydrogenated) version to limit consumption of trans fats.*

Serves 6

1. Cook pasta in boiling water according to package instructions or until firm to the bite. Drain and place in serving bowl.

2. In large nonstick skillet, melt margarine; sauté mushrooms for 5 minutes. Drain off excess liquid. Add oil; sauté garlic and onions just until tender, approximately 3 minutes. Add tomatoes; simmer on low heat for 10 minutes just until tomatoes become very soft.

3. Meanwhile, in small bowl, mix milk and flour until smooth; add to tomato mixture and simmer on medium heat for 3 minutes or until sauce thickens slightly. Pour over pasta. Sprinkle with basil and pepper, and toss.

Tips

✦ The texture and flavor of wild mushrooms warrants the expense. If they are unavailable, use regular mushrooms.

✦ Try plum tomatoes instead of field tomatoes.

Make Ahead

✦ Prepare sauce early in day, leaving at room temperature. Reheat gently, adding more milk if too thick.

Nutritional Analysis (Per Serving)

✦ Calories: 356   ✦ Protein: 14 g   ✦ Cholesterol: 3 mg
✦ Sodium: 49 mg   ✦ Fat, total: 5 g   ✦ Carbohydrates: 66 g
✦ Fiber: 7 g   ✦ Fat, saturated: 1 g

Double-Bean Chili over Rotini

12 oz	rotini	375 g
1 tbsp	vegetable oil	15 mL
2 tsp	crushed garlic	10 mL
1 cup	chopped onions	250 mL
1 cup	chopped zucchini	250 mL
1¾ cups	vegetable or chicken stock	425 mL
2½ cups	canned tomatoes, crushed	625 mL
2 tbsp	tomato paste	25 mL
1 cup	diced potatoes	250 mL
⅔ cup	canned red kidney beans, drained	150 mL
⅔ cup	canned chickpeas, drained	150 mL
1 tbsp	chili powder	15 mL
2 tsp	dried basil	10 mL
1 tsp	dried oregano	5 mL
Pinch	cayenne pepper	Pinch
¼ cup	grated Parmesan cheese	50 mL

Serves 6

1. Cook pasta in boiling water according to package instructions or until firm to the bite. Drain and place in serving bowl.
2. In large nonstick saucepan, heat oil; sauté garlic, onions and zucchini until soft, approximately 5 minutes. Add stock, tomatoes and paste, potatoes, kidney beans and chickpeas, chili powder, basil, oregano and cayenne. Cover and simmer for 40 minutes or until potatoes are tender, stirring occasionally. Pour over pasta. Sprinkle with cheese. Garnish with parsley.

Make Ahead
✦ Prepare sauce up to a day ahead. Reheat and add more stock if sauce thickens.

Nutritional Analysis (Per Serving)
✦ Calories: 394 ✦ Protein: 15 g ✦ Cholesterol: 3 mg
✦ Sodium: 629 mg ✦ Fat, total: 5 g ✦ Carbohydrates: 73 g
✦ Fiber: 8 g ✦ Fat, saturated: 1 g

Roasted Red Pepper and Ricotta Purée over Rotini

12 oz	rotini	375 g
1	medium sweet red bell pepper	1
1⅔ cups	ricotta cheese	400 mL
2 tbsp	vegetable oil	25 mL
½ cup	chicken stock	125 mL
2 tbsp	grated Parmesan cheese	25 mL
1½ tsp	crushed garlic	7 mL
½ cup	chopped basil (or 2 tsp/10 mL dried) Parsley	125 mL

The skin of sweet peppers will come off easily if, after broiling, you place the peppers in a plastic or paper bag for 10 minutes, then peel.

Serves 6
Preheat oven to broil

1. Broil pepper until charred on all sides, approximately 15 minutes. Let cool; remove top, then skin, de-seed, and cut into quarters. Set aside.
2. Cook pasta in boiling water according to package instructions or until firm to the bite. Drain and place in serving bowl.
3. In food processor, purée ricotta cheese, red pepper, oil, stock, Parmesan cheese, garlic and basil until well combined. Pour over pasta. Toss and garnish with parsley.

Make Ahead
✦ Prepare sauce early in day. Pasta must be hot before adding sauce.

Nutritional Analysis (Per Serving)
✦ Calories: 368 ✦ Protein: 18 g ✦ Cholesterol: 30 mg
✦ Sodium: 241 mg ✦ Fat, total: 10 g ✦ Carbohydrates: 51 g
✦ Fiber: 2 g ✦ Fat, saturated: 4 g

Rotini with Cauliflower, Broccoli and Goat Cheese Cream Sauce

12 oz	rotini	375 g
2½ cups	chopped broccoli	625 mL
1½ cups	chopped cauliflower	375 mL
Sauce		
1 tbsp	margarine or butter	15 mL
2 tbsp	all-purpose flour	25 mL
1½ cups	2% milk	375 mL
1 cup	chicken stock	250 mL
4 oz	crumbled goat cheese	125 g
¾ cup	diced sweet red peppers	175 mL
2 tsp	crushed garlic	10 mL

> *When using margarine, choose a soft (non-hydrogenated) version to limit consumption of trans fats.*

Serves 6

1. Cook pasta in boiling water according to package instructions or until firm to the bite. Drain and place in serving bowl.

2. Cook broccoli and cauliflower in boiling water just until tender-crisp, approximately 3 minutes; drain and rinse with cold water. Add to pasta.

3. *Make the sauce:* In small nonstick saucepan, melt margarine; add flour and cook for 1 minute, stirring constantly. Slowly add milk and stock; simmer on medium heat, stirring constantly just until thickened, for 5 to 7 minutes. Add cheese, red peppers and garlic; cook for 1 minute. Pour over pasta, and toss.

Tips

✦ Substitute feta or cheddar for goat cheese.

✦ Use more broccoli or more cauliflower according to taste, not using more than 4 cups (1L) of vegetables.

Make Ahead

✦ Prepare sauce early in day, just to the point of adding cheese. Add more stock if sauce thickens.

Nutritional Analysis (Per Serving)

✦ Calories: 376   ✦ Protein: 16 g   ✦ Cholesterol: 12 mg
✦ Sodium: 306 mg   ✦ Fat, total: 8 g   ✦ Carbohydrates: 61 g
✦ Fiber: 5 g   ✦ Fat, saturated: 3 g

Tortellini with Sweet Red Pepper and Sun-Dried Tomato Sauce

1 lb	cheese tortellini	500 g
½ cup	sun-dried tomatoes	125 mL
2 tsp	vegetable oil	10 mL
1 tsp	crushed garlic	5 mL
⅔ cup	chopped onions	150 mL
1	large sweet red pepper, chopped	1
2 cups	chopped ripe tomatoes	500 mL
¼ cup	chopped parsley	50 mL
2 tbsp	grated Parmesan cheese	25 mL
	Parsley	

Serves 5 to 6

1. Cook pasta in boiling water according to package instructions or until firm to the bite. Drain and place in serving bowl.
2. Pour boiling water over sun-dried tomatoes. Let soak for 15 minutes. Drain and chop. Set aside.
3. Meanwhile, in large nonstick skillet sprayed with vegetable spray, heat oil; add garlic, onions and red pepper and cook on medium high for 5 minutes or until tender. Add tomatoes and cook for 5 minutes.
4. Place in food processor and purée. Add sun-dried tomatoes, parsley and cheese; mix until blended. Pour over pasta. Sprinkle with parsley, and toss.

Tips
✦ Use spinach or spinach and cheese tortellini for a change.
✦ Sweet yellow or orange bell peppers can be used.
✦ Use dry sun-dried tomatoes instead of those in oil.

Make Ahead
✦ Prepare sauce up to a day ahead. Reheat gently, adding a little chicken stock or water if sauce becomes too dense.

Nutritional Analysis (Per Serving)
✦ Calories: 305   ✦ Protein: 13 g   ✦ Cholesterol: 4 mg
✦ Sodium: 259 mg   ✦ Fat, total: 9 g   ✦ Carbohydrates: 44 g
✦ Fiber: 4 g   ✦ Fat, saturated: 2 g

Fettuccine with Ricotta Cheese and Sweet Peas

8 oz	fettuccine	250 g
2 tsp	vegetable oil	10 mL
1 tsp	crushed garlic	5 mL
1 cup	chopped onions	250 mL
1 cup	frozen green peas	250 mL
1 cup	ricotta cheese	250 mL
3/4 cup	2% milk	175 mL
1/3 cup	chopped fresh tarragon or dill (or 2 tsp/10 mL dried)	75 mL
3 tbsp	grated Parmesan cheese	45 mL
	Salt and pepper	

Tarragon gives a sweet flavor to this dish. For a more subtle flavor, use dill or parsley.

Serves 4

1. Cook pasta in boiling water according to package instructions or until firm to the bite. Drain and place in serving bowl.
2. Meanwhile, in nonstick skillet, heat oil; sauté garlic and onions until soft, approximately 5 minutes. Add peas and cook for 2 more minutes. Remove from heat. Add ricotta cheese, milk, tarragon, Parmesan cheese and salt and pepper. Pour over pasta and toss well.

Make Ahead

✦ Prepare sauce early in day. While cooking pasta, add a little more milk to sauce if too thick, and immediately pour over pasta.

Nutritional Analysis (Per Serving)
✦ Calories: 421   ✦ Protein: 22 g   ✦ Cholesterol: 27 mg
✦ Sodium: 237 mg   ✦ Fat, total: 9 g   ✦ Carbohydrates: 63 g
✦ Fiber: 4 g   ✦ Fat, saturated: 4 g

Rigatoni with Sautéed Eggplant, Tomatoes and Swiss Cheese

12 oz	rigatoni	375 g
1 tbsp	olive oil	15 mL
2 tsp	crushed garlic	10 mL
3/4 cup	chopped onions	175 mL
3 cups	diced eggplant	750 mL
1	can (28 oz/796 mL) tomatoes, crushed	1
2 tsp	dried basil	10 mL
1 1/2 tsp	dried oregano	7 mL
1/2 cup	shredded Swiss cheese	125 mL

Mozzarella can replace Swiss cheese for a milder flavor, fewer calories and less fat.

Leave skin on eggplant for extra vitamins and fiber.

Serves 6

1. Cook pasta in boiling water according to package instructions or until firm to the bite. Drain and place in serving bowl.
2. In large nonstick skillet sprayed with vegetable spray, heat oil; sauté garlic and onions until soft, approximately 4 minutes. Add eggplant and sauté just until tender, approximately 8 minutes. Add tomatoes, basil and oregano; simmer on low heat for 20 minutes, stirring occasionally.
3. Pour over pasta. Sprinkle with cheese, and toss.

Make Ahead

✦ Prepare sauce up to a day ahead. Reheat gently, adding a little water if sauce is too thick.

Nutritional Analysis (Per Serving)
✦ Calories: 360   ✦ Protein: 14 g   ✦ Cholesterol: 9 mg
✦ Sodium: 252 mg   ✦ Fat, total: 6 g   ✦ Carbohydrates: 63 g
✦ Fiber: 7 g   ✦ Fat, saturated: 2 g

Penne with Zucchini, Eggplant and Tomato Ratatouille

12 oz	penne	375 g
1 tbsp	oil	15 mL
2 tsp	crushed garlic	10 mL
1 cup	diced onions	250 mL
1³/₄ cups	diced eggplant	425 mL
1³/₄ cups	diced zucchini	425 mL
1³/₄ cups	diced tomatoes	425 mL
²/₃ cup	chicken stock	150 mL
¹/₂ cup	chopped fresh basil (or 2 tsp/10 mL dried)	125 mL
1 tsp	dried oregano	5 mL
¹/₂ cup	shredded Asiago or Parmesan cheese	125 mL

Leave skin on eggplant and zucchini for extra fiber.

Serves 6

1. Cook pasta in boiling water according to package instructions or until firm to the bite. Drain and place in serving bowl.

2. In large nonstick skillet, heat oil; sauté garlic and onions until soft, approximately 4 minutes. Add eggplant and zucchini and sauté just until tender, for 5 to 8 minutes. Add tomatoes and stock and simmer on low heat for 5 minutes, stirring occasionally. Add basil and oregano; pour over pasta. Sprinkle with cheese, and toss.

Make Ahead

✦ Prepare sauce early in day. Reheat gently, adding a little stock if sauce is too thick.

Nutritional Analysis (Per Serving)
✦ Calories: 353   ✦ Protein: 14 g   ✦ Cholesterol: 7 mg
✦ Sodium: 268 mg   ✦ Fat, total: 6 g   ✦ Carbohydrates: 61 g
✦ Fiber: 7 g   ✦ Fat, saturated: 2 g

Soba Noodles with Peanut Butter Dressing

10 oz	soba noodles or fettuccine	300 g
1¹/₂ cups	snow peas, cut in half	375 mL
1¹/₂ cups	thinly sliced sweet red peppers	375 mL
¹/₂ cup	thinly sliced carrots	125 mL
¹/₃ cup	chopped green onions	75 mL
³/₄ cup	sliced water chestnuts	175 mL
Dressing		
¹/₄ cup	peanut butter	50 mL
¹/₃ cup	chicken stock	75 mL
2 tbsp	rice wine vinegar	25 mL
1 tbsp	lemon juice	15 mL
1 tbsp	soya sauce	15 mL
2 tsp	sesame oil	10 mL
2 tsp	minced gingerroot	10 mL
1¹/₂ tsp	crushed garlic	7 mL
1¹/₂ tsp	brown sugar	7 mL

Serves 4 to 5

1. Cook pasta in boiling water according to package instructions or until firm to the bite. Drain and place in serving bowl.

2. Blanch snow peas, red peppers and carrots in boiling water until barely tender, approximately 3 minutes. Drain and refresh with cold water; add to pasta along with green onions and water chestnuts.

3. *Make the dressing:* In food processor, purée peanut butter, stock, rice wine vinegar, lemon juice, soya sauce, sesame oil, ginger, garlic and brown sugar until smooth. Pour over pasta, and toss.

Nutritional Analysis (Per Serving)
✦ Calories: 364   ✦ Protein: 15 g   ✦ Cholesterol: 0 mg
✦ Sodium: 569 mg   ✦ Fat, total: 8 g   ✦ Carbohydrates: 65 g
✦ Fiber: 4 g   ✦ Fat, saturated: 1 g

Crunchy Baked Macaroni and Cheese Casserole

1 tbsp	margarine or butter	15 mL
3 tbsp	all-purpose flour	45 mL
1¼ cups	2% milk	300 mL
1⅓ cups	chicken stock	325 mL
1¼ cup	grated cheddar cheese (3½ oz/90 g)	300 mL
12 oz	macaroni	375 g

Topping

½ cup	corn flake crumbs	125 mL
3 tbsp	grated Parmesan cheese	45 mL
1 tsp	margarine or butter	5 mL

For vegetarian meals, vegetable stock can be substituted for chicken stock.

When using margarine, choose a soft (non-hydrogenated) version to limit consumption of trans fats.

Serves 8
Preheat oven to 450°F (230°C)
2-quart (2 L) casserole dish sprayed with vegetable spray

1. In saucepan over medium heat, melt margarine; add flour and cook, stirring, for 1 minute (mixture will be crumbly). Gradually add milk and stock, stirring constantly; let simmer for 5 to 8 minutes or until slightly thickened, stirring constantly. Stir in cheese and cook until melted, approximately 1 minute. Remove from heat.

2. In pot of boiling water cook the pasta according to package directions or until tender but firm; drain. Toss with cheese sauce and pour into prepared casserole dish.

3. In small bowl, combine corn flake crumbs, Parmesan and margarine. Sprinkle over casserole and bake just until top is browned, approximately 10 minutes.

Tips
+ If using whole corn flakes, use 1½ cups (375 mL) to equal ½ cup (125 mL) crumbs.
+ Bran flakes are also a delicious substitute for corn flakes.

Make Ahead
+ Can be prepared a day ahead and gently reheated in 350°F (180°C) oven.
+ Can be frozen in portions for up to 6 weeks. Great as leftovers.

Nutritional Analysis (Per Serving)
+ Calories: 288   + Protein: 12 g   + Cholesterol: 18 mg
+ Sodium: 375 mg   + Fat, total: 8 g + Carbohydrates: 41 g
+ Fiber: 1 g   + Fat, saturated: 4 g

Thai Linguine with Hoisin Sauce and Crisp Vegetables

12 oz	linguine	375 g
1 cup	diced sweet red peppers	250 mL
1 cup	sliced snow peas	250 mL
1 cup	chopped broccoli	250 mL
1/2 cup	chopped coriander or parsley	125 mL
1/4 cup	chopped green onions	50 mL
Sauce		
1/4 cup	rice wine vinegar	50 mL
1/4 cup	hoisin sauce	50 mL
2 tbsp	sesame oil	25 mL
2 tbsp	soya sauce	25 mL
2 tbsp	water	25 mL
1 1/2 tsp	grated gingerroot	7 mL
1 1/2 tsp	crushed garlic	7 mL

Try using asparagus or green or yellow sweet peppers.

Serves 5

1. Cook pasta in boiling water according to package instructions or until firm to the bite. Drain and place in serving bowl. Add red peppers.
2. Blanch snow peas for 2 minutes. Repeat with broccoli for 3 minutes. Drain and rinse both vegetables with cold water and add to pasta. Add coriander and green onions.
3. *Make the sauce:* In small bowl, combine rice wine vinegar, hoisin sauce, oil, soya sauce, water, ginger and garlic until mixed. Pour over pasta, and toss.

Make Ahead

✦ Salad can be prepared and tossed early in day. Toss again before serving.

Nutritional Analysis (Per Serving)
- ✦ Calories: 384
- ✦ Protein: 14 g
- ✦ Cholesterol: 0 mg
- ✦ Sodium: 472 mg
- ✦ Fat, total: 7 g
- ✦ Carbohydrates: 68 g
- ✦ Fiber: 3 g
- ✦ Fat, saturated: 1 g

Linguine with Smoked Salmon and Green Peas

8 oz	linguine	250 g
1 tbsp	margarine or butter	15 mL
3 1/2 tsp	all-purpose flour	17 mL
3/4 cup	2% milk	175 mL
3/4 cup	fish or chicken stock	175 mL
1 cup	frozen green peas	250 mL
4 oz	smoked salmon, chopped	125 g
1/4 cup	chopped fresh dill (or 2 tsp/10 mL dried)	50 mL

Fettuccine or penne can be substituted for linguine.

When using margarine, choose a soft (non-hydrogenated) version to limit consumption of trans fats.

Serves 4

1. Cook pasta in boiling water according to package instructions or until firm to the bite. Drain and place in serving bowl.
2. In small nonstick skillet, melt margarine; add flour and cook for 1 minute, stirring constantly. Add milk and stock; simmer just until slightly thickened, approximately 3 minutes, stirring constantly. Add peas and cook for 1 minute. Pour over pasta. Add salmon and dill, and toss.

Make Ahead

✦ Sauce can be made a day ahead and gently reheated. Add more milk if too thick.

Nutritional Analysis (Per Serving)
- ✦ Calories: 386
- ✦ Protein: 20 g
- ✦ Cholesterol: 11 mg
- ✦ Sodium: 519 mg
- ✦ Fat, total: 7 g
- ✦ Carbohydrates: 62 g
- ✦ Fiber: 3 g
- ✦ Fat, saturated: 2 g

Fettuccine with Fresh Salmon, Dill and Leeks

4 tsp	margarine	20 mL
4 tsp	all-purpose flour	20 mL
2 cups	2% milk	500 mL
1/4 cup	grated Parmesan cheese	50 mL
1/4 cup	white wine	50 mL
2 tbsp	chopped onion	25 mL
1 tsp	crushed garlic	5 mL
2	leeks, washed and sliced in thin rounds	2
12 oz	fresh salmon, boned and cubed	375 g
3 tbsp	chopped fresh dill (or 1 tsp/5 mL dried dillweed)	45 mL
10 oz	fettuccine noodles	300 g

When using margarine, choose a soft (non-hydrogenated) version to limit consumption of trans fats.

Serves 4 to 6

1. In small saucepan, melt margarine; add flour and cook, stirring, for 30 seconds. Add milk and cook, stirring constantly, until thickened, 4 to 5 minutes. Stir in cheese until melted; set aside.

2. In large skillet, combine wine, onion, garlic and leeks; cook over medium heat for approximately 10 minutes or until leeks are softened. Add white sauce along with salmon. Cook for 2 to 3 minutes or until salmon is almost opaque, stirring gently. Stir in dill.

3. Meanwhile, cook fettuccine according to package directions or until firm to the bite. Drain and place in serving bowl. Toss with sauce.

Tip
✦ Fresh tuna or swordfish is a great substitute.

Make Ahead
✦ The white sauce can be prepared early in day or up to day before, but add a little extra milk when reheating before continuing with recipe.

Nutritional Analysis (Per Serving)
✦ Calories: 372   ✦ Protein: 24 g   ✦ Cholesterol: 30 mg
✦ Sodium: 358 mg ✦ Fat: 9 g   ✦ Carbohydrates: 45 g
✦ Fiber: 2 g

Grilled Salmon Fillet with Creamy Basil-Tomato Sauce

1 cup	finely chopped onions	250 mL
1/3 cup	finely chopped carrots	75 mL
1 tsp	minced garlic	5 mL
1	can (19 oz/540 mL) tomatoes, crushed	1
1/3 cup	seafood or chicken stock or water	75 mL
1/4 cup	low-fat evaporated milk	50 mL
1 tbsp	tomato paste	15 mL
1 1/2 tsp	dried basil	7 mL
1 tsp	dried oregano	5 mL
1	bay leaf	1
8 oz	spaghetti	250 g
8 oz	salmon fillets, cut into 4 pieces	250 g
1/4 cup	grated Asiago or low-fat Parmesan cheese	50 mL
	Chopped fresh basil (optional)	

Serves 4
Preheat broiler or set grill to medium-high

1. In a nonstick saucepan sprayed with vegetable spray, cook onions, carrots and garlic over medium heat for 3 minutes or until softened. Add tomatoes, stock, evaporated milk, tomato paste, basil, oregano and bay leaf; bring to a boil. Reduce heat to medium-low; cook, stirring occasionally, for 10 minutes.

2. Meanwhile, in a large pot of boiling water, cook pasta for 8 to 10 minutes or until tender but firm; drain. Broil or grill salmon, turning once, for 10 minutes per 1-inch (2.5 cm) thickness or until cooked through.

3. In a bowl combine pasta and sauce; toss well. Divide among 4 plates; top each serving with salmon. Sprinkle with cheese and fresh basil.

Nutritional Analysis (Per Serving)
- Calories: 415
- Protein: 23 g
- Cholesterol: 49 mg
- Sodium: 90 mg
- Fat, total: 8 g
- Carbohydrates: 59 g
- Fiber: 4 g
- Fat, saturated: 2.5 g

Salmon Fettuccine

12 oz	fettuccine	375 g
1 tbsp	olive oil	15 mL
2 tsp	crushed garlic	10 mL
1/2 cup	finely diced carrots	125 mL
2/3 cup	finely diced celery	150 mL
1/3 cup	chopped green onions	75 mL
12 oz	salmon fillets, skinned, boned and cut into 1-inch (2.5 cm) cubes	375 g
1/2 cup	dry white wine	125 mL
1 1/4 cups	prepared tomato sauce or Quick Basic Tomato Sauce (see recipe, page 129)	300 mL
2/3 cup	2% milk	150 mL
1/2 cup	chopped fresh dill (or 1 tbsp/15 mL dried)	125 mL

Serves 4 to 6

1. Cook pasta in boiling water according to package instructions or until firm to the bite. Drain and place in serving bowl.

2. Meanwhile, in large nonstick skillet, heat oil; sauté garlic, carrots and celery until tender, approximately 5 minutes. Add onions and sauté for 1 minute. Add salmon and wine; simmer for 2 minutes, turning fish occasionally. Do not let salmon overcook.

3. Add tomato sauce and milk; simmer just until salmon is cooked, approximately 2 minutes, stirring often. Add dill. Pour over pasta, and gently toss.

Nutritional Analysis (Per Serving)
- Calories: 456
- Protein: 26 g
- Cholesterol: 36 mg
- Sodium: 161 mg
- Fat, total: 10 g
- Carbohydrates: 64 g
- Fiber: 3 g
- Fat, saturated: 2 g

Fettuccine with Scallops and Smoked Salmon

12 oz	fettuccine	375 g
2 tsp	crushed garlic	10 mL
12 oz	scallops, quartered	375 g
1 tbsp	margarine or butter	15 mL
2 tbsp	all-purpose flour	25 mL
1 cup	clam juice or chicken stock	250 mL
1 cup	2% milk	250 mL
2 tbsp	light sour cream	25 mL
1/3 cup	chopped fresh dill (or 2 tsp/10 mL dried)	75 mL
1/4 cup	grated Parmesan cheese	50 mL
3 oz	smoked salmon, chopped	75 g

Serves 6

1. Cook pasta in boiling water according to package instructions or until firm to the bite. Drain and place in serving bowl.

2. In large nonstick skillet sprayed with vegetable spray, sauté garlic and scallops for 2 minutes, or just until scallops are cooked. Drain and add to pasta.

3. In medium nonstick saucepan, melt margarine. Add flour and cook for 1 minute, stirring constantly. Slowly add clam juice and milk. Simmer on medium heat until slightly thickened, approximately 3 minutes, stirring constantly. Add sour cream, dill and cheese. Mix well and pour over pasta. Add smoked salmon, and toss.

Tips

✦ For a change, replace scallops with firm fish fillets such as halibut or Chilean seabass.

✦ Remove the small muscle on the side of each scallop; it toughens as it cooks.

Make Ahead

✦ Prepare sauce in Step 3 early in day. Before serving, reheat gently, adding more milk if sauce thickens.

Nutritional Analysis (Per Serving)

✦ Calories: 432	✦ Protein: 29 g	✦ Cholesterol: 35 mg
✦ Sodium: 568 mg	✦ Fat, total: 8 g	✦ Carbohydrates: 61 g
✦ Fiber: 2 g	✦ Fat, saturated: 3 g	

Fettuccine with Scallops in Tomato Sauce

12 oz	fettuccine	375 g
2 tbsp	olive oil	25 mL
1½ tsp	crushed garlic	7 mL
1 cup	thinly sliced red onions	250 mL
3 lb	tomatoes, puréed	1.5 kg
½ cup	chopped fresh basil (or 2 tsp/10 mL dried)	125 mL
	Pepper	
12 oz	medium scallops, halved	375 g
	Basil	

Remove the small muscle on the side of each scallop; it toughens as it cooks.

Firm white fish fillets such as orange roughy or grouper can be substituted for the scallops.

Serves 6

1. Cook pasta in boiling water according to package instructions or until firm to the bite. Drain and place in serving bowl.
2. In large nonstick skillet, heat oil; sauté garlic and onions until tender. Add puréed tomatoes and simmer on medium heat for 15 minutes, stirring occasionally. Add basil and pepper and cook for 2 minutes. Set aside.
3. In small nonstick skillet sprayed with vegetable spray, sauté scallops until seared on both sides and just cooked, approximately 3 minutes. Drain and add to pasta along with sauce. Toss and garnish with basil.

Make Ahead
+ Tomato sauce can be made a day ahead and gently reheated.

Nutritional Analysis (Per Serving)
+ Calories: 398   + Protein: 21 g   + Cholesterol: 21 mg
+ Sodium: 127 mg   + Fat, total: 7 g   + Carbohydrates: 65 g
+ Fiber: 8 g   + Fat, saturated: 0.9 g

Fettuccine with Scallops and Red Pepper Sauce

¾ lb	fettuccine noodles	375 g
1 tbsp	vegetable oil	15 mL
1 tsp	crushed garlic	5 mL
¾ cup	chopped onion	175 mL
1½ cups	chopped sweet red pepper	375 mL
½ cup	chicken stock	125 mL
¾ lb	raw scallops, sliced in half	375 g
1 tbsp	margarine	15 mL
¼ cup	chopped fresh dill (or 1½ tsp/7 mL dried dillweed)	50 mL
3 tbsp	grated Parmesan cheese	45 mL

When using margarine, choose a soft (non-hydrogenated) version to limit consumption of trans fats.

Serves 4 to 6

1. Cook fettuccine according to package directions or just until firm to the bite. Drain and place in serving bowl.
2. Meanwhile, in large nonstick skillet, heat oil; sauté garlic, onion and red pepper until softened, 5 to 8 minutes.
3. Add stock, scallops and margarine; cook for 2 minutes or just until scallops are opaque. Mix in dill. Pour over pasta and toss to combine. Sprinkle with cheese.

Tip
+ Shrimp can replace the scallops. However, the sweetness of red pepper goes well with the flavor of scallops.

Nutritional Analysis (Per Serving)
+ Calories: 329   + Protein: 22 g   + Cholesterol: 69 mg
+ Sodium: 532 mg   + Fat: 8 g   + Carbohydrates: 42 g
+ Fiber: 4 g

Black Bean and Mango Salsa over Swordfish and Rotini

Sauce

2 tbsp	black bean sauce	25 mL
1½ tbsp	water	20 mL
1½ tbsp	fresh lemon juice	20 mL
1½ tbsp	barbecue sauce	20 mL
1 tbsp	olive oil	15 mL
1½ tbsp	packed brown sugar	20 mL
1 tsp	minced garlic	5 mL

Salsa

2	green onions, chopped	2
1	large ripe mango, peeled and chopped	1
1 cup	canned cooked black beans, rinsed and drained	250 mL
1 cup	chopped red bell peppers	250 mL
½ cup	chopped red onions	125 mL
½ cup	chopped fresh coriander	125 mL
8 oz	rotini	250 g
6 oz	swordfish	175 g

Serves 4
Preheat broiler or set grill to medium-high

1. *Sauce:* In a bowl combine black bean sauce, water, lemon juice, barbecue sauce, olive oil, brown sugar and garlic; set aside.
2. *Salsa:* In a bowl combine green onions, mango, black beans, red peppers, red onions and coriander; set aside.
3. In a large pot of boiling water, cook rotini for 8 to 10 minutes or until tender but firm; drain. Meanwhile, broil or grill fish for 10 minutes per 1-inch (2.5 cm) thickness or until cooked through; cut into cubes.
4. In a serving bowl, combine pasta, sauce, salsa and fish; toss well. Serve immediately.

Nutritional Analysis (Per Serving)
- Calories: 432
- Protein: 21 g
- Cholesterol: 17 mg
- Sodium: 169 mg
- Fat, total: 7 g
- Carbohydrates: 71 g
- Fiber: 8 g
- Fat, saturated: 1.3 g

Angel Hair Pasta with Mushrooms and Snapper

8 oz	fine strand pasta (angel hair, capellini or spaghettini)	250 g
1 tbsp	margarine or butter	15 mL
1 tsp	crushed garlic	5 mL
8 oz	wild or regular mushrooms, finely sliced	250 g
8 oz	snapper (or any firm fish), cut into ½-inch (1 cm) pieces	250 g
2 tbsp	dry white wine	25 mL
8 oz	tomatoes, finely chopped	250 g
⅓ cup	chopped fresh basil (or 1½ tsp/7 mL dried)	75 mL
3 tbsp	grated Parmesan cheese	45 mL

Serves 4

1. Cook pasta in boiling water according to package instructions or until firm to the bite. Drain and place in serving bowl.
2. In large nonstick skillet, melt margarine; sauté garlic and mushrooms just until cooked. Add snapper and sauté until fish is still slightly underdone, for 3 to 4 minutes. Add wine and cook for 1 minute. Add tomatoes and basil and stir just until combined. Pour over pasta. Sprinkle with cheese, and toss.

Nutritional Analysis (Per Serving)
- Calories: 383
- Protein: 25 g
- Cholesterol: 27 mg
- Sodium: 180 mg
- Fat, total: 7 g
- Carbohydrates: 55 g
- Fiber: 6 g
- Fat, saturated: 2 g

Linguine with Swordfish in Tomato Basil Sauce

12 oz	linguine	375 g
1½ tsp	crushed garlic	7 mL
12 oz	swordfish, cut into 1-inch (2.5 cm) cubes	375 g
14 oz	chopped tomatoes	425 g
¾ cup	fish or chicken stock	175 mL
4 tsp	flour	20 mL
½ cup	chopped fresh basil (or 2 tsp/10 mL dried)	125 mL
3 tbsp	grated Parmesan cheese	45 mL

Be certain not to overcook fish, or it will be dry. Cook just until it is moist, tender and flaky.

Serves 6

1. Cook pasta in boiling water according to package instructions or until firm to the bite. Drain and place in serving bowl.
2. In large nonstick skillet sprayed with vegetable spray, sauté garlic and swordfish until fish is just done, approximately 3 minutes. Drain and add to pasta.
3. Add tomatoes to skillet and simmer for 2 minutes.
4. Meanwhile, in small bowl combine stock and flour until smooth. Add to tomatoes and simmer on medium heat just until slightly thickened, approximately 3 minutes. Add basil; pour over pasta. Sprinkle with cheese, and toss.

Tips
✦ Tuna or Chilean seabass are good substitutes for swordfish.
✦ Try plum tomatoes instead of field tomatoes.

Make Ahead
✦ Prepare sauce early in day. Reheat gently while preparing pasta, adding more stock if sauce is too thick.

Nutritional Analysis (Per Serving)
✦ Calories: 374   ✦ Protein: 25 g   ✦ Cholesterol: 30 mg
✦ Sodium: 311 mg   ✦ Fat, total: 6 g ✦ Carbohydrates: 54 g
✦ Fiber: 3 g   ✦ Fat, saturated: 2 g

Spaghettini with Tomatoes, Basil and Fish

12 oz	spaghettini	375 g
1/3 cup	dry white wine	75 mL
12 oz	firm white fish fillets, cut into 1-inch (2.5 cm) pieces	375 g
2 tsp	vegetable oil	10 mL
2 tsp	crushed garlic	10 mL
3/4 cup	chopped onions	175 mL
1 3/4 lb	diced tomatoes	875 g
1 tbsp	tomato paste	15 mL
2/3 cup	chopped fresh basil (or 2 tsp/10 mL dried)	150 mL
1/4 cup	grated Parmesan cheese	50 mL

Getting more omega-3s: *Eating fatty fish is a good way to add omega-3 fatty acids to your diet. But what if you don't eat a lot of fish? Try increasing your intake of alpha linolenic acid (ALA) from sources such as flaxseed, walnut and canola oil, soybeans, green leafy vegetables and omega-3 eggs. ALA is the primary member of the omega-3 family, and it's called an essential fatty acid. That means it cannot be made by the body and must be supplied from food. Omega-3s are needed for proper growth and brain development during fetal life and infancy.*

Serves 6

1. Cook pasta in boiling water according to package instructions or until firm to the bite. Drain and place in serving bowl.
2. Put wine in saucepan; add fish and simmer just until done, approximately 3 minutes. Drain and reserve liquid. Add fish to pasta.
3. In large nonstick saucepan, heat oil; sauté garlic and onions until soft, approximately 3 minutes. Add tomatoes, paste and reserved fish liquid. Simmer on low heat for 15 minutes, until the sauce thickens. Pour over pasta. Sprinkle with basil and cheese, and toss.

Tip
✦ For fish fillets, consider orange roughy, haddock or seabass.

Make Ahead
✦ Sauce in Step 3 can be made early in day but substitute 1/3 cup (75 mL) dry white wine for reserved seafood liquid. When cooking seafood, drain wine and cooking liquid.

Nutritional Analysis (Per Serving)
✦ Calories: 390   ✦ Protein: 22 g   ✦ Cholesterol: 22 mg
✦ Sodium: 185 mg   ✦ Fat, total: 7 g   ✦ Carbohydrates: 58 g
✦ Fiber: 6 g   ✦ Fat, saturated: 2 g

Tuna and Eggplant Ratatouille over Rigatoni

2 tsp	vegetable oil	10 mL
1 cup	chopped onions	250 mL
2 tsp	minced garlic	10 mL
2 cups	chopped eggplant (not peeled)	500 mL
1 cup	chopped green peppers	250 mL
1½ cups	chopped ripe plum tomatoes	375 mL
½ cup	seafood or vegetable stock	125 mL
2 tbsp	tomato paste	25 mL
2 tbsp	balsamic vinegar	25 mL
2 tsp	drained capers	10 mL
1½ tsp	dried basil	7 mL
¼ tsp	freshly ground black pepper	1 mL
1	can (6 oz/175 g) water-packed tuna, drained	1
8 oz	rigatoni	250 g
½ cup	chopped fresh parsley	125 mL

Serves 4

1. In a large nonstick saucepan sprayed with vegetable spray, heat oil over medium-high heat. Add onions and garlic; cook for 3 minutes or until softened. Add eggplant and green peppers; cook for 5 minutes or until vegetables are tender and golden. Add tomatoes, stock, tomato paste, balsamic vinegar, capers, basil and pepper; bring to a boil. Reduce heat to low; cook, covered, for 5 minutes or until tomatoes break down and sauce thickens. Add tuna, stirring to break up.

2. Meanwhile, in a large pot of boiling water, cook rigatoni for 8 to 10 minutes or until tender but firm; drain. In a serving bowl, combine pasta, sauce and parsley; toss well. Serve immediately.

Nutritional Analysis (Per Serving)
- Calories: 428
- Protein: 23 g
- Cholesterol: 18 mg
- Sodium: 530 mg
- Fat, total: 6 g
- Carbohydrates: 74 g
- Fiber: 9 g
- Fat, saturated: 0.8 g

Linguine with Baby Clams and Goat Cheese in Marinara Sauce

12 oz	linguine	375 g
2 tsp	vegetable oil	10 mL
2 tsp	crushed garlic	10 mL
1 cup	chopped onions	250 mL
¾ cup	chopped sweet green peppers	175 mL
2½ cups	crushed tomatoes (canned or fresh)	625 mL
1	can (5 oz/142 mL) baby clams, drained	1
2 tsp	dried basil	10 mL
2 tsp	dried oregano	10 mL
2 tsp	capers	10 mL
¼ tsp	chili flakes (or to taste)	1 mL
3½ oz	goat cheese, crumbled	90 g

Serves 6

1. Cook pasta in boiling water according to package instructions or until firm to the bite. Drain and place in serving bowl.

2. In large nonstick skillet, heat oil; sauté garlic and onions until soft. Add sweet peppers and sauté until tender. Add tomatoes, clams, basil, oregano, capers and chili flakes; simmer on low heat for 15 minutes, stirring occasionally. Add cheese and cook for 1 minute. Pour over pasta, and toss.

Nutritional Analysis (Per Serving)
- Calories: 368
- Protein: 18 g
- Cholesterol: 21 mg
- Sodium: 296 mg
- Fat, total: 6 g
- Carbohydrates: 61 g
- Fiber: 4 g
- Fat, saturated: 2 g

Steamed Mussels with Curried Tomatoes over Penne

12 oz	penne	375 g
1½ tsp	vegetable oil	7 mL
2 tsp	crushed garlic	10 mL
4 cups	crushed tomatoes (canned or fresh)	1 L
2 tsp	curry	10 mL
1½ tsp	minced gingerroot	7 mL
1 lb	mussels	500 g
¼ cup	dry white wine	50 mL
⅓ cup	chopped coriander or parsley	75 mL

There are few ingredients that pack so much flavor as gingerroot. As a backup to fresh ginger, keep a jar of commercially prepared minced or puréed ginger in your fridge. It's available in the vegetable section of your supermarket alongside the minced garlic. Like prepared garlic, this type of ginger is not as intense as freshly grated, so add a little more than is called for in the recipe.

Serves 6

1. Cook pasta in boiling water according to package instructions or until firm to the bite. Drain and place in serving bowl.
2. In large nonstick saucepan, heat oil; sauté garlic for 30 seconds. Add tomatoes, curry and ginger. Cover and simmer on low heat for 25 minutes. Set aside.
3. In medium saucepan, combine mussels and wine. Cover and steam just until mussels open, approximately 4 minutes. Discard any mussels that do not open. Drain and reserve mussels.
4. Add tomato sauce to pasta; toss and add mussels. Sprinkle with coriander.

Tips

✦ Adjust the curry to taste. Clams could substitute for mussels, or use a combination.

✦ Use ginger marinated in jars, available in the vegetable section of the grocery store. It keeps for months in the refrigerator.

Make Ahead

✦ Tomato sauce in Step 2 can be made a day ahead and reheated.

Nutritional Analysis (Per Serving)
✦ Calories: 368   ✦ Protein: 20 g   ✦ Cholesterol: 23 mg
✦ Sodium: 437 mg   ✦ Fat, total: 5 g   ✦ Carbohydrates: 60 g
✦ Fiber: 5 g   ✦ Fat, saturated: 0.7 g

Sweet-Sour Shrimp over Rice Fettuccine

Sauce

³⁄₄ cup	seafood or chicken stock	175 mL
2 tbsp	packed brown sugar	25 mL
2 tbsp	sweet tomato chili sauce	25 mL
2 tbsp	orange juice concentrate	25 mL
2 tbsp	light soya sauce	25 mL
1¹⁄₂ tbsp	rice wine vinegar	20 mL
1 tbsp	cornstarch	15 mL
2 tsp	sesame oil	10 mL
8 oz	wide rice noodles	250 g
2 tsp	vegetable oil	10 mL
2 tsp	minced garlic	10 mL
1 tsp	minced gingerroot	5 mL
3 cups	broccoli florets	750 mL
1 cup	sliced red bell peppers	250 mL
8 oz	medium raw shrimp, peeled	250 g
1	can (14 oz/398 mL) unsweetened pineapple chunks, drained	1

Serves 4

1. In a bowl combine stock, brown sugar, chili sauce, orange juice concentrate, soya sauce, rice wine vinegar, cornstarch and sesame oil. Set aside.

2. In a pot of boiling water, cook noodles for 5 minutes or until tender; drain. Meanwhile, in a nonstick wok or large frying pan sprayed with vegetable spray, heat oil over medium-high heat. Add garlic, ginger, broccoli and red peppers; cook for 4 minutes. Add shrimp; cook for 2 minutes or until pink. Add pineapple and sauce; cook for 1 minute or until thickened and bubbly.

3. In a serving bowl combine sauce and noodles; toss to coat well. Serve immediately.

Nutritional Analysis (Per Serving)

- Calories: 341
- Protein: 16 g
- Cholesterol: 89 mg
- Sodium: 524 mg
- Fat, total: 6 g
- Carbohydrates: 58 g
- Fiber: 4 g
- Fat, saturated: 0.7 g

Coconut Seafood Fettuccine in a Creamy Sauce

6 oz	raw shrimp, shelled (if very large, cut into halves)	175 g
1 cup	thinly sliced red bell peppers	250 mL
³⁄₄ cup	thinly sliced carrots	175 mL
1¹⁄₂ tsp	minced garlic	7 mL
1 tsp	curry powder	5 mL
²⁄₃ cup	light coconut milk	150 mL
2 tbsp	light soya sauce	25 mL
¹⁄₂ cup	chopped fresh coriander	125 mL
¹⁄₂ cup	chopped green onions	125 mL
8 oz	fettuccine	250 g

Look for light coconut milk, which has ¹⁄₃ fewer calories and ²⁄₃ less fat than regular coconut milk.

Serves 4

1. In a nonstick wok or large frying pan sprayed with vegetable spray, cook shrimp over medium-high heat for 2 minutes or just until pink. Place shrimp on a plate; respray wok. Add peppers, carrots, garlic and curry; cook for 3 minutes or until vegetables are tender-crisp. Add coconut milk and soya sauce; reduce heat to medium-low. Cook for 4 minutes or until carrots are tender. Add shrimp, coriander and green onions; reduce heat to low.

2. In a large pot of boiling water, cook pasta for 8 to 10 minutes or until tender but firm; drain. In a serving bowl, combine pasta and sauce; toss well. Serve immediately.

Nutritional Analysis (Per Serving)

- Calories: 304
- Protein: 15 g
- Cholesterol: 62 mg
- Sodium: 544 mg
- Fat, total: 2 g
- Carbohydrates: 55 g
- Fiber: 3 g
- Fat, saturated: 0.2 g

Scallops and Spinach with Yellow Peppers over Linguine

2	medium yellow bell peppers	2
1/2 cup	chopped onions	125 mL
1 tsp	minced garlic	5 mL
1/2 cup	seafood or chicken stock	125 mL
1/4 cup	low-fat evaporated milk	50 mL
1/4 tsp	freshly ground black pepper	1 mL
6 cups	packed fresh spinach leaves, rinsed and drained	1.5 L
8 oz	linguine	250 g
8 oz	scallops (if large, cut into quarters)	250 g
3 tbsp	grated low-fat Parmesan cheese	45 mL

Many of us grew up knowing that spinach makes you strong. (You only had to watch a few Popeye cartoons to realize that!) But now, as adults, we understand why: spinach is loaded with iron, as well as vitamins A and C, so use it often. In recipes where the spinach is well cooked, substitute frozen spinach. With fresh spinach, just wash it, place it in a pot and cook, covered, for 2 to 3 minutes. The moisture on the leaves is all you need to steam it.

Serves 4
Preheat broiler

1. Under the broiler or on a grill over medium-high heat, cook peppers, turning occasionally, for 15 minutes or until charred; let cool. Peel, remove stems and seeds; cut into strips. Set aside.

2. In a nonstick frying pan sprayed with vegetable spray, cook onions and garlic over medium-high heat for 4 minutes or until softened. Add peppers, stock, evaporated milk and pepper; cook for 2 minutes or until vegetables are tender. Set aside.

3. In a large saucepan over high heat, cook spinach, covered, for 1 minute; stir. Cook uncovered, stirring occasionally, just until spinach wilts. Add to sauce.

4. In a large pot of boiling water, cook linguine for 8 to 10 minutes or until tender but firm; drain. Meanwhile, in a large nonstick frying pan sprayed with vegetable spray, cook scallops over medium-high heat, stirring occasionally, for 2 minutes or until golden and cooked through. Drain any excess liquid.

5. In a serving bowl, combine pasta, sauce and scallops; toss well. Sprinkle with Parmesan cheese; serve immediately.

Tip
+ Try replacing the scallops in this recipe with shrimp or boneless chicken breast — or, to make this a vegetarian dish, with 8 oz (250 g) sautéed cubes of firm tofu.

Nutritional Analysis (Per Serving)
+ Calories: 315   + Protein: 24 g   + Cholesterol: 26 mg
+ Sodium: 400 mg   + Fat, total: 4 g   + Carbohydrates: 49 g
+ Fiber: 5 g   + Fat, saturated: 1.2 g

Lobster Alfredo over Smoked Salmon Fettuccine

8 oz	sugar snap peas or snow peas	250 g
8 oz	fettuccine	250 g
2 tsp	margarine or butter	10 mL
1 tbsp	all-purpose flour	15 mL
1 cup	seafood stock or clam juice	250 mL
3/4 cup	low-fat milk	175 mL
1/8 tsp	freshly ground black pepper	0.5 mL
2 tbsp	grated low-fat Parmesan cheese	25 mL
8 oz	chopped cooked lobster or crabmeat or shrimp	250 g
1/3 cup	chopped fresh dill (or 1 tsp/5 mL dried)	75 mL
2 oz	smoked salmon, shredded	50 g

When using margarine, choose a soft (non-hydrogenated) version.

Serves 4

1. In a large pot of boiling water, blanch sugar snap peas for 2 minutes or until tender-crisp. Remove with slotted spoon to a bowl of cold water; drain.

2. In the same pot of boiling water, cook fettuccine for 8 to 10 minutes or until tender but firm; drain. Meanwhile, in a nonstick saucepan, heat margarine over medium heat. Add flour; cook, stirring, for 1 minute. Gradually whisk in seafood stock, milk and pepper; cook, stirring constantly, for 4 minutes or until thickened and bubbly. Add peas, Parmesan cheese and lobster meat; cook for 3 minutes or until heated through.

3. In a serving bowl, combine pasta, sauce, dill and smoked salmon; toss well. Serve immediately.

Nutritional Analysis (Per Serving)
- Calories: 408
- Protein: 26 g
- Cholesterol: 28 mg
- Sodium: 384 mg
- Fat, total: 6 g
- Carbohydrates: 60 g
- Fiber: 3 g
- Fat, saturated: 2 g

Shrimp Tomato Salsa over Rice Fettuccine

8 oz	raw shrimp, peeled, deveined and cut in half	250 g
8 oz	wide rice noodles	250 g
3 cups	diced ripe plum tomatoes	750 mL
3/4 cup	diced red bell peppers	175 mL
1/2 cup	diced red onions	125 mL
1/2 cup	chopped fresh coriander	125 mL
1 1/2 tsp	minced garlic	7 mL
3 1/2 tbsp	fresh lemon juice	55 mL
2 1/2 tbsp	olive oil	35 mL
2 tsp	hot Asian chili sauce (optional)	10 mL

Serves 4

1. In a large nonstick frying pan sprayed with vegetable spray, cook shrimp over medium-high heat for 2 minutes or until cooked through; remove from pan. Set aside.

2. In a large pot of boiling water, cook rice noodles for 5 minutes or until tender; drain. Rinse under cold running water; drain. Set aside.

3. In a serving bowl combine shrimp, tomatoes, red peppers, red onions, coriander, garlic, lemon juice, olive oil, chili sauce and pasta; toss well. Serve.

Nutritional Analysis (Per Serving)
- Calories: 273
- Protein: 13 g
- Cholesterol: 89 mg
- Sodium: 121 mg
- Fat, total: 7 g
- Carbohydrates: 40 g
- Fiber: 3 g
- Fat, saturated: 1 g

Mussel Mushroom Linguine

¾ cup	water or seafood stock	175 mL
2 lbs	mussels, scrubbed and beards removed	1 kg
1 cup	chopped onions	250 mL
1½ tsp	minced garlic	7 mL
3 cups	coarsely chopped mushrooms (preferably oyster mushrooms)	750 mL
¾ cup	low-fat evaporated milk	175 mL
2 tsp	all-purpose flour	10 mL
8 oz	linguine	250 g
⅓ cup	chopped fresh dill (or 1 tsp/5 mL dried)	75 mL

Serves 4

1. In a large saucepan over medium-high heat, bring water to a boil; add mussels. Cook, covered, for 3 minutes or until mussels are opened (discard unopened ones); drain, reserving liquid. Remove mussels from shells; set aside.

2. Meanwhile, in a large nonstick frying pan sprayed with vegetable spray, cook onions and garlic over medium-high heat for 3 minutes or until softened. Add mushrooms; cook for 8 minutes or until browned. Add 1 cup (250 mL) reserved mussel cooking liquid; cook for 2 minutes.

3. In a bowl combine milk and flour; whisk well. Add flour mixture and mussels to sauce; cook for 3 minutes or until heated through and slightly thickened.

4. Meanwhile, in a large pot of boiling water, cook linguine for 8 to 10 minutes or until tender but firm; drain. In a serving bowl combine pasta, sauce and dill; toss well. Serve immediately.

Tips

✦ This recipe provides a great opportunity to experiment with different types of linguine. Try the tomato, spinach or whole wheat varieties. Keep in mind that whole wheat linguine requires a few extra minutes of cooking time.

✦ Mussels are sensational with mushrooms, but this dish also works well with clams. Buy the freshest clams you can find (Littleneck or Cherrystone are the most common varieties) and check the shells — unlike mussels, they should be almost impossible to pry open. Cook clams as you would mussels, for at least 5 minutes or until the shells open; discard any that do not.

Nutritional Analysis (Per Serving)
✦ Calories: 461 ✦ Protein: 41 g ✦ Cholesterol: 74 mg
✦ Sodium: 775 mg ✦ Fat, total: 8 g ✦ Carbohydrates: 56 g
✦ Fiber: 3 g ✦ Fat, saturated: 2.1 g

Pasta with Chicken Marsala Sauce

12 oz	fettuccine	375 g
1½ tsp	crushed garlic	7 mL
12 oz	skinless, boneless chicken breasts, cut into 1-inch (2.5 cm) strips	375 g

Sauce

2 tsp	vegetable oil	10 mL
¾ cup	chopped onions	175 mL
3½ cups	sliced mushrooms (wild or regular)	875 mL
1¼ cups	2% milk	300 mL
¾ cup	chicken stock	175 mL
⅓ cup	Marsala wine	75 mL
2½ tbsp	all-purpose flour	35 mL
	Parsley	

Serves 6

1. Cook pasta in boiling water according to package instructions or until firm to the bite. Drain and place in serving bowl.

2. In large nonstick skillet sprayed with vegetable spray, sauté garlic and chicken until chicken is no longer pink, approximately 8 minutes. Remove chicken and add to pasta.

3. Make the sauce: In same skillet, heat oil; sauté onions until tender, approximately 4 minutes. Add mushrooms and sauté until tender, approximately 5 minutes.

4. Meanwhile, in small bowl combine milk, stock, wine and flour until smooth. Add to mushroom mixture; simmer on medium heat until slightly thickened, approximately 5 minutes, stirring constantly. Pour over pasta. Sprinkle with parsley, and toss.

Tips

✦ Use oyster or portobello mushrooms if available. The texture and flavor are exceptional.

✦ Marsala is a sweet distinct wine. If a sweet flavor is not desired, use dry white wine.

Make Ahead

✦ Prepare sauce early in day. Reheat gently, adding more stock if sauce is too thick.

Nutritional Analysis (Per Serving)

✦ Calories: 419   ✦ Protein: 28 g   ✦ Cholesterol: 40 mg
✦ Sodium: 168 mg   ✦ Fat, total: 5 g   ✦ Carbohydrates: 63 g
✦ Fiber: 6 g   ✦ Fat, saturated: 1 g

Chicken Cacciatore over Penne

12 oz	penne	375 g
2 tsp	vegetable oil	10 mL
2 tsp	crushed garlic	10 mL
1⅓ cups	chopped onions	325 mL
1¼ cups	chopped sweet red peppers	300 mL
1½ cups	sliced mushrooms	375 mL
1 lb	skinless, boneless chicken breasts, cubed	500 g
½ cup	dry red wine	125 mL
⅓ cup	chicken stock	75 mL
2¾ cups	fresh or canned tomatoes, crushed	675 mL
1 tbsp	tomato paste	15 mL
2 tsp	dried basil	10 mL
1 tsp	dried oregano	5 mL
¼ cup	chopped parsley	50 mL

Serves 6

1. Cook pasta in boiling water according to package instructions or until firm to the bite. Drain and place in serving bowl.

2. In large nonstick skillet, heat oil; sauté garlic, onions and red peppers until soft, approximately 5 minutes. Add mushrooms and sauté until soft, approximately 5 minutes. Add chicken and sauté on medium heat until just no longer pink, approximately 5 minutes.

3. Add wine and stock; simmer for 2 minutes. Add tomatoes, tomato paste, basil and oregano; simmer for 15 minutes, covered, on low heat, stirring occasionally. Pour over pasta. Add parsley, and toss.

Tip

+ Dark chicken meat can be used, but the calories and fat will increase slightly.

Make Ahead

+ Prepare sauce up to a day ahead. Reheat gently, adding more stock if sauce is too thick.

Nutritional Analysis (Per Serving)
+ Calories: 441
+ Protein: 32 g
+ Cholesterol: 48 mg
+ Sodium: 283 mg
+ Fat, total: 5 g
+ Carbohydrates: 66 g
+ Fiber: 6 g
+ Fat, saturated: 0.7 g

Creamy Tomato Pesto and Chicken over Fettuccine

Sun-dried Tomato Pesto

1½ oz	dry-packed sun-dried tomatoes	40 g
¼ cup	chopped fresh parsley	50 mL
2 tbsp	grated low-fat Parmesan cheese	25 mL
1 tbsp	toasted pine nuts	15 mL
1 tsp	minced garlic	5 mL
½ cup	chicken stock	125 mL
¼ cup	low-fat evaporated milk	50 mL
2 tbsp	olive oil	25 mL
8 oz	skinless boneless chicken breast	250 g
12 oz	fettuccine or rice noodles	375 g

> Getting more iron: *Calorie for calorie, parsley is higher in iron than almost any other food. One cup (250 mL) of the green stuff has only 22 calories, yet provides almost 4 mg of iron. (See pages 88 and 191 for more info on iron.) Unfortunately, much of this iron is unusable because it's chemically bonded to oxalic acid, which carries the iron out of the body with other wastes. To increase iron absorption from plant foods, include a small portion of meat, poultry or fish in the same meal.*

Serves 6

1. In a bowl cover sun-dried tomatoes with boiling water. Let stand for 15 minutes or until softened; drain.
2. In a food processor or blender, combine sun-dried tomatoes, parsley, 1 tbsp (15 mL) Parmesan cheese, pine nuts and garlic; process until finely chopped. Add stock, evaporated milk and olive oil; purée until smooth. Set aside.
3. In a nonstick skillet sprayed with vegetable spray or on a preheated grill, cook chicken over medium-high heat, turning once, for 12 minutes or until cooked through. Cut into chunks. Meanwhile, in a large pot of boiling water, cook fettuccine for 8 to 10 minutes or until tender but firm; drain.
4. In a serving bowl, combine chicken, pesto, pasta and remaining Parmesan cheese; toss to coat well. Serve immediately.

Tip

✦ Skinless boneless chicken breasts are tender, delicious and, best of all, really low in fat! In fact, a 4-oz (125 g) serving contains only 130 calories and only 2.5 g fat. If you're ever tempted to try skin-on chicken breasts, just consider that the skin will add 60 calories and increase the fat by nearly 400% to 12 g. And if you like dark meat? Sorry, but one serving contains a whopping 250 calories and 18 g fat!

Nutritional Analysis (Per Serving)

✦ Calories: 330 ✦ Protein: 20 g ✦ Cholesterol: 25 mg
✦ Sodium: 240 mg ✦ Fat, total: 4 g ✦ Carbohydrates: 54 g
✦ Fiber: 2 g ✦ Fat, saturated: 1.4 g

Bow-Tie Pasta with Chicken Alfredo Sauce

12 oz	skinless boneless chicken breasts	375 g
Sauce		
1 tbsp	margarine or butter	15 mL
2 tbsp	all-purpose flour	25 mL
1 cup	2% milk	250 mL
1 cup	chicken stock	250 mL
2 tsp	dried tarragon	10 mL
¼ cup	grated Parmesan cheese	50 mL
2 tsp	vegetable oil	10 mL
2 tsp	minced garlic	10 mL
1 cup	chopped onions	250 mL
1 cup	chopped red or green peppers	250 mL
12 oz	bow-tie pasta	375 g

When using margarine, choose a soft (non-hydrogenated) version to limit consumption of trans fats.

Serves 6

1. In nonstick skillet sprayed with vegetable spray, cook whole chicken breasts over medium-high heat until browned; turn over and cook for 3 minutes more, or until just done at center. Let cool slightly and slice into thin strips. Set aside.

2. In small saucepan, melt margarine over medium heat; add flour and cook, stirring, for 1 minute. Gradually add milk and stock, stirring constantly, just until mixture thickens slightly (approximately 5 minutes). Add tarragon and cook for 2 more minutes. Add Parmesan and remove from heat.

3. Meanwhile, in saucepan, heat vegetable oil over medium heat; add garlic and onions and sauté for 4 minutes until browned. Add red peppers and sauté for 4 minutes or until softened. Set aside. In large pot of boiling water, cook pasta according to package directions or until tender but firm; drain. Put pasta, chicken and cooked vegetables in serving bowl. Add sauce, toss and serve.

Tips

✦ Cooking the entire chicken breast before slicing gives a moister piece.

✦ If using fresh tarragon, chop ⅓ cup (75 mL) and add just before tossing entire pasta dish. Basil can replace tarragon.

Make Ahead

✦ Prepare sauce up to a day ahead. Reheat gently, adding more stock if too thick.

Nutritional Analysis (Per Serving)

✦ Calories: 365   ✦ Protein: 24 g   ✦ Cholesterol: 37 mg
✦ Sodium: 307 mg ✦ Fat, total: 7 g ✦ Carbohydrates: 50 g
✦ Fiber: 2 g   ✦ Fat, saturated: 2 g

Savory Chicken Fagioli over Rigatoni

1/2 cup	chopped carrots	125 mL
1/2 cup	chopped onions	125 mL
1/3 cup	chopped celery	75 mL
1 1/2 tsp	minced garlic	7 mL
1	can (19 oz/540 mL) red kidney beans, rinsed and drained, half the amount mashed	1
1	can (19 oz/540 mL) tomatoes, with juice	1
2/3 cup	chicken stock	150 mL
2 tsp	packed brown sugar	10 mL
1 1/2 tsp	dried basil	7 mL
1 tsp	chili powder	5 mL
1 tsp	dried oregano	5 mL
1	bay leaf	1
12 oz	skinless boneless chicken breast, diced	375 g
12 oz	rigatoni	375 g
1/4 cup	grated low-fat Parmesan cheese	50 mL
1/4 cup	chopped fresh parsley	50 mL

Serves 6

1. In a large nonstick saucepan sprayed with vegetable spray, cook carrots, onions, celery and garlic over medium-high heat for 4 minutes or until softened. Add mashed beans, whole beans, tomatoes, chicken stock, brown sugar, basil, chili powder, oregano and bay leaf. Bring to a boil; reduce heat to medium-low. Cook for 20 minutes or until vegetables are tender, stirring occasionally to break up tomatoes. Add chicken; cook for 3 minutes or until cooked through.

2. Meanwhile, in a large pot of boiling water, cook rigatoni for 10 to 12 minutes or until tender but firm; drain.

3. In a serving bowl, combine pasta and sauce; toss well. Sprinkle with Parmesan cheese and parsley. Serve immediately.

Tips

+ Ever wonder what goes into chili powder? Well, there's ground chilies (no surprise there), but also a number of other spices common to Southwestern-style cooking. These often include cumin, ginger, cayenne, oregano and dried mustard. But since there is no one formula for chili powder, the actual ingredients vary with different brands. Those from the smallest producers are often the most flavorful.

+ *That was then, this is now:* Hard to believe, but today's chicken is about 40% leaner than it was as recently as 15 years ago. A 4-oz (125 g) skinless roasted chicken breast now contains a meager 2.1 g fat, down from 3.6 g in the old days. And a serving of chicken leg, with the back attached, has 6.9 g fat, down from almost 11 g.

Nutritional Analysis (Per Serving)
+ Calories: 464   + Protein: 30 g   + Cholesterol: 37 mg
+ Sodium: 122 mg   + Fat, total: 4 g   + Carbohydrates: 76 g
+ Fiber: 12 g   + Fat, saturated: 1.3 g

Teriyaki Chicken with Sesame Seeds over Rotini

Sauce

1/4 cup	rice wine vinegar	50 mL
1/4 cup	packed brown sugar	50 mL
1/4 cup	water	50 mL
1/4 cup	light soya sauce	50 mL
1 tbsp	sesame oil	15 mL
2 1/2 tsp	cornstarch	12 mL
1 1/2 tsp	minced garlic	7 mL
1 1/2 tsp	minced gingerroot	7 mL
12 oz	skinless boneless chicken breast	375 g
12 oz	rotini	375 g
1 cup	thinly sliced red bell peppers	250 mL
1 cup	thinly sliced yellow peppers	250 mL
1 cup	snow peas, trimmed and halved	250 mL
2 tsp	sesame seeds	10 mL

Chances are you've heard of (if not actually tasted) Teriyaki chicken, beef or vegetables. But what is it that makes a dish Teriyaki? It's the Japanese technique of marinating and/or cooking food in a mixture of soya sauce, vinegar, sugar, ginger and seasonings. The sugar gives the food its distinctive glazed appearance.

Serves 6

1. In a bowl combine rice wine vinegar, brown sugar, water, soya sauce, sesame oil, cornstarch, garlic and ginger; set aside.

2. In a nonstick skillet sprayed with vegetable spray or on a preheated grill, cook chicken over medium-high heat, turning once, for 12 minutes or until cooked through. Slice chicken into thin strips; set aside.

3. In a large pot of boiling water, cook rotini for 8 to 10 minutes or until tender but firm; drain.

4. Meanwhile, in a large nonstick frying pan or wok sprayed with vegetable spray, cook red peppers, yellow peppers, snow peas and sesame seeds over medium-high heat for 4 minutes or until tender-crisp. Add sauce; cook for 2 minutes or until thickened and bubbly.

5. In a serving bowl, combine pasta, sauce and chicken strips; toss well. Serve immediately.

Tip

+ Rice vinegar or rice wine vinegar is made from fermented rice, which gives it a milder flavor than North American vinegars. (These are typically made from grains, wine or cider.) Typically, you'll find two types of rice vinegar — pale yellow or darker brown. The lighter variety has a smoother flavor. And if you can't find any rice wine vinegar? Just substitute sherry or white wine.

Nutritional Analysis (Per Serving)
+ Calories: 371   + Protein: 22 g   + Cholesterol: 34 mg
+ Sodium: 396 mg   + Fat, total: 5 g   + Carbohydrates: 59 g
+ Fiber: 3 g   + Fat, saturated: 1 g

Creamy Paprika Sauté with Grilled Chicken and Egg Noodles

8 oz	skinless boneless chicken breast	250 g
8 oz	broad egg noodles	250 g
½ cup	chopped red onions	125 mL
1½ tsp	minced garlic	7 mL
1½ cups	chopped oyster mushrooms	375 mL
1 tbsp	all-purpose flour	15 mL
1½ cups	chicken stock	375 mL
2 tsp	paprika	10 mL
½ cup	low-fat sour cream	125 mL
¼ cup	chopped fresh dill (or 1 tsp/5 mL dried)	50 mL

Egg noodles are slightly richer tasting than other noodles — that's because of the eggs — and are therefore somewhat higher in fat and calories. (So live a little!) Egg noodles are available in a variety of widths; the thin variety are commonly used in soups, while broad noodles are used with sauces.

Serves 4

1. In a nonstick saucepan sprayed with vegetable spray or on a preheated grill, cook chicken over medium-high heat, turning once, for 12 minutes or until cooked through; slice thinly.

2. In a large pot of boiling water, cook noodles for 8 minutes or until tender but firm; drain.

3. Meanwhile, in a nonstick frying pan sprayed with vegetable spray, cook onions and garlic over medium-high heat for 3 minutes or until softened. Add mushrooms; cook for 4 minutes, stirring occasionally. Add flour; cook, stirring, for 1 minute. Add chicken stock and paprika; cook for 2 minutes or until thickened. Remove from heat; add sour cream and dill.

4. In a serving bowl combine sauce, noodles and chicken; toss well. Serve immediately.

Tip

✦ Regular fettuccine can replace the egg noodles. For a change, try seafood or steak instead of chicken; or replace oyster mushrooms with any other wild variety.

Nutritional Analysis (Per Serving)
✦ Calories: 384   ✦ Protein: 26 g   ✦ Cholesterol: 105 mg
✦ Sodium: 127 mg   ✦ Fat, total: 7 g   ✦ Carbohydrates: 53 g
✦ Fiber: 3 g   ✦ Fat, saturated: 3.2 g

Curried Vegetable Chicken Fettuccine

8 oz	skinless boneless chicken breast	250 g
8 oz	fettuccine	250 g
3/4 cup	chopped onions	175 mL
3/4 cup	chopped green bell peppers	175 mL
1/2 cup	finely chopped carrots	125 mL
1 tsp	minced garlic	5 mL
1 1/2 tbsp	all-purpose flour	20 mL
2 tsp	curry powder	10 mL
1 cup	chicken stock	250 mL
3/4 cup	low-fat milk	175 mL
1 1/2 tsp	packed brown sugar	7 mL
1/4 tsp	freshly ground black pepper	1 mL

Curry powder isn't a spice in itself, but a blend of up to 20 spices and herbs — typically including cardamom, chilies, cinnamon, cloves, coriander, cumin, fennel seed, saffron, tamarind and turmeric. Depending on the balance of ingredients, curry powder can be mild or mouth-scorching! So be sure to adjust the amount you use according to your taste.

Serves 4

1. In a nonstick frying pan sprayed with vegetable spray or on a preheated grill, cook chicken over medium-high heat, turning once, for 12 minutes or until cooked through. Cut into thin slices; set aside.

2. In a large pot of boiling water, cook fettuccine for 8 to 10 minutes or until tender but firm; drain. Meanwhile, in a large nonstick frying pan sprayed with vegetable spray, cook onions, green peppers, carrots and garlic over medium-high heat for 5 minutes or until softened. Add flour and curry powder; cook for 30 seconds. Add stock, milk, brown sugar and pepper; reduce heat to medium. Cook for 2 minutes or until thickened.

3. In a serving bowl, combine pasta, sauce and chicken; toss well. Serve immediately.

Tips

✦ When it comes to choosing milk, what's a percentage point here or there? A lot! Just consider that a 1-cup (250 mL) serving of homogenized (3.3%) milk contains 150 calories and 8 g fat, while the same amount of 1% milk has only 102 calories and 2.5 g fat. (As you might expect, 2% milk falls in the middle, with 121 calories and 4.7 g fat.) And the fact is that for many sauces (like the one here), 1% milk delivers all the taste and texture you want. You can substitute low-fat milk in any recipe that calls for homogenized — although, for some sauces, you may need to increase the amount of flour.

✦ It's easy to transform this recipe into a vegetarian or kosher dish: just substitute firm tofu for the chicken (grill or sauté it for 5 minutes or just until lightly browned); use soya milk instead of dairy milk; and, replace chicken stock with vegetable stock.

Nutritional Analysis (Per Serving)
- ✦ Calories: 369
- ✦ Protein: 23 g
- ✦ Cholesterol: 37 mg
- ✦ Sodium: 102 mg
- ✦ Fat, total: 3 g
- ✦ Carbohydrates: 60 g
- ✦ Fiber: 3 g
- ✦ Fat, saturated: 0.9 g

Cranberry Chicken over Penne

1 cup	chopped onions	250 mL
¾ cup	chopped red bell peppers	175 mL
1 cup	canned whole cranberry sauce	250 mL
3 tbsp	light soya sauce	45 mL
2 tbsp	orange juice concentrate	25 mL
1 tbsp	sesame oil	15 mL
1 tbsp	fresh lemon juice	15 mL
1½ tsp	minced garlic	7 mL
1 tsp	minced gingerroot	5 mL
8 oz	skinless boneless chicken breast	250 g
12 oz	penne	375 g
⅓ cup	dried cranberries or dried cherries	75 mL
⅓ cup	chopped green onions	75 mL

Liquid plumber: *Does a glass of cranberry juice a day keep bladder infections away? There is scientific evidence to suggest that this home remedy is indeed effective in preventing and treating such infections. A Tufts University study found that bacterial urinary tract infections could be reduced by 50% in older women who drank 1¼ cups (300 mL) of cranberry juice each day. It seems that cranberries contain a natural antibiotic substance that prevents bacteria from adhering to the bladder wall.*

Serves 6

1. In a nonstick saucepan sprayed with vegetable spray, cook onions and red peppers over medium-high heat for 5 minutes or until softened; set aside.

2. In another saucepan combine cranberry sauce, soya sauce, orange juice concentrate, sesame oil, lemon juice, garlic and ginger. Cook over medium heat, stirring, for 4 minutes or until heated through and smooth. Add red pepper mixture.

3. In a nonstick skillet sprayed with vegetable spray, cook chicken over medium-high heat, turning once, for 12 minutes or until cooked through; slice thinly.

4. In a large pot of boiling water, cook penne for 8 to 10 minutes or until tender but firm; drain. In a serving bowl combine pasta, sauce, chicken, dried cranberries and green onions; toss well.

Tips

✦ When shopping for canned cranberry sauce for this recipe, be sure to get the type that contains whole berries. Avoid jellied cranberry sauce; in this variety, the berries have been puréed.

✦ While commercially prepared cranberry sauce is the most convenient, it's actually quite easy to make your own. Just combine 1 lb (500 g) cranberries, 2 cups (500 mL) sugar and 1 cup (250 mL) water. Cook, uncovered, over medium heat for 10 minutes.

Nutritional Analysis (Per Serving)

✦ Calories: 423   ✦ Protein: 18 g   ✦ Cholesterol: 23 mg
✦ Sodium: 563 mg   ✦ Fat, total: 4 g   ✦ Carbohydrates: 78 g
✦ Fiber: 4 g   ✦ Fat, saturated: 0.8 g

Pasta with Spicy Turkey Tomato Sauce

12 oz	rotini	375 g
2 tsp	vegetable oil	10 mL
2 tsp	crushed garlic	10 mL
1 cup	diced red onions	250 mL
1 cup	diced red or green peppers	250 mL
12 oz	ground turkey	375 g
3 cups	crushed tomatoes (canned or fresh)	750 mL
1½ tsp	dried basil	7 mL
1 tsp	dried oregano	5 mL
2 tsp	chili powder	10 mL
Pinch	cayenne pepper	Pinch
½ cup	coriander leaves or parsley, chopped	125 mL

Serves 6

1. Cook pasta in boiling water according to package instructions or until firm to the bite. Drain and place in serving bowl.

2. In large nonstick saucepan sprayed with vegetable spray, heat oil; sauté garlic, onions and red peppers until soft, approximately 5 minutes. Add turkey and sauté on medium heat until cooked, approximately 5 minutes.

3. Add tomatoes, basil, oregano, chili powder and cayenne. Cover and simmer on low heat for 15 minutes, stirring occasionally. Add coriander. Pour over pasta, and toss.

Tip

✦ As a substitute for the turkey, try using ground veal, beef or chicken.

✦ Rotini can be replaced with any medium-sized pasta.

Make Ahead

✦ Sauce can be prepared up to 2 days before and gently reheated before serving. Do not add coriander or parsley until ready to serve.

Nutritional Analysis (Per Serving)

✦ Calories: 382 ✦ Protein: 26 g ✦ Cholesterol: 39 mg
✦ Sodium: 221 mg ✦ Fat, total: 4 g ✦ Carbohydrates: 61 g
✦ Fiber: 4 g ✦ Fat, saturated: 0.5 g

Calves' Liver with Caramelized Onions over Linguine

4 cups	thinly sliced sweet white onions (Spanish, Bermuda or Vidalia)	1 L
2 tsp	minced garlic	10 mL
2 tbsp	packed brown sugar	25 mL
1½ cups	cold beef stock or chicken stock	375 mL
1 tbsp	all-purpose flour	15 mL
8 oz	linguine (regular or whole wheat)	250 g
8 oz	calves' liver, cut into ¼-inch (5 mm) strips	250 g
	Freshly ground black pepper	

Serves 4

1. In a large nonstick frying pan sprayed with vegetable spray, cook onions, garlic and brown sugar over medium heat, stirring occasionally, for 20 minutes or until soft and golden. Remove from pan; set aside.

2. In a bowl whisk together stock and flour; set aside.

3. In a large pot of boiling water, cook linguine for 8 to 10 minutes or until tender but firm; drain. Meanwhile, in the same frying pan used in Step 1 (wiped clean and sprayed with vegetable spray), cook liver over medium-high heat, stirring, for 1 minute or until just pink inside. Add stock and flour mixture; cook, stirring, for 2 minutes or until bubbly and slightly thickened.

4. In a serving bowl, combine sauce, caramelized onions and pasta; toss well. Season to taste with pepper. Serve immediately.

Tips

✦ Yes, it's more expensive, but calves' liver really is the best choice for this recipe. Not only is it more delicately flavored and tender than beef liver, but it's higher in nutrients — a good source of protein, iron and vitamin A. You can use beef liver in this recipe (and save a few dollars), but it will have a stronger taste and odor, and will be less tender. Of course, no matter what type of liver you use, be sure you don't overcook it — otherwise you'll end up with something resembling shoe leather!

✦ For a change of pace, try this recipe with chicken livers. They're very economical and provide a mild (yet distinctive) taste. The key to success here is in cooking the livers — cut them into quarters and cook in small batches in a hot pan.

Nutritional Analysis (Per Serving)
✦ Calories: 327 ✦ Protein: 21 g ✦ Cholesterol: 226 mg
✦ Sodium: 330 mg ✦ Fat, total: 4 g ✦ Carbohydrates: 54 g
✦ Fiber: 4 g ✦ Fat, saturated: 0.1 g

Rose's Hearty Pasta Sauce with Beef and Sausage

½ cup	chopped onions	125 mL
¼ cup	finely chopped carrots	50 mL
1 tsp	minced garlic	5 mL
6 oz	lean ground beef	175 g
4 oz	Italian sausage, casings removed	125 g
1½ lbs	ripe plum tomatoes, chopped	750 g
2 tbsp	tomato paste	25 mL
1	bay leaf	1
1½ tsp	dried basil	7 mL
1 tsp	chili powder	5 mL
¼ tsp	salt	1 mL
¼ tsp	freshly ground black pepper	1 mL
1 lb	rigatoni	500 g
¼ cup	grated low-fat Parmesan cheese	50 mL

Sweet and mild or spicy and hot, sausages add a wonderful flavor to meat dishes. Although traditionally made from beef and/or pork, they're now made with other (often leaner) meats, including chicken and turkey. So experiment — and use whatever type of sausage you prefer. Just remember that all sausages have extra fat added, so use them in moderate quantities and be sure to drain the fat after sautéeing.

Serves 6

1. In a nonstick saucepan sprayed with vegetable spray, cook onions, carrots and garlic over medium-high heat for 3 minutes or until onions are softened. Add beef and sausage; cook, stirring to break up meat, for 4 minutes or until no longer pink. Add tomatoes, tomato paste, bay leaf, basil and chili powder. Season to taste with salt and pepper. Reduce heat to medium; cook, covered, for 20 minutes or until thickened.

2. Meanwhile, in a large pot of boiling water, cook rigatoni for 8 to 10 minutes or until tender but firm; drain. In a serving bowl combine pasta and sauce; sprinkle with Parmesan cheese. Serve immediately.

Tip

✦ This tomato sauce is so good that you can keep it on hand for all kinds of dishes. Make up a large batch in the late summer, when plum tomatoes are their peak, and preserve it in sterilized jars. Alternatively, you can freeze the sauce in airtight containers and defrost as needed. If the defrosted sauce appears too watery, add 1 to 2 tbsp (15 to 25 mL) tomato paste and simmer for 10 minutes.

Nutritional Analysis (Per Serving)
✦ Calories: 319   ✦ Protein: 14 g   ✦ Cholesterol: 14 mg
✦ Sodium: 135 mg   ✦ Fat, total: 5 g ✦ Carbohydrates: 53 g
✦ Fiber: 3 g   ✦ Fat, saturated: 2 g

Beef Pad Thai with Bell Peppers and Snow Peas

8 oz	wide rice noodles	250 g
Sauce		
½ cup	beef or chicken stock	125 mL
¼ cup	oyster sauce or fish sauce	50 mL
3 tbsp	ketchup	45 mL
2 tbsp	fresh lime or lemon juice	25 mL
2 tsp	packed brown sugar	10 mL
1½ tsp	cornstarch	7 mL
1½ tsp	minced garlic	7 mL
1 tsp	minced gingerroot	5 mL
12 oz	boneless beef sirloin	375 g
1 cup	sliced green bell peppers	250 mL
1 cup	sliced red bell peppers	250 mL
1 cup	halved snow peas	250 mL
½ cup	chopped green onions	125 mL
⅓ cup	chopped fresh coriander	75 mL
3 tbsp	chopped cashews	45 mL

Perhaps the best known (and loved) of Thai dishes, pad thai is typically made with rice noodles and a combination of ingredients that can include seafood, tofu, eggs, chicken, pork, beef — plus a mixture of vegetables flavored with fish sauce. This low-fat version has no eggs, more vegetables and a choice of fish sauce or oyster sauce. This is a wonderful dish — best prepared just before serving.

Serves 4

1. In a bowl cover rice noodles with boiling water; let stand for 15 minutes. Drain.

2. Meanwhile, in a bowl combine stock, oyster sauce, ketchup, lime juice, brown sugar, cornstarch, garlic and ginger. Set aside.

3. In a large nonstick frying pan sprayed with vegetable spray or on a preheated grill, cook beef over high heat for 6 minutes or until medium-rare; remove from pan. Slice thinly; set aside. Respray pan; cook green peppers and red peppers over medium-high heat, stirring, for 3 minutes. Add snow peas; cook, stirring, for 1 minute. Add sauce, beef and rice noodles; cook for 1 minute or until noodles are tender. Add green onions, coriander and cashews; serve immediately.

Tip

✦ If you have an intolerance to the gluten contained in wheat-based pasta, then rice noodles are an ideal substitute. You can either soak them in boiling water (about 15 minutes), or boil them until tender (about 8 minutes). Avoid excessive rinsing, or the noodles will become starchy.

Nutritional Analysis (Per Serving)

✦ Calories: 350 ✦ Protein: 25 g ✦ Cholesterol: 45 mg
✦ Sodium: 345 mg ✦ Fat, total: 7 g ✦ Carbohydrates: 46 g
✦ Fiber: 3 g ✦ Fat, saturated: 1.9 g

Savory Cabbage with Steak over Rigatoni

1 cup	chopped onions	250 mL
2/3 cup	chopped red bell peppers	150 mL
1/2 cup	chopped carrots	125 mL
2 tsp	minced garlic	10 mL
3 cups	shredded green cabbage	750 mL
1	can (19 oz/540 mL) tomatoes, with juice	1
1 cup	beef or chicken stock	250 mL
2/3 cup	diced peeled potatoes	150 mL
2 tsp	fresh lemon juice	10 mL
1 1/2 tsp	caraway seeds	7 mL
1/4 tsp	salt	1 mL
1/4 tsp	freshly ground black pepper	1 mL
8 oz	boneless beef steak, such as top sirloin	250 g
12 oz	rigatoni	375 g

Serves 6

1. In a large nonstick saucepan sprayed with vegetable spray, cook onions, red peppers, carrots and garlic over medium heat, stirring occasionally, for 5 minutes or until softened. Add cabbage; cook for 3 minutes. Add tomatoes, stock, potatoes, lemon juice, caraway seeds, salt and pepper; bring to a boil. Reduce heat to low; cook, covered, for 25 minutes, breaking up tomatoes occasionally with the back of a spoon.

2. Meanwhile, in a nonstick frying pan sprayed with vegetable spray or on a preheated grill, cook steak, turning once, over medium-high heat for 5 minutes or until medium-rare; slice thinly. Set aside.

3. In a large pot of boiling water, cook rigatoni for 8 to 10 minutes or until tender but firm; drain. In a serving bowl combine pasta, sauce and beef; toss well. Serve.

Tips

✦ Use the best (which is to say, most tender) steak you can afford. If using sirloin or rib-eye, be sure to cut away the visible fat.

✦ Traditionally, this type of dish calls for regular green cabbage. But it's even better with savoy cabbage, which has a milder flavor, and retains its texture and color better than regular cabbage. Definitely worth a try!

Nutritional Analysis (Per Serving)
✦ Calories: 345 ✦ Protein: 19 g ✦ Cholesterol: 20 mg
✦ Sodium: 182 mg ✦ Fat, total: 3 g ✦ Carbohydrates: 60 g
✦ Fiber: 5 g ✦ Fat, saturated: 0.8 g

Pork Tenderloin with Apricots and Bok Choy over Fettuccine

Sauce

1 cup	beef or chicken stock	250 mL
¼ cup	Asian plum sauce	50 mL
3 tbsp	sweet tomato chili sauce	45 mL
1½ tbsp	light soya sauce	20 mL
2 tsp	cornstarch	10 mL
8 oz	pork tenderloin	250 g
1 cup	chopped onions	250 mL
1½ tsp	minced garlic	7 mL
1 tsp	minced gingerroot	5 mL
5 cups	sliced bok choy	1.25 L
¾ cup	chopped dried apricots	175 mL
12 oz	fettuccine	375 g

Another white meat? *Looking for a low-fat alternative to chicken breast? Think pork! Here's a comparison chart for a 3½ oz (90 g) serving of cooked meat:*

	fat (g)	*calories*
Chicken breast	*2.0*	*156*
Pork tenderloin	*3.6*	*162*
Pork loin, center-cut chop	*6.6*	*162*
Chicken leg, with back	*6.3*	*150*
Chicken drumstick, no skin	*6.3*	*148*

Serves 6

1. In a bowl combine stock, plum sauce, chili sauce, soya sauce and cornstarch. Set aside.
2. In a nonstick frying pan sprayed with vegetable spray or on a preheated grill, cook pork tenderloin over medium-high heat, turning once, for 15 minutes or until cooked through.
3. Meanwhile, in a large nonstick frying pan sprayed with vegetable spray, cook onions, garlic and ginger over medium-high heat for 5 minutes or until softened. Add bok choy and apricots; cook for 3 minutes or until bok choy wilts. Add sauce; reduce heat to medium-low. Cook for 2 minutes or until thickened; remove from heat.
4. In a large pot of boiling water, cook fettuccine for 8 to 10 minutes or until tender but firm; drain. Slice pork tenderloin thinly crosswise. In a large serving bowl, combine pasta, sauce and pork; toss well. Serve immediately.

Tip

✦ The good news about pork tenderloin is that it's very low in fat. The bad news is that its low fat content makes it susceptible to drying out when cooked. That's why you should always cook tenderloin quickly over high heat. Use it whole, sliced into medallions and pounded for scallopini, or cut into strips or cubes for stir-fries or kebabs. Keep in mind when shopping that the smaller the tenderloin, the more tender the meat.

Nutritional Analysis (Per Serving)
✦ Calories: 379 ✦ Protein: 21 g ✦ Cholesterol: 25 mg
✦ Sodium: 246 mg ✦ Fat, total: 2 g ✦ Carbohydrates: 68 g
✦ Fiber: 4 g ✦ Fat, saturated: 0.6 g

Rotini with Sausages and Mushrooms

12 oz	rotini (twisted pasta)	375 g
1 tsp	vegetable oil	5 mL
1½ tsp	crushed garlic	7 mL
½ cup	chopped onions	125 mL
8 oz	skinless sausages, chopped	250 g
¾ cup	chopped mushrooms	175 mL
⅓ cup	dry red or white wine	75 mL
¾ cup	prepared tomato sauce or Quick Basic Tomato Sauce (see recipe, page 129)	175 mL
⅔ cup	2% milk	150 mL
1½ tsp	dried basil	7 mL
¼ cup	grated Parmesan cheese	50 mL

Use either spicy or mild sausages.

Serves 6

1. Cook pasta in boiling water according to package instructions or until firm to the bite. Drain and place in serving bowl.
2. In nonstick skillet sprayed with vegetable spray, heat oil; sauté garlic and onions until tender, approximately 4 minutes. Add sausages; sauté until no longer pink, approximately 4 minutes. Add mushrooms and sauté until soft, approximately 2 minutes. Add wine and simmer for 2 minutes.
3. Add tomato sauce, milk and basil; simmer on low heat for 10 minutes, stirring occasionally. Pour over pasta. Add cheese and toss.

Nutritional Analysis (Per Serving)
- ✦ Calories: 452
- ✦ Protein: 18 g
- ✦ Cholesterol: 36 mg
- ✦ Sodium: 364 mg
- ✦ Fat, total: 17 g
- ✦ Carbohydrates: 54 g
- ✦ Fiber: 3 g
- ✦ Fat, saturated: 6 g

Linguine with Spicy Italian Sausage in a Red Wine Tomato Sauce

12 oz	linguine	375 g
Sauce		
2 tsp	vegetable oil	10 mL
1 tsp	crushed garlic	5 mL
1 cup	diced onions	250 mL
8 oz	spicy sausages, skinned and chopped	250 g
½ cup	dry red wine	125 mL
2 cups	prepared tomato sauce or Quick Basic Tomato Sauce (see page 129)	500 mL
3 tbsp	grated Parmesan cheese	45 mL

This dish can be turned into a sweet pasta by replacing spicy sausage with sweet sausage.

White wine can replace red wine.

Serves 6

1. Cook pasta in boiling water according to package instructions or until firm to the bite. Drain and place in serving bowl.
2. *Make the sauce:* In large nonstick skillet, heat oil; sauté garlic and onions just until soft. Add sausages and sauté until meat loses its pinkness, approximately 5 minutes.
3. Add wine and tomato sauce to sausage mixture; simmer over low heat for 15 minutes, just until sauce thickens, stirring occasionally. Pour over pasta. Sprinkle with cheese, and toss.

Make Ahead
- ✦ Prepare sauce early in day and reheat gently, adding more tomato sauce if it becomes too thick.

Nutritional Analysis (Per Serving)
- ✦ Calories: 493
- ✦ Protein: 19 g
- ✦ Cholesterol: 35 mg
- ✦ Sodium: 578 mg
- ✦ Fat, total: 19 g
- ✦ Carbohydrates: 58 g
- ✦ Fiber: 4 g
- ✦ Fat, saturated: 6 g

Rotini with Radicchio, Ham, Tomatoes and Cheese

12 oz	rotini	375 g
Sauce		
2 tsp	vegetable oil	10 mL
1 tsp	crushed garlic	5 mL
½ cup	diced onions	125 mL
1½ cups	coarsely sliced radicchio	375 mL
¾ cup	dry white wine	175 mL
3 cups	chopped tomatoes	750 mL
2 tbsp	tomato paste	25 mL
4 oz	diced ham	125 g
½ cup	shredded mozzarella cheese	125 mL

Serves 6

1. Cook pasta in boiling water according to package instructions or until firm to the bite. Drain and place in serving bowl.
2. *Make the sauce:* In large nonstick skillet, heat oil; sauté garlic and onions just until tender, approximately 4 minutes. Add radicchio and simmer until wilted, approximately 3 minutes. Add wine and simmer for 3 minutes.
3. Add tomatoes and paste. Simmer over low heat for 10 minutes, stirring occasionally. Add ham. Pour sauce over pasta. Sprinkle with cheese, and toss.

Tips

+ The radicchio can be increased to 1¾ cups (425 mL) if desired.
+ For a stronger flavor, use Swiss cheese or 3 oz (75 g) of goat or feta cheese.
+ If you don't care for the bitter flavor of radicchio, use romaine or Bibb lettuce instead.

Make Ahead

+ Prepare sauce early in day and reheat gently, adding a little wine if sauce thickens.

Nutritional Analysis (Per Serving)

+ Calories: 333
+ Protein: 14 g
+ Cholesterol: 10 mg
+ Sodium: 317 mg
+ Fat, total: 4 g
+ Carbohydrates: 56 g
+ Fiber: 5 g
+ Fat, saturated: 0.7 g

Rigatoni with Artichokes, Mushrooms and Ham

12 oz	rigatoni (wide tube pasta)	375 g
1 tsp	vegetable oil	5 mL
1½ tsp	crushed garlic	7 mL
1 cup	diced onions	250 mL
1 cup	sliced mushrooms	250 mL
½ cup	sliced sweet red peppers	125 mL
1½	cans (14 oz/390 mL) artichokes, drained and diced	1½
⅔ cup	frozen green peas	150 mL
2 oz	ham, chopped	50 g
Sauce		
1 tbsp	margarine or butter	15 mL
2 tbsp	all-purpose flour	25 mL
1¼ cups	chicken or beef stock	300 mL
½ cup	dry white wine	125 mL
½ cup	2% milk	125 mL
¼ cup	grated Parmesan cheese	50 mL

Fresh or frozen? Have you always thought that frozen vegetables were inferior to fresh? Well they're not! In fact, they're often more nutritious than fresh because they're processed immediately after harvest and their nutrients are "locked in." As a result, there's no change to their nutrient content over their shelf life — whereas that bunch of broccoli sitting in your crisper might have been picked 2 or 3 weeks ago, during which time the vitamins and minerals have diminished steadily.

When using margarine, choose a soft (non-hydrogenated) version to limit consumption of trans fats.

Serves 4 to 6

1. Cook pasta in boiling water according to package instructions or until firm to the bite. Drain and place in serving bowl.

2. Meanwhile, in large skillet, heat oil; sauté garlic and onions until soft, approximately 4 minutes. Add mushrooms and red peppers and sauté for 2 minutes. Add artichokes and peas and cook just until peas are soft, approximately 2 minutes. Add to pasta along with ham.

3. *Make the sauce:* In small nonstick saucepan, melt margarine; add flour and cook for 1 minute, stirring constantly. Add stock, wine and milk, and cook on a medium heat, stirring constantly until thickened, approximately 3 minutes. Pour over pasta. Sprinkle with Parmesan cheese, and toss.

Tip

✦ Use smoked or Black Forest ham. For a change, try using prosciutto.

Make Ahead

✦ Prepare sauce early in day, adding more stock if sauce thickens.

Nutritional Analysis (Per Serving)

✦ Calories: 390   ✦ Protein: 17 g   ✦ Cholesterol: 8 mg
✦ Sodium: 639 mg   ✦ Fat, total: 6 g   ✦ Carbohydrates: 66 g
✦ Fiber: 4 g   ✦ Fat, saturated: 2 g

Baked Beans with Molasses and Ham over Small Shell Pasta

1 cup	dried navy or pea beans, rinsed and drained or 2¾ cups/675 mL canned cooked beans, drained	250 mL
1 cup	chopped onions	250 mL
1½ tsp	minced garlic	7 mL
4 oz	cooked ham, chopped	125 g
1¼ cups	beef or chicken stock	300 mL
½ cup	tomato pasta sauce	125 mL
¼ cup	ketchup	50 mL
⅓ cup	molasses	75 mL
¼ cup	packed brown sugar	50 mL
8 oz	small shell pasta	250 g

Iron and brain power: *Did you know that iron deficiency can affect attention span, learning ability and intellectual performance in adolescents and children? Well, according to a number of studies, it's true. With less iron available to transport oxygen to body cells, less energy is produced for concentration, thinking and learning. Iron is also used to make brain compounds called neurotransmitters, in particular the ones that regulate the ability to pay attention. So focus on this recipe for baked beans — it'll give you 5 mg iron per serving! For more on iron, see pages 88 and 175.*

Serves 4
Preheat oven to 400°F (200°C)
Small baking dish

1. If using cooked beans, proceed to step 2. Otherwise, in a saucepan over medium-high heat, cover uncooked beans with cold water; bring to a boil. Reduce heat; simmer for 5 minutes. Remove from heat; let stand, covered, for 1 hour. Drain beans. Return to saucepan; cover with cold water. Bring to a boil; reduce heat to medium. Cook, covered, for 1 hour or until tender; drain.

2. In a nonstick saucepan sprayed with vegetable spray, cook onions and garlic over medium-high heat for 3 minutes or until softened. Add ham, stock, pasta sauce, ketchup, molasses and brown sugar; bring to a boil. Pour ham mixture and beans into baking dish; bake, covered, in preheated oven for 20 minutes.

3. Meanwhile, in a large pot of boiling water, cook pasta for 8 to 10 minutes or until tender but firm; drain. In a serving bowl combine pasta and bean mixture; toss well. Serve immediately.

Tip

✦ If you've got 2 or 3 hours to spare, you can make a tasty pot of old-fashioned baked beans. Or you can take a few shortcuts and still end up with a great result! Store-bought cooked ham gives this dish a smoky-salty flavor that's delicious with the beans-and-molasses combination. Who needs all the fatty bacon that comes with traditional baked beans?

Nutritional Analysis (Per Serving)
✦ Calories: 440 ✦ Protein: 20 g ✦ Cholesterol: 12 mg
✦ Sodium: 375 mg ✦ Fat, total: 3 g ✦ Carbohydrates: 88 g
✦ Fiber: 10 g ✦ Fat, saturated: 0.7 g

Hoisin Lamb Stew with Tomato over Rotini

12 oz	boneless stewing lamb, cut into 3/4-inch (4 cm) cubes	375 g
3 tbsp	all-purpose flour	45 mL
3 cups	coarsely chopped oyster mushrooms or regular mushrooms	750 mL
2 tsp	minced garlic	10 mL
20	baby carrots	20
16	pearl onions, peeled	16
2/3 cup	beef or chicken stock	150 mL
1	can (19 oz/540 mL) tomatoes, with juice	1
3 tbsp	hoisin sauce	45 mL
3 tbsp	oyster sauce	45 mL
	Freshly ground black pepper	
1 lb	rotini	500 g
1/2 cup	chopped fresh parsley	125 mL

Lighter lamb: *Think lamb contains more fat than beef? Wrong! When lean cuts are selected, lamb and beef are almost identical. Just compare a 3-oz (85 g) serving of leg of lamb (lean only) with the same amount of lean-only sirloin steak. The lamb contains 168 calories and 7 g fat, compared to 160 calories and 6 g fat for the beef.*

Serves 6

1. In a bowl dust lamb with flour; coat well. In a large nonstick saucepan sprayed with vegetable spray, cook lamb over medium-high heat, stirring occasionally, for 5 minutes or until browned on all sides. Remove lamb from pan; set aside.

2. Respray saucepan; cook mushrooms and garlic over medium-high heat for 5 minutes or until browned. Add carrots, onions, stock, tomatoes, hoisin sauce, oyster sauce and lamb; bring to a boil. Reduce heat to low; cook, covered, for 45 minutes or until lamb and vegetables are tender, breaking tomatoes with back of a spoon. Season to taste with pepper.

3. In a large pot of boiling water, cook rotini for 8 to 10 minutes or until tender but firm; drain. Pour stew over pasta; garnish with parsley. Serve immediately.

Tips

✦ Stewing lamb usually comes from the shoulder, neck, breast, shanks or leg. And while the best-tasting meat comes from the shoulder and neck, you get a milder flavor with leg of lamb. The only disadvantage of leg meat is that it dries out easily while cooking. Remember that stewing lamb is different from beef: you need to cook it on a lower heat in a lot of liquid; the longer you cook it, the more tender it will become.

Nutritional Analysis (Per Serving)
✦ Calories: 437   ✦ Protein: 26 g   ✦ Cholesterol: 41 mg
✦ Sodium: 307 mg   ✦ Fat, total: 5 g   ✦ Carbohydrates: 70 g
✦ Fiber: 4 g   ✦ Fat, saturated: 1.5 g

Pork Fajitas with Salsa, Onions and Rice Noodles (page 210) ➤

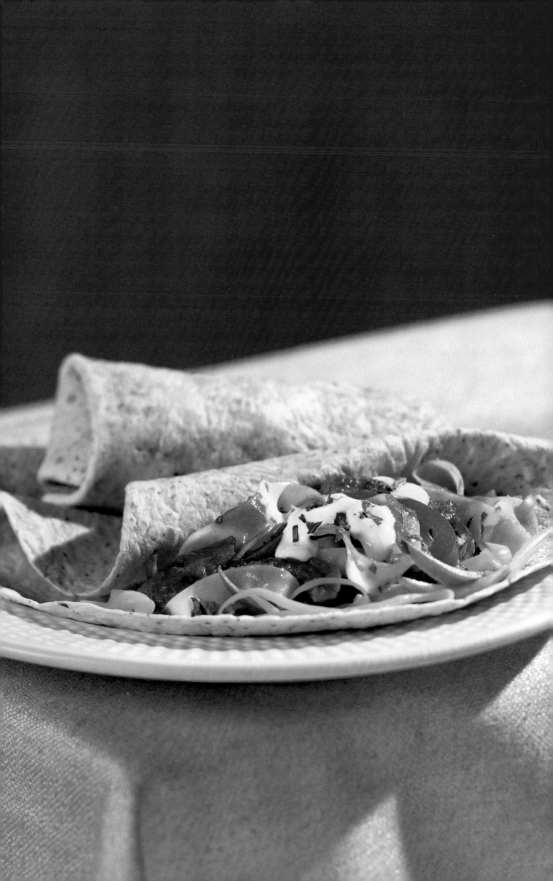

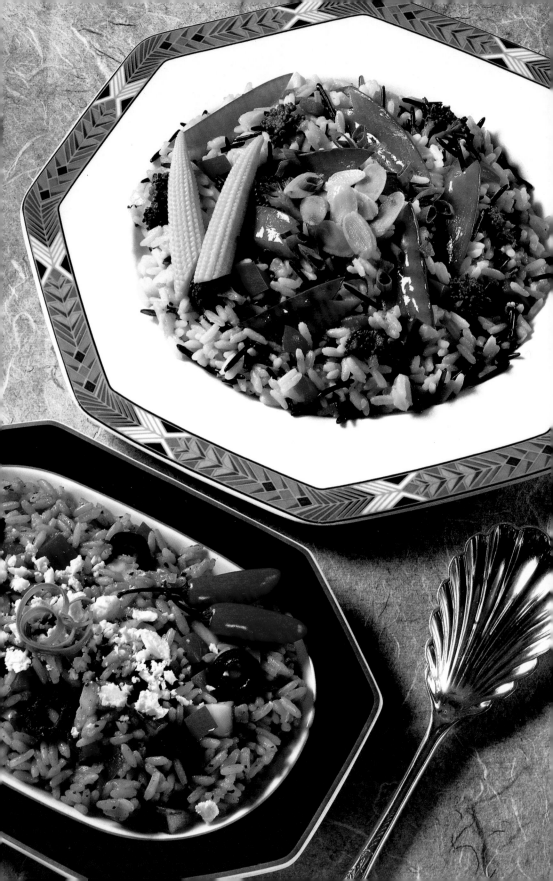

Vegetarian Cheese Pizza Pasta

1/2 cup	sun-dried tomatoes	125 mL
6 oz	small shell pasta	170 g
1	egg	1
1/3 cup	2% milk	75 mL
3 tbsp	grated Parmesan cheese	45 mL
2 tsp	vegetable oil	10 mL
2 tsp	crushed garlic	10 mL
1/2 cup	chopped red onions	125 mL
1 cup	chopped green beans	250 mL
2/3 cup	chopped sweet red peppers	150 mL
1 cup	vegetable stock	250 mL
1 cup	2% milk	250 mL
3 tbsp	all-purpose flour	45 mL
1/3 cup	chopped fresh oregano (or 1 1/2 tsp/7 mL dried)	125 mL
1/2 cup	shredded cheddar cheese	125 mL
2 oz	crumbled goat cheese	50 g

Serves 8
Preheat oven to 350°F (180°C)
10- to 11-inch (3 L) springform pan sprayed
  with vegetable spray

1. Pour boiling water over sun-dried tomatoes. Let soak for 15 minutes. Drain and chop.

2. Cook pasta in boiling water according to package instructions or until firm to the bite. Drain and place in mixing bowl. Add egg, milk and Parmesan. Mix and pour into baking pan. Bake for 20 minutes.

3. In large nonstick skillet sprayed with vegetable spray, heat oil; sauté garlic, red onions, green beans and red peppers for 8 minutes. Add sun-dried tomatoes and cook on medium heat for 2 minutes.

4. Meanwhile, in small bowl, combine stock, milk and flour until smooth. Add to vegetables and simmer on medium heat until slightly thickened, approximately 4 minutes. Add oregano; pour into pasta crust. Sprinkle with cheeses and bake for 10 minutes. Let rest for 10 minutes before serving.

Tips

+ Other vegetables of your choice can be substituted.

+ Other cheeses can replace cheddar and goat cheese.

+ Replace oregano with basil, dill, coriander or tarragon.

Make Ahead

+ The crust and vegetable sauce can be made early in day, but do not pour sauce over crust until ready to bake and serve. If the sauce thickens too much, add stock to thin slightly.

Nutritional Analysis (Per Serving)
+ Calories: 195   + Protein: 9 g   + Cholesterol: 20 mg
+ Sodium: 298 mg   + Fat: 7 g   + Carbohydrates: 23 g
+ Fiber: 2 g

◄ Wild Rice with Sautéed Oriental Vegetables (page 213) /
Spicy Rice with Feta Cheese and Black Olives (page 214)

Sautéed Potato Pesto Pita Pizzas

2 tsp	vegetable oil	10 mL
1 cup	chopped red onions	250 mL
2 tsp	minced garlic	10 mL
1/2 tsp	dried oregano	2 mL
8 oz	potatoes, peeled and shredded (about 2)	250 g
	Freshly ground black pepper to taste	
3	6-inch (15 cm) pita breads	3
1/4 cup	Creamy Pesto Sauce (see recipe, page 128)	50 mL
1/3 cup	chopped softened sun-dried tomatoes (see tip, page 91)	75 mL
1/4 cup	sliced black olives	50 mL
1/2 cup	shredded part-skim mozzarella cheese (about 2 oz/50 g)	125 mL

Serves 4 to 6
Preheat oven to 400°F (200°C)
Baking sheet sprayed with vegetable spray

1. In a large nonstick frying pan sprayed with vegetable spray, heat oil over medium-high heat. Add onions, garlic and oregano; cook 5 minutes or until onions are softened. Stir in potatoes; cook, stirring often and scraping bottom of pan, until potatoes are browned and tender, about 25 to 30 minutes. Season to taste with pepper. Remove from heat.

2. Spread each pita with pesto and place on baking sheet. Divide potato mixture evenly among pitas. Sprinkle sun-dried tomatoes and black olives evenly over pitas; top with mozzarella.

3. Bake 10 minutes, or until cheese is melted.

Nutritional Analysis (Per Serving)
- Calories: 299
- Protein: 9 g
- Cholesterol: 7 mg
- Sodium: 217 mg
- Fat, total: 10 g
- Carbohydrates: 44 g
- Fiber: 3 g
- Fat, saturated: 2.5 g

Polenta Pizza with Mushrooms, Olives and Goat Cheese

2 1/4 cups	chicken stock	550 mL
3/4 cup	yellow cornmeal	175 mL
1 tsp	minced garlic	5 mL
1/3 cup	tomato pasta sauce	75 mL
1/2 cup	sliced mushrooms	125 mL
1/3 cup	sliced black olives	75 mL
2 tbsp	chopped green onions (about 1 medium)	25 mL
1 oz	goat cheese	25 g

For a change, use 3 tbsp (45 mL) pesto sauce instead of tomato sauce. Use feta, mozzarella or cheddar instead of goat cheese.

Serves 6
Preheat oven to 400°F (200°C)
8-inch (2 L) square baking dish sprayed with vegetable spray

1. Bring stock to a boil in small saucepan; gradually add cornmeal and garlic, stirring constantly. Reduce heat to low and cook for 10 minutes, stirring frequently. Pour into prepared pan and smooth with the back of a wet spoon. Let cool for 10 minutes.

2. Spread tomato sauce over top. Sprinkle with mushrooms, olives and green onions; dot with goat cheese. Bake for 12 to 15 minutes or until heated through.

Nutritional Analysis (Per Serving)
- Calories: 104
- Protein: 3 g
- Cholesterol: 0 mg
- Sodium: 497 mg
- Fat, total: 3 g
- Carbohydrates: 17 g
- Fiber: 1 g
- Fat, saturated: 0.3 g

Potato Crust Pesto Pizza

3 cups	diced potatoes	750 mL
2 tbsp	olive oil	25 mL
1 cup	all-purpose flour	250 mL
2 tbsp	grated Parmesan cheese	25 mL
1 tsp	dried basil	5 mL
¼ tsp	salt	1 mL
¼ tsp	freshly ground black pepper	1 mL
⅓ cup	Creamy Pesto Sauce (see recipe, page 128)	75 mL
¼ cup	sliced black olives	50 mL
¼ cup	thinly sliced red bell peppers	50 mL
½ cup	shredded part-skim mozzarella cheese (about 2 oz/50 g)	125 mL

Using potatoes for a pizza crust instead of bread is unusual and delicious.

Serves 6
Preheat oven to 425°F (220°C)
10-inch (3 L) springform pan sprayed with vegetable spray

1. In a saucepan add cold water to cover to potatoes. Bring to a boil; cook 10 minutes or until tender when pierced with the tip of a knife. Drain; mash with oil. Stir in flour, Parmesan, basil, salt and pepper until well mixed. Do not overmix. Press onto bottom of prepared pan. Bake 15 minutes or until golden at edges.

2. Spread with pesto. Sprinkle with black olives, red peppers and mozzarella. Return to oven; bake 10 minutes.

Make Ahead
✦ Prepare pizza up to 1 day in advance. Bake just before serving.

Nutritional Analysis (Per Serving)
✦ Calories: 299   ✦ Protein: 9 g   ✦ Cholesterol: 7 mg
✦ Sodium: 217 mg   ✦ Fat, total: 10 g   ✦ Carbohydrates: 44 g
✦ Fiber: 4 g   ✦ Fat, saturated: 3 g

Mini Pesto Shrimp Tortilla Pizzas

4	small flour tortillas	4
⅓ cup	pesto	75 mL
½ cup	finely chopped red peppers	125 mL
½ cup	finely chopped cooked shrimp	125 mL
⅔ cup	shredded part-skim mozzarella cheese	150 mL

Using store-bought pesto adds more calories and fat. The sauce recipe on page 128 is delicious, and the unused portion can be used over pasta. It can be frozen for up to 3 weeks.

Serves 8
Preheat oven to 400°F (200°C)
Baking sheet sprayed with vegetable spray

1. Place tortillas on baking sheet. Divide pesto among tortillas; spread evenly.

2. Top tortillas with red peppers, shrimp and mozzarella.

3. Bake for 12 to 15 minutes or until cheese has melted and tortillas are crisp. Cut each into 4 pieces.

Make Ahead
✦ Prepare the pizzas early in day. Keep covered and refrigerated until ready to bake.
✦ Pizzas can also be prepared and frozen for up to 6 weeks.

Nutritional Analysis (Per Serving)
✦ Calories: 131   ✦ Protein: 6 g   ✦ Cholesterol: 23 mg
✦ Sodium: 159 mg   ✦ Fat, total: 7 g   ✦ Carbohydrates: 11 g
✦ Fiber: 1 g   ✦ Fat, saturated: 2 g

Turkey and Dill Pizza Pasta

6 oz	broken spaghetti	170 g
1	egg	1
1/3 cup	2% milk	75 mL
3 tbsp	grated Parmesan cheese	45 mL
1 cup	chopped asparagus	250 mL
1 1/2 tsp	crushed garlic	7 mL
8 oz	skinless, boneless turkey breasts, cut into 1-inch (2 cm) cubes	250 g
2/3 cup	diced sweet red peppers	150 mL
2/3 cup	diced onions	150 mL
1 cup	cold chicken stock	250 mL
1 cup	2% milk	250 mL
3 tbsp	all-purpose flour	45 mL
1/3 cup	chopped fresh dill (or 1 tbsp/15 mL dried)	75 mL
2 1/2 oz	grated cheddar cheese	60 g

Serves 6

Preheat oven to 350°F (180°C)

10- to 11-inch (3 L) pizza or springform baking pan sprayed with vegetable spray

1. Cook pasta in boiling water according to package instructions or until firm to the bite. Drain and place in mixing bowl. Add egg, milk and Parmesan; mix well and pour in pan. Bake for 20 minutes.

2. Blanch asparagus in boiling water just until tender. Drain, rinse with cold water, and set aside

3. In large nonstick skillet sprayed with vegetable spray, sauté garlic and turkey until turkey is no longer pink, approximately 4 minutes. Set aside.

4. Spray skillet again with vegetable spray; sauté red peppers and onions for 4 minutes. In small bowl, mix stock, milk and flour until smooth. Add to skillet with asparagus, turkey and dill. Simmer on low heat until sauce thickens, approximately 4 minutes, stirring constantly. Pour into pan; sprinkle with cheese. Bake for 10 minutes. Let sit for 10 minutes before cutting.

Tips

✦ Macaroni or small shell pasta can replace spaghetti.

✦ Another fresh herb can replace dill, such as oregano, basil or coriander.

✦ Pork or boneless chicken can replace turkey.

Make Ahead

✦ Crust and filling can be made early in day. Keep separate. Add more stock to filling if it thickens.

Nutritional Analysis (Per Serving)

✦ Calories: 304　✦ Protein: 24 g　✦ Cholesterol: 44 mg
✦ Sodium: 377 mg　✦ Fat: 8 g　✦ Carbohydrates: 36 g
✦ Fiber: 3 g

Pita or Tortilla Pizzas

³/₄ cup	tomato sauce	175 mL
4	flour tortillas or pita breads (preferably whole wheat)	4
8	small mushrooms, thinly sliced	8
¼ cup	diced sweet red or green pepper	50 mL
1 tbsp	chopped fresh basil (or 1 tsp/5 mL dried)	15 mL
½ tsp	dried oregano	2 mL
1 cup	shredded mozzarella cheese	250 mL
¼ cup	chopped feta cheese (optional)	50 mL

Get out of the habit of eating in front of the TV. It's too easy to lose track of how much you have eaten and when you are full. Keep in mind, too, that eating after dinner can add a significant amount of extra calories to your day.

Serves 6 to 8 or makes 16 hors d'oeuvres
Preheat oven to 400°F (200°C)

1. Divide tomato sauce among breads; spread evenly.
2. Top with mushrooms, red pepper, basil and oregano. Sprinkle with cheese.
3. Bake for 12 minutes or until crisp and cheese is melted. Cut each into 4 pieces.

Tips
✦ Try ¼ cup (50 mL) chopped sun-dried tomatoes.
✦ Any combination of vegetables can be used, as well as any type of cheese. Goat cheese is exceptional on pizzas.

Make Ahead
✦ Prepare pizzas early in day and refrigerate. Bake just before serving.

Nutritional Analysis (Per Serving)
✦ Calories: 180 ✦ Protein: 9 g ✦ Cholesterol: 11 mg
✦ Sodium: 504 mg ✦ Fat: 4 g ✦ Carbohydrates: 26 g
✦ Fiber: 4 g

Chicken and Tarragon Pasta Pizza

6 oz	broken fettuccine	150 g
1	egg	1
1/3 cup	2% milk	75 mL
3 tbsp	grated Parmesan cheese	45 mL
1 cup	chopped broccoli	250 mL
1½ tsp	crushed garlic	7 mL
8 oz	skinless boneless chicken breasts, cut into 1-inch (2.5 cm) cubes	250 g
2/3 cup	diced sweet green peppers	150 mL
2/3 cup	diced red onions	150 mL
1 cup	cold chicken stock	250 mL
1 cup	2% milk	250 mL
3 tbsp	all-purpose flour	45 mL
1/4 cup	chopped fresh tarragon (or 3 tsp/ 15 mL dried)	50 mL
2½ oz	shredded Swiss or mozzarella cheese	60 g

Serves 6
Preheat oven to 350°F (180°C)
10-inch (3 L) springform pan sprayed with vegetable spray

1. Cook pasta in boiling water according to package instructions or until firm to the bite. Drain and place in mixing bowl. Add egg, milk and cheese; mix well and pour in pan. Bake for 20 minutes.

2. Blanch broccoli in boiling water just until tender. Drain, rinse with cold water, and set aside.

3. In large nonstick skillet sprayed with vegetable spray, sauté garlic and chicken until chicken is no longer pink, approximately 4 minutes. Set chicken aside.

4. Spray skillet again with vegetable spray; sauté green peppers and onions for 4 minutes. In small bowl, mix stock, milk and flour until smooth. Add to skillet with broccoli, chicken and tarragon. Simmer on low heat until sauce thickens, approximately 4 minutes, stirring constantly. Pour into pan, sprinkle with cheese. Bake for 10 minutes.

Tips

✦ Macaroni or small shell pasta can replace fettuccine.

✦ Asparagus is a tasty substitute for the broccoli.

Make Ahead

✦ Crust and filling can be made early in day. Keep separate. Add more stock to filling if it thickens.

Nutritional Analysis (Per Serving)
✦ Calories: 304   ✦ Protein: 24 g   ✦ Cholesterol: 44 mg
✦ Sodium: 377 mg   ✦ Fat, total: 8 g   ✦ Carbohydrates: 36 g
✦ Fiber: 3 g   ✦ Fat, saturated: 4 g

Beef and Sausage Cheese Pizza Pasta

6 oz	small shell pasta	170 g
1	egg	1
1/3 cup	2% milk	75 mL
3 tbsp	grated Parmesan cheese	45 mL
1 tsp	vegetable oil	5 mL
2 tsp	crushed garlic	10 mL
2/3 cup	finely chopped onions	150 mL
1/3 cup	finely chopped celery	75 mL
1/3 cup	finely chopped carrots	75 mL
4 oz	ground beef	125 g
4 oz	spicy sausage, chopped, casing removed	125 g
1	can (19 oz/540 mL) tomatoes, crushed	1
2 tbsp	tomato paste	25 mL
1½ tsp	Italian seasoning	7 mL
½ cup	shredded mozzarella cheese	125 mL
1/3 cup	grated cheddar cheese	75 mL

> Same great taste, less fat: *You know that sausages are high in fat: a 1-oz (28 g) serving of beef or pork sausage has 9.3 g saturated fat. But you also know how much flavor they can add to a hearty bean soup or spicy tomato sauce. Try removing the casing before browning and drain all the fat afterwards to remove extra fat.*

Serves 8
Preheat oven to 350°F (180°C)
10- to 11-inch (3 L) pizza or springform baking pan sprayed with vegetable spray

1. Cook pasta in boiling water according to package instructions or until firm to the bite. Drain and place in serving bowl. Add egg, milk and Parmesan. Mix well. Place in baking pan as a crust and bake for 20 minutes.

2. Meanwhile, in medium nonstick saucepan sprayed with vegetable spray, heat oil; sauté garlic, onions, celery and carrots until tender, approximately 5 minutes. Add beef and sausage and sauté until no longer pink, approximately 4 minutes. Add tomatoes, tomato paste and Italian seasoning. Cover and simmer on low heat for 15 minutes, stirring occasionally, until thickened.

3. Pour sauce into pasta crust. Sprinkle with both cheeses; bake for 10 minutes or until cheese melts. Let sit for 10 minutes before cutting.

Tips

+ Any combination of different vegetables can be used.
+ Any pasta can be substituted. If using long pasta, break into pieces.
+ Stronger cheeses can be used.

Make Ahead

+ Prepare pasta crust and sauce early in day. Do not pour sauce over top until ready to bake. Great to reheat.

Nutritional Analysis (Per Serving)
+ Calories: 247   + Protein: 13 g   + Cholesterol: 29 mg
+ Sodium: 320 mg   + Fat: 9 g   + Carbohydrates: 23 g
+ Fiber: 3 g

Pizza Pasta with Beef-Tomato Sauce and Cheese

6 oz	macaroni	150 g
1	egg	1
1/3 cup	2% milk	75 mL
3 tbsp	grated Parmesan cheese	45 mL
1 tsp	vegetable oil	5 mL
2 tsp	crushed garlic	10 mL
3/4 cup	finely chopped onions	175 mL
1/2 cup	finely chopped sweet green peppers	125 mL
1/3 cup	finely chopped carrots	75 mL
8 oz	ground beef or chicken	250 g
1	can (19 oz/540 mL) tomatoes, crushed	1
2 tbsp	tomato paste	25 mL
1 1/2 tsp	dried basil	7 mL
1 tsp	dried oregano	5 mL
1 cup	low-fat mozzarella cheese, shredded	250 mL

Serves 8
Preheat oven to 350°F (180°C)
10- to 11-inch (25- to 28-cm) pizza or springform baking pan sprayed with vegetable spray

1. Cook pasta in boiling water according to package instructions or until firm to the bite. Drain and place in serving bowl. Add egg, milk and cheese. Mix well. Place in baking pan as a crust and bake for 20 minutes.

2. Meanwhile, in medium nonstick saucepan sprayed with vegetable spray, heat oil; sauté garlic, onions, green peppers and carrots until tender, approximately 5 minutes. Add beef and sauté until no longer pink, approximately 4 minutes. Add tomatoes, paste, basil and oregano. Cover and simmer on low heat for 15 minutes, stirring occasionally.

3. Pour sauce into pasta crust. Sprinkle with cheese; bake for 10 minutes or until cheese melts.

Tip
+ Any combination of different vegetables can be used as long as you do not exceed 2 1/4 cups (550 mL).

Make Ahead
+ Prepare pasta crust and sauce early in day. Do not pour sauce over top until ready to bake.

Nutritional Analysis (Per Serving)
+ Calories: 247   + Protein: 15 g   + Cholesterol: 29 mg
+ Sodium: 264 mg   + Fat, total: 9 g   + Carbohydrates: 23 g
+ Fiber: 3 g   + Fat, saturated: 4 g

Pesto and Red Pepper Tortilla Bites

3 tbsp	pesto sauce (store-bought or see recipe, page 128)	45 mL
3 oz	goat cheese 75 g	
1/4 cup	5% ricotta cheese	50 mL
1	large red pepper	1
3	10-inch (25 cm) flour tortillas or six 6-inch (15 cm) flour tortillas	3

Traditional pesto, whether store-bought or homemade, is laden with fat and calories because of all the oil, nuts and cheese. In fact, 2 tbsp (30 mL) can contain as much as 150 calories and 15 g fat. The low-fat recipe on page 128 uses stock to replace some of the oil, and contains less cheese and fewer nuts. The results are delicious, and the fat and calories are reduced by more than half. Freeze leftover pesto in ice cube trays and use one cube per plate of pasta.

Serves 6 to 8
Preheat broiler

1. In bowl or food processor, combine pesto, goat cheese and ricotta; mix until well combined.

2. Roast pepper under the broiler for 15 to 20 minutes, turning several times until charred on all sides; place in a bowl covered tightly with plastic wrap; let stand until cool enough to handle. Remove skin, stem and seeds; cut roasted pepper into thin strips.

3. If using larger tortillas, spread 1/4 cup (50 mL) filling on each tortilla; if using smaller tortillas, spread 2 tbsp (25 mL) on each tortilla. Spread filling to edges of tortillas, scatter red pepper strips on top, and roll tightly. Chill, wrapped in plastic wrap, for an hour. Cut into 1-inch (2.5 cm) pieces and serve.

Tips

✦ If you're using a store-bought pesto sauce, the calories and fat will be higher. Prepare sauce recipe on page 128 and freeze unused sauce for another purpose.

✦ If in a hurry, you don't need to chill the tortilla before cutting. Just use a sharp knife.

✦ If tortillas are very small, increase the number to 8.

✦ Try 4 oz (125 g) of roasted sweet peppers in a jar to replace fresh pepper. Use those which are packed in water.

Make Ahead

✦ Prepare up to a day ahead, keeping tightly wrapped in refrigerator.

Nutritional Analysis (Per Serving)
✦ Calories: 142 ✦ Protein: 5 g ✦ Cholesterol: 3 mg
✦ Sodium: 156 mg ✦ Fat, total: 7 g ✦ Carbohydrates: 16 g
✦ Fiber: 1 g ✦ Fat, saturated: 1 g

Cheese and Vegetable Stuffed Tortillas

1 tbsp	margarine	15 mL
1 tsp	crushed garlic	5 mL
1 cup	finely chopped onions	250 mL
1 cup	finely chopped sweet green or red pepper	250 mL
2/3 cup	finely chopped broccoli	150 mL
	Salt and pepper	
1	large green onion, sliced	1
4	tortillas	4
1/2 cup	shredded cheddar cheese	125 mL

When using margarine, choose a soft (non-hydrogenated) version to limit consumption of trans fats.

Serves 8
Preheat oven to 400°F (200°C)

1. In nonstick skillet, melt margarine; sauté garlic, onions, green pepper, broccoli, and salt and pepper to taste until just tender. Add green onion and mix.
2. Divide vegetables among tortillas and spread over top; sprinkle with cheese. Roll up and place on baking sheet. Bake for 3 to 5 minutes or until hot and cheese melts. Cut in half to serve.

Tips
+ These tortillas can be served as an appetizer or side dish.
+ Serve with salsa, yogurt or light sour cream.
+ Vary the vegetables if desired.

Nutritional Analysis (Per Serving)
+ Calories: 119   + Protein: 4 g   + Cholesterol: 9 mg
+ Sodium: 146 mg + Fat: 5 g   + Carbohydrates: 15 g
+ Fiber: 1 g

Bean and Cheese Tortilla Slices

1 cup	canned red kidney beans, rinsed and drained	250 mL
1 tbsp	freshly squeezed lemon juice	15 mL
1/2 tsp	chili powder	2 mL
1/2 tsp	minced garlic	2 mL
3/4 cup	5% smooth ricotta cheese	175 mL
3 tbsp	chopped green onions	45 mL
3 tbsp	chopped fresh coriander	45 mL
2 tbsp	light sour cream	25 mL
1 tbsp	light mayonnaise	15 mL
4	small 6-inch (15 cm) flour tortillas	4

For a more decorative look, add a lettuce leaf to top of filling before rolling.

Serves 4 to 6

1. In a food processor or with a fork in a bowl, mash together beans, lemon juice, chili powder and garlic. In a separate bowl, combine ricotta, green onions, coriander, sour cream and mayonnaise; stir until well mixed.
2. Divide ricotta mixture among tortillas and spread over surface. Top with bean mixture. Roll tightly, cover and chill 30 minutes.
3. Cut each roll into 6 pieces and serve.

Tip
+ Serve as an appetizer or as a side dish.

Make Ahead
+ Prepare up to 1 day in advance; cut just before serving.

Nutritional Analysis (Per Serving)
+ Calories: 132   + Protein: 9 g   + Cholesterol: 9 mg
+ Sodium: 208 mg + Fat, total: 3 g   + Carbohydrates: 17 g
+ Fiber: 3 g   + Fat, saturated: 2 g

Quinoa Wraps with Hoisin Vegetables

1 cup	quinoa, rinsed	250 mL
2 cups	vegetable or chicken stock	500 mL
1 tsp	minced garlic	5 mL
1 tsp	minced gingerroot	5 mL
1/2 cup	diced red bell peppers	125 mL
1/2 cup	diced snow peas	125 mL
1/2 cup	diced water chestnuts	125 mL
1/4 cup	chopped green onions	50 mL
1/4 cup	hoisin sauce	50 mL
1/4 cup	light mayonnaise	50 mL
2 tbsp	honey	25 mL
1/4 cup	chopped fresh coriander or parsley	50 mL
8	6-inch (15 cm) flour tortillas	8

An iron-rich grain or a vegetable? *Although widely considered a grain, quinoa is actually related to the spinach family. And like spinach, quinoa is a good source of iron. While the iron in grains and vegetables is not as well absorbed as the iron in animal foods, you can enhance the amount of iron your body absorbs from plant foods by eating them with a source of vitamin C, such as the red peppers in this recipe.*

Serves 8

1. In a small nonstick skillet, toast quinoa over medium-high heat for 2 minutes.
2. In a saucepan over medium-high heat, bring stock to a boil. Add quinoa; reduce heat to medium-low. Cook, covered, for 15 minutes or until grain is tender and liquid is absorbed. Set aside.
3. In a nonstick frying pan sprayed with vegetable spray, cook garlic, ginger, red peppers, snow peas and water chestnuts over medium-high heat for 3 minutes or until softened. Add green onions; cook for 1 minute. Remove from heat; add to quinoa.
4. In a bowl combine hoisin sauce, mayonnaise, honey and coriander; spread over tortillas. Place about 1/3 cup (75 mL) quinoa mixture in center of each tortilla. Fold right side over filling; roll up from the bottom. Serve.

Tips

✦ Quinoa (pronounced KEEN-wah) may be unfamiliar to many North Americans, but it's not exactly new. In fact, it was a staple of the ancient Incas, who described it as the "mother grain." And it seems that they were right! Quinoa contains more protein than any other grain. Use it in soups, as part of a main or side dish, in salads or as a substitute for rice.

✦ While it's incredibly nutritious, quinoa can have a slightly bitter taste. But you can eliminate the bitterness by rinsing the quinoa thoroughly, drying it and then toasting it lightly in a nonstick skillet.

Nutritional Analysis (Per Serving)
✦ Calories: 264   ✦ Protein: 7 g   ✦ Cholesterol: 0 mg
✦ Sodium: 213 mg ✦ Fat, total: 6 g   ✦ Carbohydrates: 46 g
✦ Fiber: 3 g   ✦ Fat, saturated: 0.8 g

Vermicelli Sesame Oriental Vegetable Wraps

2 tbsp	light mayonnaise	25 mL
4 tsp	soya sauce	20 mL
1 tbsp	water	15 mL
1 tbsp	sesame oil	15 mL
1½ tsp	honey	7 mL
1 tsp	minced garlic	5 mL
¾ tsp	minced gingerroot	4 mL
¼ cup	sliced carrots	50 mL
½ cup	halved snow peas	125 mL
⅓ cup	sliced baby corn cobs	75 mL
⅓ cup	chopped red or green bell peppers	75 mL
⅓ cup	chopped fresh coriander	75 mL
1	green onion, chopped	1
4 oz	vermicelli or capellini, broken into thirds	125 g
4	10-inch (25 cm) flour tortillas, preferably different flavors, if available	4

Serves 4

1. In a food processor, combine mayonnaise, soya sauce, water, sesame oil, honey, garlic and ginger; process until smooth. Set aside.

2. Boil or steam carrots for 3 minutes or until tender-crisp; rinse with cold water, drain and put in serving bowl. Boil or steam snow peas for 1 minute or until tender-crisp; rinse with cold water, drain and add to serving bowl. Add baby corn, peppers, coriander and green onion.

3. In a large pot of boiling water, cook vermicelli 8 to 10 minutes until tender but firm. Drain and add to serving bowl. Add sauce; toss all ingredients until well mixed.

4. Divide pasta mixture between tortillas. Form each tortilla into a packet by folding bottom edge over filling, then sides, then top, to enclose filling completely.

Tips

+ Flavored tortillas — such as pesto, sun-dried tomato, herb or whole wheat — are now appearing in many supermarkets. Using different flavors will add taste and variety, as well as visual interest, to these wraps.

+ Substitute other vegetables of your choice.

+ Fresh parsley or dill can replace coriander.

+ Any thin-strand pasta will work well.

Make Ahead

+ Prepare filling up to 1 day in advance.

+ Tortillas are best filled just before serving, but can be filled 1 or 2 hours ahead.

Nutritional Analysis (Per Serving)
+ Calories: 319 + Protein: 9 g + Cholesterol: 0 mg
+ Sodium: 594 mg + Fat, total: 8 g + Carbohydrates: 52 g
+ Fiber: 3 g + Fat, saturated: 1.8 g

Seafood Tortilla Pinwheels

3 oz	light cream cheese, softened	75 g
½ cup	5% ricotta cheese	125 mL
2 tbsp	chopped fresh dill (or 1 tsp/5 mL dried)	
2 tbsp	chopped green onions (1 medium)	25 mL
1 tbsp	light mayonnaise	15 mL
2 tsp	lemon juice	10 mL
4 oz	chopped cooked shrimp	125 g
¼ cup	chopped red peppers	50 mL
4	small flour tortillas	4
	Lettuce leaves (optional)	

The curly edges of green or red leaf lettuce are especially attractive in these pinwheels.

Serves 6 or makes 24 pinwheels

1. Place cream cheese, ricotta, dill, green onions, mayonnaise and lemon juice in a bowl; combine thoroughly. Stir in shrimp and red peppers.
2. Divide shrimp mixture among tortillas and spread to the edges; top with lettuce leaves (if using), overlapped to cover entire tortilla. Roll up tightly, cover and refrigerate for an hour to chill.
3. Cut each roll crosswise into 6 pieces and serve.

Tip
✦ You may substitute crab legs (surimi, or imitation crab) for the shrimp.

Make Ahead
✦ Prepare tortillas early in the day and keep tightly covered in refrigerator.

Nutritional Analysis (Per Serving)
✦ Calories: 158 ✦ Protein: 11 g ✦ Cholesterol: 51 mg
✦ Sodium: 304 mg ✦ Fat, total: 6 g ✦ Carbohydrates: 15 g
✦ Fiber: 1 g ✦ Fat, saturated: 3 g

Ricotta and Smoked Salmon Tortilla Bites

1 cup	ricotta cheese	250 mL
1 tbsp	light mayonnaise or light sour cream	15 mL
2 tbsp	chopped fresh dill (or ½ tsp/2 mL dried dillweed)	25 mL
2 tbsp	finely chopped chives or green onions	25 mL
2 oz	smoked salmon, diced	50 g
4	flour tortillas	4
	Lettuce leaves	

Serves 4 to 6 or makes 24 hors d'oeuvres

1. In bowl or food processor, combine ricotta and light mayonnaise until smooth. Gently stir in dill, chives and smoked salmon until combined.
2. Divide filling among tortillas, spreading evenly. Roll up jelly roll style. Cut each tortilla into 6 pieces. Arrange on lettuce-lined plate.

Tip
✦ These are best served at room temperature.

Make Ahead
✦ Make early in day and refrigerate. Arrange on lettuce-lined plate just before serving.

Nutritional Analysis (Per Serving)
✦ Calories: 160 ✦ Protein: 8 g ✦ Cholesterol: 17 mg
✦ Sodium: 247 mg ✦ Fat: 6 g ✦ Carbohydrates: 18 g
✦ Fiber: 1 g

Shrimp Potstickers with Peanut Sauce

Peanut sauce

2 tbsp	peanut butter	25 mL
2 tbsp	water	25 mL
2 tbsp	chopped fresh coriander	25 mL
1 tbsp	honey	15 mL
1 tbsp	rice wine vinegar	15 mL
2 tsp	light soya sauce	10 mL
1 tsp	sesame oil	5 mL
½ tsp	minced gingerroot	2 mL
½ tsp	minced garlic	2 mL

Filling

8 oz	raw shrimp, peeled, deveined and diced	250 g
1	clove garlic, minced	1
1	medium green onion, chopped	1
2 tbsp	chopped fresh coriander	25 mL
26	3-inch (8 cm) square small egg roll wrappers	26
¾ cup	seafood or chicken stock	175 mL

Watch those fast-food sandwiches! *Looking for a quick sandwich when you're on the road? Keep in mind that a typical fast-food fillet of fish sandwich packs 23 g fat. You can improve on this by holding the tartar sauce and looking for fish that's breaded, not deep-fried. Also, some deli tuna sandwiches can come to 600 calories and 40 g fat. Look for outlets that use low-fat dressings, or ask for plain tuna and spread each slice of bread with only a little mayonnaise.*

Serves 6

1. *Peanut sauce:* In a food processor or in a bowl with a whisk, combine peanut butter, water, coriander, honey, vinegar, soya sauce, sesame oil, ginger and garlic; set aside.

2. *Filling:* In a food processor combine shrimp, garlic, green onion, coriander and 2 tbsp (25 mL) of the peanut sauce; pulse on and off 10 times or until well-mixed.

3. Place 2 tsp (10 mL) filling in center of each wrapper. Pull edges up, pleating and bunching; press together to seal.

4. In a large nonstick frying pan sprayed with vegetable spray, cook potstickers, flat-side down, over medium-high heat for 3 minutes or until golden brown on bottom. Add stock; reduce heat to low. Cook, covered, for 2 minutes or until cooked through. Remove from pan; discard any remaining liquid. Serve with remaining peanut sauce for dipping.

Tips

✦ Fresh coriander leaves — also known as cilantro or Chinese parsley — has an intense flavor that is common in Indian, Mexican, Caribbean and Asian cuisine. It's a flavor you either love or hate. And if you love it, chances are you can't get enough. If it's not to your taste, substitute fresh parsley, dill or basil.

✦ When you purchase frozen shrimp in the shell, be sure to buy a little more than is called for in the recipe. By the time you defrost and devein the shrimp, it will weigh less.

Nutritional Analysis (Per Serving)

✦ Calories: 496	✦ Protein: 22 g	✦ Cholesterol: 72 mg
✦ Sodium: 753 mg	✦ Fat, total: 6 g	✦ Carbohydrates: 88 g
✦ Fiber: 0 g	✦ Fat, saturated: 1 g	

Chicken Tortillas

6 oz	skinless, boneless chicken breast, diced	150 g
1 tsp	vegetable oil	5 mL
1 tsp	crushed garlic	5 mL
1 cup	chopped onions	250 mL
1/2 cup	finely chopped carrots	125 mL
1 cup	tomato pasta sauce	250 mL
1 cup	canned red kidney beans, drained	250 mL
1/2 cup	chicken stock	125 mL
1 tsp	chili powder	5 mL
8	small 6-inch (15 cm) flour tortillas	8
1/2 cup	shredded cheddar cheese (optional)	125 mL

Serves 4
Preheat oven to 375°F (190°C)
Baking sheet sprayed with vegetable spray

1. In nonstick skillet sprayed with vegetable spray, cook chicken over high heat for 2 minutes, or until done at center. Remove from skillet and set aside.

2. Reduce heat to medium and add oil to pan. Respray with vegetable spray and cook garlic, onions, and carrots for 10 minutes, or until browned and softened, stirring often. Add some water if vegetables start to burn. Add tomato sauce, beans, stock and chili powder and cook for 10 to 12 minutes or until carrots are tender, mixture has thickened and most of the liquid is absorbed. Stir in chicken and remove from heat.

3. Put 1/3 cup (75 mL) of mixture on each tortilla, sprinkle with cheese (if using) and roll up. Put on prepared baking sheet and bake for 10 minutes or until heated through.

Tips
✦ Boneless turkey breast, pork or veal scallopini can replace chicken.
✦ The cheese adds a creamy texture to the tortillas. Mozzarella can also be used.

Make Ahead
✦ Prepare filling early in the day and gently reheat before stuffing tortillas. Add extra stock if sauce is too thick.

Nutritional Analysis (Per Serving)
✦ Calories: 438 ✦ Protein: 21 g ✦ Cholesterol: 25 mg
✦ Sodium: 884 mg ✦ Fat, total: 10 g ✦ Carbohydrates: 65 g
✦ Fiber: 7 g ✦ Fat, saturated: 2 g

Beef Potstickers with Coconut Sauce

6 oz	lean ground beef	175 g
1/4 cup	finely chopped green onions	50 mL
1 tbsp	oyster sauce	15 mL
2 tsp	rice wine vinegar	10 mL
1 tsp	sesame oil	5 mL
1 tsp	minced garlic	5 mL
1/2 tsp	minced gingerroot	2 mL
18 to 20	small (3-inch/8 cm) egg roll wrappers	18 to 20

Sauce

1/3 cup	light coconut milk	75 mL
1/4 cup	chopped green onions	50 mL
3 tbsp	water	45 mL
2 tbsp	chopped fresh coriander	25 mL
1 tbsp	rice wine vinegar	15 mL
1 tbsp	oyster sauce	15 mL

Serves 6

1. In a bowl combine ground beef, green onions, oyster sauce, rice wine vinegar, sesame oil, garlic and ginger. Place 2 tsp (10 mL) filling in center of each wrapper. Pull edges up, pleating and bunching. Press edges together to seal.

2. In another bowl, combine coconut milk, green onions, water, coriander, rice wine vinegar and oyster sauce; whisk well.

3. In a large nonstick frying pan sprayed with vegetable spray, cook potstickers, flat-side down, over medium-high heat for 3 minutes or until golden brown on bottom. Add sauce; reduce heat to low. Cook, covered, for 3 minutes or until cooked through. Serve with sauce remaining in pan.

Tips

✦ Oyster sauce is a dark brown sauce made from oysters (big surprise there), brine seasoning and soya sauce, which is cooked until thick. It's a staple of Asian cooking and adds richness to any dish.

✦ *A high-fat milk:* It sure pays to use light coconut milk when you consider that 1/2 cup (125 mL) of the regular stuff packs 307 calories and 30 g fat! That's equivalent to 7 1/2 tsp (38 mL) of added fat. And here's more bad news: 90% of the oil in coconut milk is saturated. The good news is that you'll save 20 g fat by substituting light coconut milk. And use a little less. After all, who needs a lot when it adds so much flavor?

Nutritional Analysis (Per Serving)
✦ Calories: 330 ✦ Protein: 16 g ✦ Cholesterol: 25 mg
✦ Sodium: 654 mg ✦ Fat, total: 2 g ✦ Carbohydrates: 57 g
✦ Fiber: 3 g ✦ Fat, saturated: 1.1 g

Beef-Pepper Wraps with Rice Vermicelli

3 oz	wide rice noodles	75 g
8 oz	boneless steak (such as striploin)	250 g
1 cup	julienned red bell peppers	250 mL
1 cup	julienned snow peas	250 mL
1/3 cup	beef or chicken stock	75 mL
2 tbsp	packed brown sugar	25 mL
1 1/2 tbsp	light soya sauce	22 mL
1 tbsp	rice wine vinegar	15 mL
1 tbsp	orange juice concentrate	15 mL
2 1/2 tsp	cornstarch	12 mL
2 tsp	sesame oil	10 mL
1 1/2 tsp	minced garlic	7 mL
1 1/2 tsp	minced gingerroot	7 mL
6	8-inch (20 cm) flour tortillas	6

If you have an intolerance to the gluten contained in wheat-based pasta, then rice noodles are an ideal substitute. You can either soak them in boiling water (about 15 minutes), or boil them until tender (about 8 minutes). Avoid excessive rinsing or the noodles will become starchy.

Serves 6

1. In a pot of boiling water, cook rice noodles for 5 minutes or until tender; drain. Rinse under cold running water. Set aside.

2. In a nonstick frying pan sprayed with vegetable spray, cook beef over medium-high heat, turning once, for 3 to 5 minutes or until medium-rare. Slice thinly; set aside. Respray frying pan; cook red peppers and snow peas over medium-high heat, stirring, for 4 minutes or until tender-crisp.

3. In a bowl combine stock, brown sugar, soya sauce, rice vinegar, orange juice concentrate, cornstarch, sesame oil, garlic and ginger. Add to vegetables along with beef. Simmer for 1 minute or until thickened.

4. Place about 1/2 cup (125 mL) filling in center of each tortilla. Fold bottom end up over filling; tuck sides in. Roll up tightly. Serve.

Tips

+ Move over sandwiches — here comes the wrap! This innovation in portable eating is wonderfully versatile. Basically, it's just a flour tortilla (plain or colored and flavored) wrapped around any combination of vegetable, chicken, fish or meat and a tasty sauce. Try these wraps for lunch, or a light, nutritious snack.

+ *Vitamin C and the common cold:* As you might expect, these wraps are low in fat. But thanks to the red peppers, snow peas and orange juice, they're also high in vitamin C, providing 125% of your daily requirement. An important nutrient for immunity, vitamin C is able to reduce the severity and duration of cold symptoms. It does this, in part, by enhancing the body's production of interferon, a natural antiviral agent. While supplements are handy, you can get all the vitamin C you need through your diet.

Nutritional Analysis (Per Serving)
+ Calories: 274   + Protein: 14 g   + Cholesterol: 28 mg
+ Sodium: 350 mg   + Fat, total: 7 g   + Carbohydrates: 37 g
+ Fiber: 2 g   + Fat, saturated: 1.9 g

Pork Fajitas with Salsa, Onions and Rice Noodles

3 oz	wide rice noodles	75 g
8 oz	pork or beef tenderloin	250 g
2 tsp	vegetable oil	10 mL
1 cup	thinly sliced red onions	250 mL
2 tsp	minced garlic	10 mL
1 cup	thinly sliced green bell peppers	250 mL
1 cup	thinly sliced red bell peppers	250 mL
1	large green onion, sliced	1
¾ cup	medium salsa	175 mL
⅓ cup	chopped fresh coriander	75 mL
8	8-inch (20 cm) flour tortillas	8
¾ cup	shredded low-fat cheddar cheese	175 mL
⅓ cup	low-fat sour cream	75 mL

Pork and B vitamins: *Is true that B vitamins give you more energy? Sorry, but they don't — at least, not directly. Rather, B vitamins serve as coenzymes in the release of energy from the carbohydrates, fat and protein in foods. But if you're looking for a good source of these vitamins (and they are important), you can't do much better than pork. Pork's nutritional claim to fame is its high thiamin (vitamin B₁) content — in fact, it's the best dietary source available; it's also a great source of other B vitamins, including niacin, riboflavin, B₆ and B₁₂. For more on B vitamins, see page 277.*

Serves 8

1. In a pot of boiling water, cook rice noodles for 5 minutes or until tender; drain. Rinse under cold running water; drain. Set aside.

2. In a nonstick frying pan sprayed with vegetable spray or on a preheated grill, cook pork tenderloin over medium-high heat, turning once, for 15 minutes or until just cooked through. Slice thinly.

3. In a nonstick frying pan sprayed with vegetable spray, heat oil over medium-high heat; add red onions and garlic. Cook for 2 minutes or until softened. Add green peppers and red peppers; cook, stirring frequently, for 2 minutes or until tender-crisp. Add green onion, rice noodles and pork; remove from heat. Add salsa and coriander; combine well.

4. Sprinkle tortillas with cheddar cheese. Place about ½ cup (125 mL) filling in center of each tortilla. Add sour cream; fold bottom end up over filling. Tuck sides in; roll up tightly. Serve immediately.

Tip

✦ Order fajitas from a fast-food restaurant and chances are you'll feel pretty good about your choice. After all, they contain meat, vegetables and cheese — pretty much a complete, healthy meal, right? Don't kid yourself! Most fast-food fajitas are loaded with fatty cuts of meat, oil used to fry the vegetables, as well sour cream and cheese. These fajitas use lean pork tenderloin (5 g fat per 4 oz [125 g]) as well as low-fat sour cream and a small amount of light cheddar cheese. Add in plenty of great vegetables and salsa, and you get all the flavor without the fat!

Nutritional Analysis (Per Serving)

✦ Calories: 249   ✦ Protein: 14 g   ✦ Cholesterol: 29 mg
✦ Sodium: 292 mg   ✦ Fat, total: 8 g   ✦ Carbohydrates: 30 g
✦ Fiber: 2 g   ✦ Fat, saturated: 3 g

Grains and Legumes

Wild Rice, Snow Peas and Almond Casserole

2 tsp	margarine	10 mL
1/2 cup	chopped onion	125 mL
1 tsp	crushed garlic	5 mL
1/2 cup	wild rice	125 mL
1/2 cup	white rice	125 mL
3 1/4 cups	chicken stock	800 mL
3/4 cup	chopped snow peas	175 mL
1/4 cup	diced sweet red pepper	50 mL
1/4 cup	toasted sliced almonds	50 mL
1 tbsp	grated Parmesan cheese	15 mL

Toast almonds in small skillet on top of stove or in 400°F (200°C) oven for 2 minutes.

When using margarine, choose a soft (non-hydrogenated) version.

Serves 4

1. In large nonstick saucepan, melt margarine; sauté onion and garlic until softened. Add wild and white rice; stir for 2 minutes.
2. Add stock; reduce heat, cover and simmer just until rice is tender and liquid is absorbed, 30 to 40 minutes.
3. Add snow peas, red pepper and almonds; cook for 2 minutes. Place in serving bowl and sprinkle with cheese.

Make Ahead

✦ If serving cold, prepare early in day and stir just prior to serving.

Nutritional Analysis (Per Serving)
✦ Calories: 305   ✦ Protein: 13 g   ✦ Cholesterol: 1 mg
✦ Sodium: 1425 mg ✦ Fat: 8 g   ✦ Carbohydrates: 43 g
✦ Fiber: 3 g

Wild Rice with Feta Cheese Dressing

3 cups	chicken stock or water	750 mL
1/2 cup	wild rice	125 mL
1/2 cup	white rice	125 mL
3	medium asparagus, chopped	3
1/2 cup	chopped broccoli	125 mL
1	stalk celery, chopped	1
1/3 cup	chopped carrot	75 mL
2	green onions, chopped	2
1/2 cup	chopped sweet red or green pepper	125 mL
3/4 cup	chopped tomato	175 mL

Dressing

1/2 tsp	crushed garlic	2 mL
1 tbsp	lemon juice	15 mL
1 1/2 tsp	red wine vinegar	7 mL
3 tbsp	crumbled feta cheese	45 mL
3/4 tsp	dried oregano (or 1 tbsp/15 mL chopped fresh)	4 mL
3 tbsp	olive oil	45 mL

Serves 4 to 6

1. In saucepan, bring stock to boil; add wild and white rice and reduce heat. Cover and simmer for 25 to 30 minutes or until just tender. Drain, rinse with cold water and place in serving bowl.
2. Blanch asparagus and broccoli in boiling water until still crisp. Drain and rinse with cold water. Add to bowl along with celery, carrot, green onions, red pepper and tomato; mix well.
3. *Dressing:* In small bowl, whisk together garlic, lemon juice, vinegar, cheese, oregano and oil until well combined. Pour over rice mixture and mix well. Serve at room temperature or chilled.

Make Ahead

✦ Make early in the day and stir well before serving.

Nutritional Analysis (Per Serving)
✦ Calories: 224   ✦ Protein: 7 g   ✦ Cholesterol: 4 mg
✦ Sodium: 809 mg ✦ Fat: 9 g   ✦ Carbohydrates: 29 g
✦ Fiber: 2 g

Wild Rice with Sautéed Oriental Vegetables

1 tbsp	margarine	15 mL
½ cup	chopped onion	125 mL
1 tsp	crushed garlic	5 mL
⅓ cup	wild rice	75 mL
⅓ cup	white rice	75 mL
1¾ cups	chicken stock	425 mL
½ cup	chopped broccoli	125 mL
½ cup	chopped sweet red pepper	125 mL
1 cup	snow peas, cut in half	250 mL
2 tbsp	chicken stock	25 mL
2½ tsp	soya sauce	12 mL
2 tbsp	sliced almonds, toasted	25 mL
¼ cup	chopped green onions	50 mL

When using margarine, choose a soft (non-hydrogenated) version to limit consumption of trans fats.

1. In medium nonstick saucepan, melt half of the margarine; sauté onion and garlic for 3 minutes or until softened. Add wild and white rice; sauté just until golden, approximately 3 minutes.

2. Add 1¾ cups (425mL) stock; cover and simmer for approximately 40 minutes or just until rice is tender and liquid absorbed, adding more stock if mixture dries out too quickly. Place in serving bowl.

3. In large nonstick skillet, melt remaining margarine; sauté broccoli, red pepper and snow peas just until tender-crisp. Add remaining 2 tbsp (25 mL) stock and soya sauce; cook for 1 minute. Pour over rice and mix well. Sprinkle with almonds and green onions.

Tips

✦ Although wild rice is expensive, it's worth every penny if the occasion is right.

✦ Asparagus and yellow pepper are good substitutes for the broccoli and red pepper.

✦ Serve warm or cold.

✦ Toast almonds in skillet on top of stove until brown or in 400°F (200°C) oven for 2 minutes.

Make Ahead

✦ If serving cold, refrigerate until chilled and stir just before serving. Add almonds and green onions at last minute.

Nutritional Analysis (Per Serving)
✦ Calories: 217 ✦ Protein: 8 g ✦ Cholesterol: 0 mg
✦ Sodium: 980 mg ✦ Fat: 6 g ✦ Carbohydrates: 32 g
✦ Fiber: 3 g

Rice with Pine Nuts and Spinach

3½ cups	fresh spinach	875 mL
1 tbsp	vegetable oil	15 mL
⅓ cup	chopped onion	75 mL
1 cup	rice	250 mL
3 cups	chicken stock	750 mL
1½ tsp	margarine	7 mL
¼ cup	grated Parmesan cheese	50 mL
2 tbsp	toasted pine nuts	25 mL

Freshly grated Parmesan cheese will make this dish outstanding.

Toast nuts in skillet on top of stove just until browned or in 400°F (200°C) oven for 2 minutes.

When using margarine, choose a soft (non-hydrogenated) version to limit consumption of trans fats.

Serves 4 to 6

1. Rinse spinach under cold water and shake off excess water. With just the water clinging to leaves, cook spinach just until wilted. Drain well and squeeze out moisture; chop and set aside.

2. In medium nonstick saucepan, heat oil; sauté onion for 3 minutes. Add rice; sauté until browned, approximately 3 minutes. Add stock; cover and simmer for 15 to 20 minutes or until rice is tender and liquid absorbed.

3. Add spinach, margarine, cheese and pine nuts; mix well.

Make Ahead

✦ Make and refrigerate up to a day in advance, then reheat over low heat.

Nutritional Analysis (Per Serving)
✦ Calories: 210 ✦ Protein: 7 g ✦ Cholesterol: 3 mg
✦ Sodium: 852 mg ✦ Fat: 7 g ✦ Carbohydrates: 29 g
✦ Fiber: 2 g

Spicy Rice with Feta Cheese and Black Olives

1 tbsp	vegetable oil	15 mL
2 tsp	crushed garlic	10 mL
½ cup	chopped onion	125 mL
½ cup	chopped zucchini	125 mL
¼ cup	chopped sweet red pepper	50 mL
1 cup	rice	250 mL
1½ cups	chicken stock	375 mL
1 tsp	dried oregano	5 mL
1 tsp	dried basil	5 mL
1 tsp	chili powder	5 mL
¼ cup	sliced pitted black olives	50 mL
2 oz	feta cheese, crumbled	50 g

Instead of zucchini, try chopped broccoli. Try goat cheese instead of feta for a change.

Serves 4

1. In large nonstick saucepan, heat oil; sauté garlic, onion, zucchini and red pepper until softened, approximately 5 minutes. Add rice and brown for 2 minutes, stirring constantly.

2. Add stock, oregano, basil, chili powder and olives; cover and simmer for approximately 20 minutes or until rice is tender. Pour into serving dish and sprinkle with cheese.

Tip

✦ This can be served either warm or cold.

Make Ahead

✦ Prepare and refrigerate early in day. Reheat gently until just warm. If serving cold, stir well before serving.

Nutritional Analysis (Per Serving)
✦ Calories: 291 ✦ Protein: 8 g ✦ Cholesterol: 12 mg
✦ Sodium: 1067 mg ✦ Fat: 8 g ✦ Carbohydrates: 44 g
✦ Fiber: 2 g

Sautéed Rice with Almonds, Curry and Ginger

1 tbsp	vegetable oil	15 mL
1 tsp	crushed garlic	5 mL
1½ cups	thinly sliced bok choy or nappa cabbage	375 mL
1 cup	snow peas	250 mL
½ cup	chopped sweet red pepper	125 mL
⅓ cup	chopped carrot	75 mL
1 tsp	ground ginger	5 mL
1 tsp	curry powder	5 mL
¾ cup	chicken stock	175 mL
4 tsp	soya sauce	20 mL
1	egg	1
2 cups	cooked rice	500 mL
2 tbsp	toasted chopped almonds (see tip, page 212)	25 mL
2 tbsp	chopped green onion	25 mL

Serves 4

1. In large nonstick skillet, heat oil; sauté garlic, cabbage, snow peas, red pepper and carrot for 3 minutes or just until tender, stirring constantly. Add ginger, curry powder, stock and soya sauce; cook for 1 minute.
2. Add egg and rice; cook for 1 minute or until egg is well incorporated. Place in serving dish and sprinkle with almonds and green onions.

Make Ahead

✦ Prepare and refrigerate early in day. Just prior to serving, reheat on low heat.

Nutritional Analysis (Per Serving)
✦ Calories: 248 ✦ Protein: 8 g ✦ Cholesterol: 53 mg
✦ Sodium: 950 mg ✦ Fat: 8 g ✦ Carbohydrates: 36 g
✦ Fiber: 3 g

Vegetable Hoisin Fried Rice

1 cup	white rice	250 mL
¼ cup	chicken stock	50 mL
2 tbsp	soya sauce	25 mL
2 tbsp	hoisin sauce	25 mL
½ cup	chopped carrots	125 mL
1 tbsp	vegetable oil	15 mL
1 tsp	minced garlic	5 mL
1 tsp	minced gingerroot	5 mL
¾ cup	chopped red peppers	175 mL
¾ cup	chopped snow peas	175 mL
2	green onions, chopped	2

Serves 4

1. Bring 2 cups (500 mL) water to a boil in a saucepan; stir in rice, cover, reduce heat to medium and cook for 20 minutes or until liquid is absorbed. Remove from heat.
2. In small bowl, whisk together stock, soya sauce and hoisin sauce; set aside.
3. Cook carrots in boiling water or microwave for 4 minutes or until tender-crisp. Drain. Heat oil in wok or skillet over high heat. Add garlic, ginger, red peppers, snow peas and carrots; cook, stirring, for 2 minutes. Add rice; cook, stirring, 2 minutes longer. Add hoisin-soya mixture and cook for 1 minute longer. Serve garnished with green onions.

Make Ahead

✦ Prepare early in the day and gently reheat before serving.

Nutritional Analysis (Per Serving)
✦ Calories: 261 ✦ Protein: 5 g ✦ Cholesterol: 0 mg
✦ Sodium: 578 mg ✦ Fat, total: 4 g ✦ Carbohydrates: 50 g
✦ Fiber: 2 g ✦ Fat, saturated: 0.4 g

Zucchini Stuffed with Rice and Mushrooms

3 cups	Basic Vegetable Stock (see recipe, page 52)	750 mL
½ cup	wild rice	125 mL
2	large zucchini (each about 8 oz/250 g)	2
1 tsp	vegetable oil	5 mL
2 tsp	minced garlic	10 mL
¾ cup	chopped onions	175 mL
2 cups	sliced mushrooms	500 mL
1½ tsp	drained capers	7 mL
1 tsp	dried basil	5 mL
½ tsp	dried oregano	2 mL
¾ cup	prepared tomato pasta sauce	175 mL
3 tbsp	grated Parmesan cheese (optional)	45 mL

> *Wild rice is expensive, so you may want to use it only for special meals — or use less by combining it with white rice, brown rice or mixed greens.*

Serves 4 as a side dish
Preheat oven to 350°F (180°C)
13- by 9-inch (3 L) baking dish sprayed with vegetable spray

1. In a small saucepan, bring stock to a boil; stir in rice, cover, reduce heat to low and cook 35 to 40 minutes or until rice is tender. Drain excess liquid.

2. Meanwhile, cut each zucchini in half lengthwise. In a large pot of boiling water, cook zucchini 4 minutes; drain. When cool enough to handle, carefully scoop out pulp, leaving shells intact. Chop pulp and set aside. Put zucchini shells into prepared baking dish.

3. In a large nonstick frying pan sprayed with vegetable spray, heat oil over medium-high heat. Add garlic and onions; cook 3 minutes or until softened. Stir in mushrooms, capers, basil and oregano; cook 5 minutes or until mushrooms are browned. Stir in zucchini pulp; cook 2 minutes. Remove from heat.

4. Stir cooked rice, tomato sauce and 1 tbsp (15 mL) of the Parmesan cheese, if desired, into vegetable mixture. Stuff mixture evenly into zucchini boats, mounding filling high. Sprinkle with remaining Parmesan, if desired. Cover dish tightly with foil.

5. Bake 15 minutes or until heated through.

Tips

+ Wild rice can be replaced with brown or white rice or a combination. Cook white rice for only 15 to 20 minutes; allow 35 minutes for brown rice.

+ For a spicier version of this dish, try adding ½ tsp (2 mL) chili powder

Make Ahead

+ Prepare up to 1 day in advance and bake just before serving.

Nutritional Analysis (Per Serving)
+ Calories: 135
+ Protein: 6 g
+ Cholesterol: 0 mg
+ Sodium: 404 mg
+ Fat, total: 2 g
+ Carbohydrates: 27 g
+ Fiber: 5 g
+ Fat, saturated: 0.2 g

Rice Cakes with Tomato Purée (page 217) ➤
Overleaf: Potato Crust Pesto Pizza (page 195)

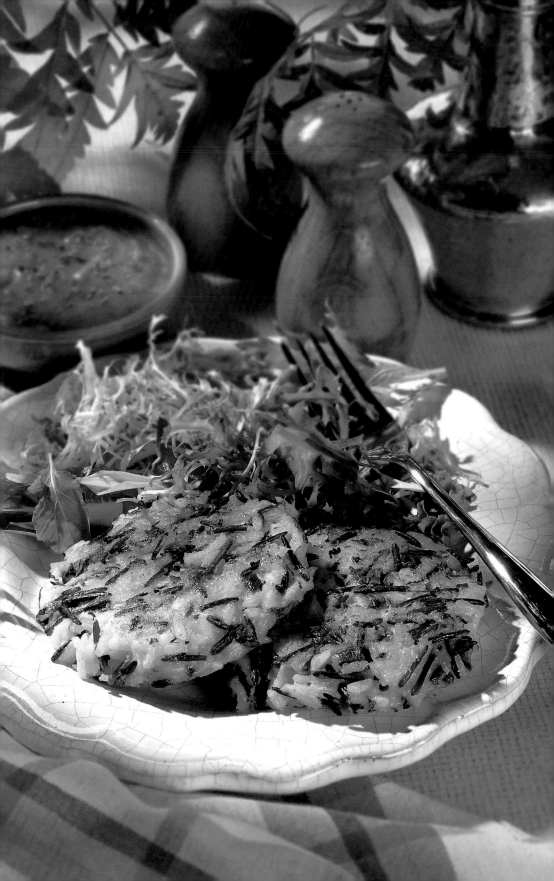

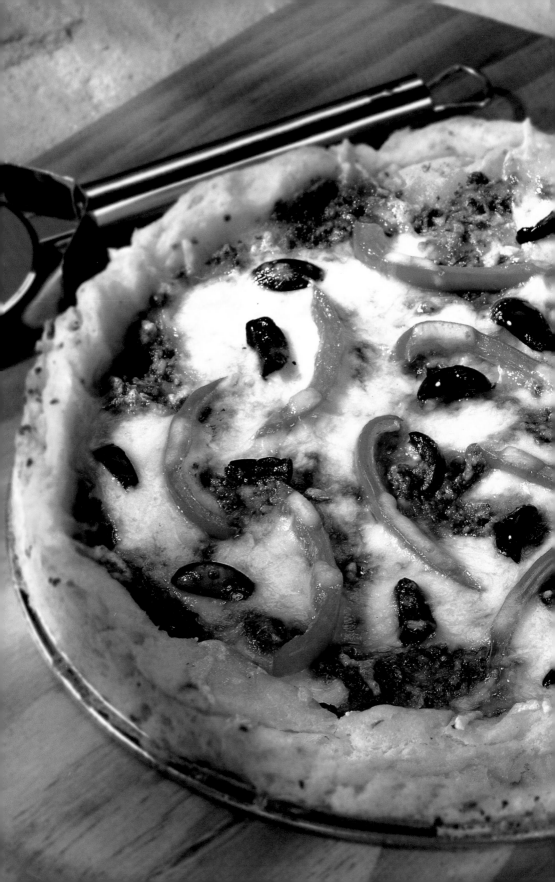

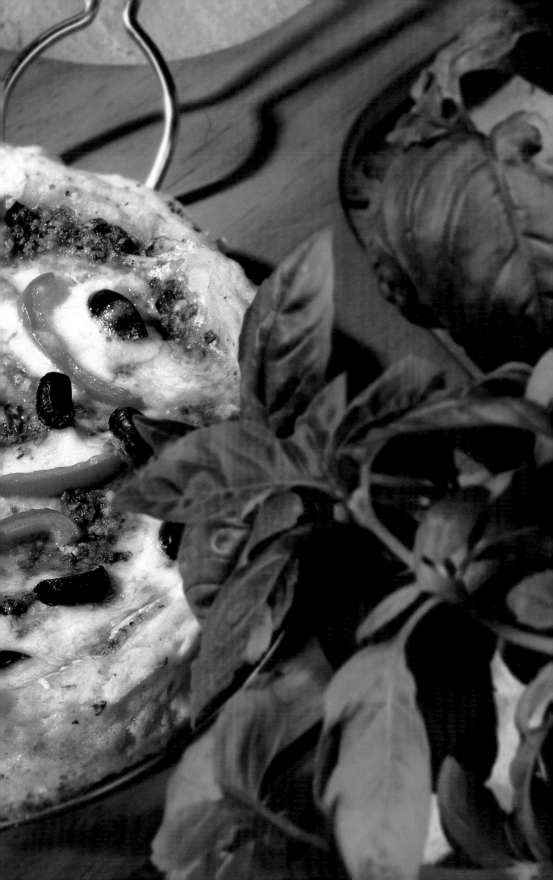

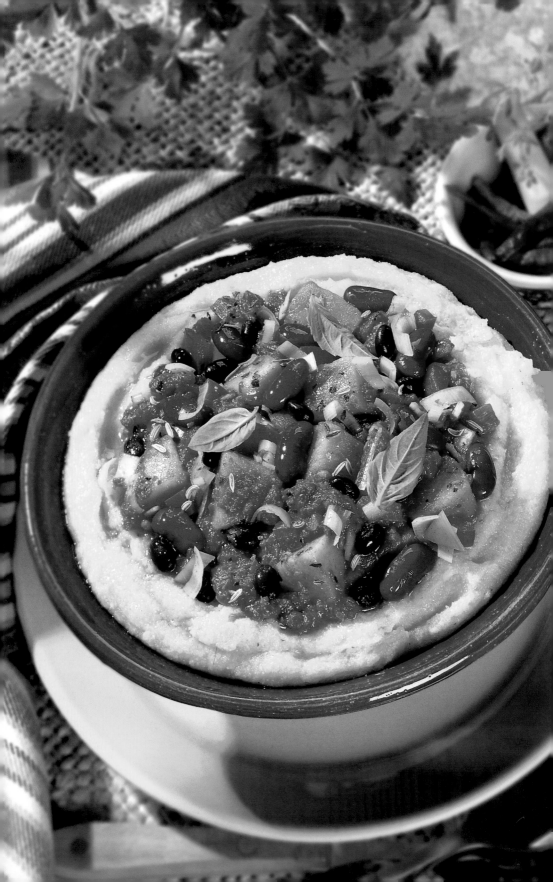

Rice Cakes with Tomato Purée

Rice Cakes

4 cups	Basic Vegetable Stock (see recipe, page 52)	1 L
½ cup	wild rice	125 mL
½ cup	white rice	125 mL
1 tsp	minced garlic	5 mL
½ cup	shredded part-skim mozzarella cheese (about 2 oz/50 g)	125 mL
¼ cup	shredded Swiss cheese (about ½ oz/15 g)	50 mL
¼ cup	chopped green onions	50 mL
2 tbsp	grated Parmesan cheese	25 mL
1 tsp	dried basil	5 mL
1	egg	1
2	egg whites	2

Sauce

½ cup	prepared tomato pasta sauce	125 mL
2 tbsp	2% milk	25 mL
¼ tsp	dried basil	1 mL

Makes 10 cakes
Preheat oven to 425°F (220°C)
Baking sheet sprayed with vegetable spray

1. In a saucepan bring stock to a boil; stir in wild rice and white rice; cover, reduce heat to medium-low and cook 35 minutes or until rice is tender. Let rice cool slightly. Drain any excess liquid. Rinse with cold water.

2. In a bowl stir together cooled rice, garlic, mozzarella, Swiss, green onions, Parmesan, basil, whole egg and egg whites until well mixed. Using a ¼ cup (50 mL) measure, form mixture into 10 patties.

3. Place on prepared baking sheet. Bake approximately 10 minutes per side until browned.

4. Meanwhile, in a small saucepan, heat tomato sauce, milk and basil. Serve with rice cakes.

Tips

✦ Serve these with soup and salad for an excellent complete meal. Or serve as a side dish.

✦ These cakes can also be sautéed in a nonstick skillet sprayed with vegetable spray.

✦ Try brown rice. Cook 35 minutes or until tender, adding more stock if necessary.

Make Ahead

✦ Prepare cakes up to 1 day in advance; keep refrigerated until ready to bake.

Nutritional Analysis (Per Serving)

✦ Calories: 114 ✦ Protein: 6 g ✦ Cholesterol: 27 mg
✦ Sodium: 149 mg ✦ Fat, total: 3 g ✦ Carbohydrates: 16 g
✦ Fiber: 1 g ✦ Fat, saturated: 1 g

◄ Bean and Sweet Potato Chili on Garlic Polenta (page 231)

Spicy Rice, Bean and Lentil Casserole

2 tsp	vegetable oil	10 mL
2 tsp	minced garlic	10 mL
1 cup	chopped onions	250 mL
3/4 cup	chopped green peppers	175 mL
3 3/4 cups	Basic Vegetable Stock (see recipe, page 52)	950 mL
3/4 cup	brown rice	175 mL
1/2 cup	green lentils	125 mL
1 tsp	dried basil	5 mL
1 tsp	chili powder	5 mL
1	can (19 oz/540 mL) red kidney beans, rinsed and drained	1
1 cup	canned or frozen corn kernels, drained	250 mL
1 cup	medium salsa	250 mL

An excellent total meal for vegetarians!

1. In a nonstick saucepan, heat oil over medium-high heat. Add garlic, onions and green peppers; cook 3 minutes. Stir in stock, brown rice, lentils, basil and chili powder; bring to a boil, cover, reduce heat to medium-low and cook 30 to 40 minutes, stirring occasionally, until rice and lentils are tender and liquid is absorbed.

2. Stir in beans, corn and salsa; cover and cook 5 minutes or until heated through.

Tips

✦ Instead of lentils, substitute green or yellow split peas.

✦ Grilled or barbecued corn is excellent in this dish.

✦ Any type of bean can replace the red kidney beans.

✦ This dish is a great source of fiber.

Make Ahead

✦ Prepare up to 2 days in advance and reheat gently.

Nutritional Analysis (Per Serving)

✦ Calories: 278 ✦ Protein: 14 g ✦ Cholesterol: 0 mg
✦ Sodium: 361 mg ✦ Fat, total: 3 g ✦ Carbohydrates: 52 g
✦ Fiber: 9 g ✦ Fat, saturated: 0.4 g

Curried Squash Risotto with Apricots and Dates

1 tsp	vegetable oil	5 mL
2 tsp	minced garlic	10 mL
3/4 cup	chopped onions	175 mL
1 1/2 tsp	curry powder	7 mL
3/4 cup	wild rice	175 mL
3/4 cup	white rice	175 mL
3 1/2 cups	Basic Vegetable Stock (see recipe, page 52)	875 mL
1 cup	diced butternut squash	250 mL
1/3 cup	chopped dried apricots	75 mL
1/3 cup	chopped dates	75 mL

> *True risotto requires that you add hot liquid in small amounts, stirring constantly until absorbed. Use this technique (if you have time) for a creamier texture. (Keep in mind that you'll also need to add a larger quantity of stock.)*

Serves 4 to 6

1. In a nonstick saucepan sprayed with vegetable spray, heat oil over medium heat. Add garlic, onions and curry powder; cook 4 minutes or until softened. Add wild rice and white rice; cook, stirring, 2 minutes.

2. Add the stock; bring to a boil. Reduce heat to low, cover and cook 20 minutes. Stir in squash. Increase heat to medium; cover and cook another 10 minutes or until liquid is absorbed and rice and squash are tender.

3. Stir in apricots and dates. Let stand, covered, 10 minutes before serving.

Tips

+ Try any dried fruit in place of apricots and dates.
+ Try replacing squash with diced sweet potatoes.
+ Try brown rice instead of white; cook the rice separately in stock until tender, about 40 minutes.

Make Ahead

+ Prepare up to 1 day in advance. Reheat gently.

Nutritional Analysis (Per Serving)

+ Calories: 223
+ Protein: 6 g
+ Cholesterol: 0 mg
+ Sodium: 10 mg
+ Fat, total: 1 g
+ Carbohydrates: 49 g
+ Fiber: 3 g
+ Fat, saturated: 0.1 g

Feta Grain Burgers with Dijon Sauce

3 cups	vegetable or chicken stock	750 mL
1/3 cup	pearl barley	75 mL
1/3 cup	brown rice	75 mL
1/3 cup	wild rice	75 mL
1/2 cup	diced mushrooms	125 mL
1/2 cup	diced red bell peppers	125 mL
1/2 cup	diced red onions	125 mL
1 tsp	minced garlic	5 mL
1/4 cup	dry seasoned bread crumbs	50 mL
2 oz	light feta cheese, crumbled	50 g
1 tbsp	fresh lemon juice	15 mL
1 tsp	dried oregano	5 mL
1	large egg	1
1	large egg white	1
Sauce		
1/3 cup	low-fat sour cream	75 mL
2 tsp	Dijon mustard	10 mL

Makes about 7 burgers
Preheat oven to 425°F (220°C)
Baking sheet sprayed with vegetable spray

1. In a saucepan over medium-high heat, bring stock to a boil. Add barley, brown rice and wild rice; reduce heat to medium-low. Cook, covered and stirring occasionally, for 45 minutes or until grains are tender and liquid is absorbed.

2. Meanwhile, in a nonstick frying pan sprayed with vegetable spray, cook mushrooms, red peppers, red onions and garlic over medium-high heat for 5 minutes or until tender. In a bowl combine vegetables and grains.

3. In a food processor combine grain mixture, bread crumbs, feta cheese, lemon juice, oregano, egg and egg white; pulse on and off just until combined.

4. Using wet hands, form each 1/2 cup (125 mL) of mixture into a patty (makes about 7 patties). Transfer to prepared baking sheet. Bake in preheated oven, turning halfway, for 15 minutes or until golden and heated through.

5. In a bowl combine sour cream and mustard; add a dollop of sauce to each burger. Serve.

Tip

✦ The secret to these burgers is in the combination of barley, brown rice and wild rice. Try them in a pita, loaded with tomatoes, onions, lettuce and alfalfa sprouts and drizzled with sauce.

Complementary proteins: *A diet that includes meat, chicken and milk provides "complete proteins," since these foods have all the amino acids the body requires. But this is not the case for vegetarian diets, since plant foods (including beans, grains and vegetables) are missing one or more of these essential amino acids (thus providing "incomplete proteins"). At one time, it was believed that vegetarians had to combine grains with beans at the same meal to "complete" the protein. We now know that this is not necessary. As long as vegetarians eat a variety of protein foods throughout the day, they'll meet their amino acid requirements.*

Nutritional Analysis (Per Serving)

✦ Calories: 295   ✦ Protein: 13 g   ✦ Cholesterol: 74 mg
✦ Sodium: 263 mg   ✦ Fat, total: 8 g   ✦ Carbohydrates: 44 g
✦ Fiber: 5 g   ✦ Fat, saturated: 4.2 g

Chickpea Tofu Burgers with Coriander Mayonnaise

1 cup	canned chickpeas, rinsed and drained	250 mL
8 oz	firm tofu	250 g
1/3 cup	dry bread crumbs	75 mL
2 tbsp	tahini	25 mL
1 1/2 tbsp	freshly squeezed lemon juice	20 mL
1 tsp	minced garlic	5 mL
1	egg	1
1/4 tsp	freshly ground black pepper	1 mL
1/4 tsp	salt	1 mL
1/3 cup	chopped fresh coriander	75 mL
1/4 cup	chopped green onions	50 mL
1/4 cup	chopped red bell peppers	50 mL

Sauce

1/4 cup	2% plain yogurt	50 mL
1/4 cup	light sour cream	50 mL
1/4 cup	chopped fresh coriander	50 mL
1 tbsp	light mayonnaise	15 mL
1/2 tsp	minced garlic	2 mL

Soy protein and heart health:
If your blood cholesterol is high, consider adding soy foods — such as tofu, texturized soy protein, soy beverages and soy flour — to your diet. Diets low in saturated fat and cholesterol that include 25 g of soy protein a day may reduce the risk of heart disease. Soy's protective power comes from natural chemicals called isoflavones, which are found inside soybeans.

Serves 4 to 5
Preheat oven to 425°F (220°C)
Baking sheet sprayed with vegetable spray

1. In a food processor, combine chickpeas, tofu, bread crumbs, tahini, lemon juice, garlic, egg, pepper and salt; process until smooth. Add coriander, green onions and red peppers; pulse on and off until well-mixed. With wet hands, scoop up 1/4 cup (50 mL) of mixture and form into a patty. Put on prepared baking sheet. Repeat procedure for remaining patties. Bake 20 minutes, turning burgers at halfway point.

2. Meanwhile, make the sauce: In a small bowl, stir together yogurt, sour cream, coriander, mayonnaise and garlic; set aside.

3. Serve burgers hot with sauce on side.

Tips

✦ Serve in pita breads or on rolls, with lettuce, tomatoes and onions.

✦ Tofu is found in the vegetable section of your grocery store. If desired, it can be replaced with 5% ricotta cheese.

✦ Tahini is a sesame paste, usually found in the international section of your grocery store. If unavailable, try peanut butter.

✦ The combination of chickpeas and tofu gives a rich texture to these unusual burgers.

Make Ahead

✦ Prepare patties and sauce up to 1 day advance. Bake just before serving.

Nutritional Analysis (Per Serving)
✦ Calories: 226 ✦ Protein: 15 g ✦ Cholesterol: 44 mg
✦ Sodium: 280 mg ✦ Fat, total: 10 g ✦ Carbohydrates: 21 g
✦ Fiber: 3 g ✦ Fat, saturated: 2 g

Falafel Burgers with Creamy Sesame Sauce

2 cups	drained canned chickpeas	500 mL
1/4 cup	chopped green onions	50 mL
1/4 cup	chopped fresh coriander	50 mL
1/4 cup	finely chopped carrots	50 mL
1/4 cup	bread crumbs	50 mL
3 tbsp	lemon juice	45 mL
3 tbsp	water	45 mL
2 tbsp	tahini (puréed sesame seeds)	25 mL
2 tsp	minced garlic	10 mL
1/4 tsp	ground black pepper	1 mL
2 tsp	vegetable oil	10 mL

Sauce

1/4 cup	light sour cream	50 mL
2 tbsp	tahini	25 mL
2 tbsp	chopped fresh coriander	25 mL
2 tbsp	water	25 mL
2 tsp	lemon juice	10 mL
1/2 tsp	minced garlic	2 mL

Tahini is used in Middle Eastern cooking. Its texture is very much like peanut butter — in fact, peanut butter or any nut butter can be used as a replacement. You can usually find tahini in health food stores, Middle Eastern groceries or in the specialty section of larger supermarkets.

Serves 4

1. Put chickpeas, green onions, coriander, carrots, bread crumbs, lemon juice, water, tahini, garlic and black pepper in food processor; pulse on and off until finely chopped. With wet hands, form each 1/4 cup (50 mL) into a patty.

2. In small bowl, whisk together sour cream, tahini, coriander, water, lemon juice and garlic.

3. In nonstick skillet sprayed with vegetable spray, heat 1 tsp (5 mL) of oil over medium heat. Add 4 patties and cook for 3 1/2 minutes or until golden; turn and cook 3 1/2 minutes longer or until golden and hot inside. Remove from pan. Heat remaining 1 tsp (5 mL) oil and cook remaining patties. Serve with sesame sauce.

Tip

✦ Replace coriander with dill or parsley.

Make Ahead

✦ Prepare burgers early in the day and refrigerate until ready to cook. Prepare sauce to up a day ahead.

Nutritional Analysis (Per Serving)
✦ Calories: 285   ✦ Protein: 12 g   ✦ Cholesterol: 5 mg
✦ Sodium: 276 mg   ✦ Fat, total: 12 g   ✦ Carbohydrates: 35 g
✦ Fiber: 7 g   ✦ Fat, saturated: 2 g

Falafel with Tahini Lemon Dressing

1	can (19 oz/540 mL) chickpeas, rinsed and drained	540 mL
1/4 cup	chopped green onions	50 mL
1/4 cup	chopped fresh coriander	50 mL
1/4 cup	bread crumbs	50 mL
2 tbsp	tahini	25 mL
1 tbsp	freshly squeezed lemon juice	15 mL
1 1/2 tsp	minced garlic	7 mL
1/4 tsp	baking powder	1 mL
1/4 tsp	ground cumin	1 mL
1	egg	1
	Freshly ground black pepper, to taste	
4	small pita breads	4
Half	recipe Creamy Tahini Lemon Dressing (see recipe, below)	Half

Garnish (optional)

Tomato slices

Lettuce leaves

Serves 4 to 6
Preheat oven to 400°F (200°C)
Baking sheet sprayed with vegetable spray

1. In a food processor, combine chickpeas, green onions, coriander, bread crumbs, tahini, lemon juice, garlic, baking powder, cumin, egg and pepper. Pulse on and off until well-mixed. Form into 16 balls of 2 tbsp (25 mL) each; flatten slightly. Put on prepared baking sheet.
2. Bake chickpea balls 20 minutes, turning at halfway point, or until golden.
3. Serve in pita breads with Creamy Tahini Lemon Dressing and, if desired, tomato slices and lettuce.

Tip

✦ *Nutritional note:* Values given below are for each of 6 servings, with each serving accompanied by 2 tsp (10 mL) dressing.

Nutritional Analysis (Per Serving)
✦ Calories: 264 ✦ Protein: 11 g ✦ Cholesterol: 36 mg
✦ Sodium: 415 mg ✦ Fat, total: 6 g ✦ Carbohydrates: 41 g
✦ Fiber: 5 g ✦ Fat, saturated: 1 g

Creamy Tahini Lemon Dressing

1/3 cup	Basic Vegetable Stock (see recipe, page 52)	75 mL
1/3 cup	5% ricotta or 2% cottage cheese	75 mL
2 tbsp	tahini	25 mL
2 tbsp	light mayonnaise	25 mL
2 tbsp	olive oil	25 mL
1 tbsp	freshly squeezed lemon juice	15 mL
1 tbsp	soya sauce	15 mL
1 tsp	minced garlic	5 mL
1/4 cup	chopped fresh coriander	50 mL

Makes 1 cup (250 mL)

1. In a food processor combine stock, ricotta, tahini, mayonnaise, olive oil, lemon juice, soya sauce and garlic; process until smooth. Stir in coriander.

Tips

✦ Toss a combination of cooked beans together and use this as a dressing.

✦ If tahini is not available, substitute creamy peanut butter.

Make Ahead

✦ Prepare up to 2 days in advance. Stir well before using.

Nutritional Analysis (Per Tablespoon/15 mL)
✦ Calories: 33 ✦ Protein: 1 g ✦ Cholesterol: 1 mg
✦ Sodium: 84 mg ✦ Fat, total: 3 g ✦ Carbohydrates: 1 g
✦ Fiber: 0 g ✦ Fat, saturated: 1 g

Couscous Salad with Tomatoes, Feta Cheese and Olives

1³/₄ cups	chicken stock	425 mL
1¹/₄ cups	couscous	300 mL
2 cups	chopped tomatoes	500 mL
³/₄ cup	chopped cucumbers	175 mL
³/₄ cup	chopped red or green peppers	175 mL
¹/₂ cup	crumbled feta cheese	125 mL
¹/₃ cup	sliced red onions	75 mL
¹/₃ cup	sliced black olives	75 mL
¹/₄ cup	chopped green onions (about 2 medium)	50 mL
¹/₂ cup	chopped fresh parsley (or 1 tbsp/15 mL dried)	125 mL
¹/₂ cup	chopped fresh basil (or 1 tbsp/15 mL dried)	125 mL

Dressing

3 tbsp	lemon juice	45 mL
2 tbsp	vegetable oil	25 mL
2 tsp	minced garlic	10 mL
¹/₄ tsp	ground black pepper	1 mL

Serves 4 to 6

1. Bring stock to boil in a saucepan. Add couscous and stir; cover and remove from heat. Let stand for 5 minutes.
2. In large serving bowl, combine tomatoes, cucumbers, red peppers, feta cheese, onions, olives, green onions, parsley and basil.
3. In small bowl, whisk together lemon juice, oil, garlic and pepper. Add to bowl along with couscous and toss.

Make Ahead

✦ Prepare entire salad early in the day and toss well before serving.

Nutritional Analysis (Per Serving)
✦ Calories: 283 ✦ Protein: 10 g ✦ Cholesterol: 20 mg
✦ Sodium: 603 mg ✦ Fat, total: 10 g ✦ Carbohydrates: 39 g
✦ Fiber: 2 g ✦ Fat, saturated: 4 g

Couscous with Raisins, Dates and Curry

1¹/₄ cups	chicken stock	300 mL
³/₄ cup	couscous	175 mL
1 tbsp	margarine	15 mL
³/₄ cup	finely chopped onions	175 mL
1 tsp	crushed garlic	5 mL
1 cup	finely chopped sweet red pepper	250 mL
¹/₄ cup	raisins	50 mL
1 tsp	curry powder	5 mL
5	dried dates or apricots, chopped	5

Try adding ¹/₄ cup (50 mL) diced carrots to vegetables. Bulger can replace couscous.

When using margarine, choose a soft (non-hydrogenated) version to limit consumption of trans fats.

Serves 4

1. In small saucepan, bring chicken stock to boil. Stir in couscous and remove from heat. Cover and let stand until liquid is absorbed, 5 to 8 minutes. Place in serving bowl.
2. Meanwhile, in nonstick saucepan, melt margarine; sauté onions, garlic and red pepper until softened, approximately 5 minutes. Add raisins, curry powder and dates; mix until combined. Add to couscous and mix well.

Make Ahead

✦ Prepare up to the day before, then gently reheat over low heat.

Nutritional Analysis (Per Serving)
✦ Calories: 243 ✦ Protein: 6 g ✦ Cholesterol: 0 mg
✦ Sodium: 239 mg ✦ Fat: 3 g ✦ Carbohydrates: 47 g
✦ Fiber: 3 g

Curried Couscous with Tomatoes and Chickpeas

2 cups	Basic Vegetable Stock (see recipe, page 52)	500 mL
1½ cups	couscous	375 mL
1 tsp	vegetable oil	5 mL
3 cups	chopped plum tomatoes	750 mL
½ cup	Basic Vegetable Stock	125 mL
2 tsp	curry powder	10 mL
2 tsp	minced garlic	10 mL
2 cups	canned chickpeas, rinsed and drained	500 mL
¾ cup	chopped fresh coriander	175 mL
½ cup	chopped green onions	125 mL

Couscous is available in the rice section of grocery stores.

Serves 4 to 6

1. In a saucepan bring stock to a boil; stir in couscous, cover and remove from heat. Let stand 5 minutes; transfer to a serving bowl.
2. Meanwhile, in a large nonstick saucepan, heat oil over medium-high heat. Add tomatoes, stock, curry and garlic; cook, stirring, 5 minutes or until tomatoes begin to break up. Stir in chickpeas; cook 2 minutes or until heated through. Add to couscous along with coriander and green onions; toss to combine. Serve immediately.

Tip
✦ Great source of nutrition for vegetarians.

Make Ahead
✦ Prepare up to 2 days in advance. Reheat gently.

Nutritional Analysis (Per Serving)
✦ Calories: 309 ✦ Protein: 12 g ✦ Cholesterol: 0 mg
✦ Sodium: 154 mg ✦ Fat, total: 3 g ✦ Carbohydrates: 59 g
✦ Fiber: 6 g ✦ Fat, saturated: 0.3 g

Barley with Sautéed Vegetables and Feta Cheese

1 tbsp	vegetable oil	15 mL
2 tsp	crushed garlic	10 mL
¾ cup	chopped sweet green pepper	175 mL
¾ cup	chopped mushrooms	175 mL
¾ cup	pot barley	175 mL
1½ cups	crushed canned tomatoes	375 mL
3 cups	chicken stock	750 mL
1½ tsp	dried basil (or 2 tbsp/25 mL chopped fresh)	7 mL
½ tsp	dried oregano	2 mL
3 oz	feta cheese, crumbled	75 g

Although barley is rarely used this way, this dish proves how wonderful it is with tomatoes and feta cheese.

Serves 5 to 6

1. In large nonstick saucepan, heat oil; sauté garlic, green pepper and mushrooms until softened, approximately 5 minutes. Add barley and sauté for 2 minutes, stirring constantly.
2. Add tomatoes, stock, basil and oregano; cover and simmer for approximately 30 minutes or until barley is tender. Pour into serving dish and sprinkle with cheese.

Make Ahead
✦ Make early in day and refrigerate; reheat on low to serve. Also delicious at room temperature.

Nutritional Analysis (Per Serving)
✦ Calories: 185 ✦ Protein: 8 g ✦ Cholesterol: 12 mg
✦ Sodium: 646 mg ✦ Fat: 6 g ✦ Carbohydrates: 25 g
✦ Fiber: 4 g

Barley, Tomato and Olive Casserole

1 tsp	vegetable oil	5 mL
2 tsp	minced garlic	10 mL
1 cup	chopped red peppers	250 mL
1 cup	chopped green peppers	250 mL
3 cups	chicken stock	750 mL
¾ cup	barley	175 mL
⅓ cup	sliced black olives	75 mL
1 tbsp	drained capers	15 mL
1½ tsp	dried basil	7 mL
¾ tsp	dried oregano	4 mL
1	dried bay leaf	1
1½ cups	chopped plum tomatoes	375 mL
¼ cup	chopped fresh coriander	50 mL
¼ cup	chopped green onions (about 2 medium)	50 mL

If plum tomatoes are not available, use field tomatoes — deseeded to eliminate excess liquid.

Serves 4 to 6

1. In large nonstick saucepan, heat oil over medium heat; add garlic and red and green peppers and cook for 5 minutes, or until softened. Add stock, barley, olives, capers, basil, oregano and bay leaf; bring to a boil and cover. Reduce heat to low and cook covered for 35 minutes or until barley is tender. Add tomatoes, coriander and green onions and cook for 5 minutes longer.

Tip

✦ If you don't like the taste of coriander (chinese parsley), substitute basil or dill.

Make Ahead

✦ Prepare early in the day and reheat gently before serving. Tastes great next day.

Nutritional Analysis (Per Serving)
✦ Calories: 140 ✦ Protein: 5 g ✦ Cholesterol: 0 mg
✦ Sodium: 761 mg ✦ Fat, total: 3 g ✦ Carbohydrates: 27 g
✦ Fiber: 6 g ✦ Fat, saturated: 0.4 g

Barley with Tomato, Red Onion, Goat Cheese and Basil

3 cups	vegetable or chicken stock	750 mL
¾ cup	pearl barley	175 mL
3 cups	chopped ripe plum tomatoes	750 mL
1 cup	chopped red onions	250 mL
¾ cup	chopped fresh basil (or ⅕ mL dried)	175 mL
2 oz	goat cheese, crumbled	50 g
Dressing		
1 tbsp	olive oil	15 mL
1 tbsp	fresh lemon juice	15 mL
1 tbsp	balsamic vinegar	15 mL
1 tsp	minced garlic	5 mL

Serves 4

1. In a saucepan over medium-high heat, bring stock to a boil. Add barley; reduce heat to medium-low. Cook, covered, for 45 minutes or until tender and liquid is absorbed. Transfer to a large serving bowl. Add tomatoes, red onions, basil and goat cheese; toss well.

2. In a bowl combine olive oil, lemon juice, balsamic vinegar and garlic. Pour over barley mixture; toss to coat well. Serve warm or at room temperature.

Nutritional Analysis (Per Serving)
✦ Calories: 253 ✦ Protein: 10 g ✦ Cholesterol: 9 mg
✦ Sodium: 270 mg ✦ Fat, total: 8 g ✦ Carbohydrates: 38 g
✦ Fiber: 9 g ✦ Fat, saturated: 3 g

Barley Cabbage Rolls in Tomato Basil Sauce

2½ cups	Basic Vegetable Stock (see recipe, page 52)	625 mL
½ cup	barley	125 mL
1	bay leaf	1
1½ tsp	dried basil	7 mL
1	large green cabbage	1
1 tsp	vegetable oil	5 mL
2 tsp	minced garlic	10 mL
½ cup	chopped onions	125 mL
½ cup	chopped green peppers	125 mL
1 cup	chopped plum tomatoes	250 mL
¼ cup	chopped black olives	50 mL
2 tsp	drained capers	10 mL
1	can (19 oz/540 mL) tomatoes	1
1 tbsp	packed brown sugar	15 mL
1 tbsp	tomato paste	15 mL
1 tsp	dried basil	5 mL

Makes 8 to 10

1. In a saucepan bring stock to a boil. Stir in barley, bay leaf and basil; cover, reduce heat to medium-low and cook 40 minutes or until barley is tender. Remove bay leaf.
2. Meanwhile, remove as much of cabbage core as possible. In a large pot of boiling water, cook cabbage 20 to 25 minutes. Drain. When cool enough to handle, separate leaves carefully.
3. In a nonstick frying pan, heat oil over medium-high heat. Add garlic, onions and green peppers; cook 4 minutes or until softened. Stir in tomatoes, black olives and capers. Cook 2 minutes or until tomatoes start to break up. Stir into cooked barley.
4. Put approximately ⅓ cup (75 mL) barley filling in center of cabbage leaf; fold in sides and roll up. Repeat with remaining filling.
5. In a food processor, purée tomatoes, sugar, tomato paste and basil. Transfer to a large saucepan. Bring tomato sauce to a boil; reduce heat to low and place cabbage rolls into simmering sauce. Cover and cook 1¼ hours, turning rolls over at halfway point.

Tips

+ Here's a fabulous variation of traditional cabbage rolls. The nutritious barley is well suited to a vegetarian diet.
+ Barley is available in "pearl" and "pot" varieties; whichever you use, cook until tender.
+ If you like extra sauce, double the tomato sauce recipe.

Make Ahead

+ Prepare filled rolls up to 2 days in advance.
+ Can be reheated.
+ Freeze up to 3 weeks

Nutritional Analysis (Per Serving)
+ Calories: 88
+ Protein: 3 g
+ Cholesterol: 0 mg
+ Sodium: 185 mg
+ Fat, total: 2 g
+ Carbohydrates: 17 g
+ Fiber: 4 g
+ Fat, saturated: 0.2 g

Barley Risotto with Grilled Peppers

1	medium red bell pepper	1
1	medium yellow bell pepper	1
3½ to 4 cups	vegetable or chicken stock	875 mL to 1 L
1 cup	pearl barley	250 mL
1 cup	chopped onions	250 mL
2 tsp	minced garlic	10 mL
3 tbsp	grated low-fat Parmesan cheese	45 mL
¼ tsp	freshly ground black pepper	1 mL

Serves 4
Preheat broiler
Baking sheet

1. Place red pepper and yellow pepper on baking sheet. Cook under preheated broiler, turning occasionally, for 20 minutes or until charred on all sides; remove from oven. When cool enough to handle, peel, stem and core peppers. Cut into chunks; set aside.

2. In a saucepan over medium-high heat, combine 2 cups (500 mL) stock with barley. Bring to a boil; reduce heat to low. Cook, stirring occasionally, for 30 minutes or until tender but firm. Set aside.

3. In a large nonstick frying pan sprayed with vegetable spray, cook onions and garlic over medium-high heat for 4 minutes or until softened. Add 1½ cups (375 mL) remaining stock; bring to a boil. Add cooked barley and roasted peppers; bring to a boil, stirring often. Reduce heat to medium-low; cook, stirring often, for 10 minutes or until barley is creamy. Add extra stock as needed. Add Parmesan cheese and pepper. Serve immediately.

Tip

✦ To ensure that you always have some roasted peppers on hand, prepare them in large batches. When cool enough to handle, remove the skin and seeds, slice the peppers, and freeze them in airtight containers. When needed, they defrost quickly. This is a real time-saver — and much more economical than commercially prepared roasted peppers in a jar.

Nutritional Analysis (Per Serving)
✦ Calories: 253 ✦ Protein: 10 g ✦ Cholesterol: 5 mg
✦ Sodium: 327 mg ✦ Fat, total: 4 g ✦ Carbohydrates: 47 g
✦ Fiber: 10 g ✦ Fat, saturated: 1.5 g

Tomatoes with Barley and Pesto Stuffing

2 cups	vegetable or chicken stock	500 mL
½ cup	pearl barley	125 mL
Pesto		
½ cup	tightly packed fresh basil leaves	125 mL
1½ tbsp	grated low-fat Parmesan cheese	20 mL
1 tbsp	toasted pine nuts	15 mL
½ tsp	minced garlic	2 mL
2 tbsp	water	25 mL
1½ tbsp	olive oil	20 mL
4	large ripe tomatoes	4
¼ cup	chopped bottled roasted red bell peppers	50 mL
1 tbsp	grated low-fat Parmesan cheese	15 mL

Shades of vegetarianism: *Being a vegetarian these days doesn't always mean swearing off all animal products. For many people, it simply means changing to a diet that focuses on plant foods. Here's a quick summary of the most common types of vegetarianism:*

- *Semi-vegetarians avoid red meat.*
- *Pesco-vegetarians avoid red meat and poultry.*
- *Lacto-ovo-vegetarians avoid meat, poultry and fish, but eat dairy and eggs.*
- *Vegans avoid all animal products, including dairy and eggs — even honey, in some cases!*

Serves 4
Preheat oven to 425°F (220°C)
Baking sheet

1. In a nonstick saucepan over medium-high heat, bring stock to a boil. Add barley; reduce heat to medium-low. Cook, covered, for 45 minutes or until grain is tender and liquid is absorbed.

2. Meanwhile, in a small food processor or blender, combine basil, Parmesan cheese, pine nuts and garlic; process until finely chopped. Add water and olive oil; process until smooth, adding a little more water if necessary. Set aside.

3. Slice top ½ inch (1 cm) off tomatoes; reserve tops. Scoop out tomato shells. Save pulp for another use.

4. In a bowl combine roasted red peppers, pesto and cooked barley. Stuff tomato shells with mixture, mounding high. Sprinkle with Parmesan cheese; place stuffed tomatoes on baking sheet. Bake in preheated oven for 15 minutes. Serve hot, with tomato "lids" on, if desired.

Tip

✦ Barley is a nutty, versatile grain (not just for soups anymore!) that makes a nice change from traditional accompaniments like rice or pasta. Pearl barley has the husk, bran and germ ground away and cooks in only 40 to 45 minutes. Scotch (or pot) barley has more of the bran left on — so it contains more fiber — but it must be soaked and left to simmer for at least 1½ hours.

Nutritional Analysis (Per Serving)
- ✦ Calories: 183
- ✦ Sodium: 79 mg
- ✦ Fiber: 6 g
- ✦ Protein: 7 g
- ✦ Fat, total: 7 g
- ✦ Fat, saturated: 1.6 g
- ✦ Cholesterol: 3 mg
- ✦ Carbohydrates: 25 g

Bean Burgers with Dill Sauce

Burgers

2 cups	canned black beans, rinsed and drained	500 mL
1/2 cup	dry seasoned bread crumbs	125 mL
1/3 cup	chopped fresh dill	75 mL
1/3 cup	chopped red onions	75 mL
1/4 cup	finely chopped carrots	50 mL
2 tbsp	cornmeal	25 mL
1	egg	1
1 1/2 tsp	minced garlic	7 mL
1/4 tsp	salt	1 mL

Sauce

3 tbsp	light sour cream	45 mL
2 tbsp	light mayonnaise	25 mL
2 tsp	freshly squeezed lemon juice	10 mL
1/4 to 1/2 tsp	minced garlic	1 to 2 mL
1 tbsp	chopped fresh dill (or 1/2 tsp/2 mL dried)	15 mL

Serves 8 or 9
Preheat oven to 425°F (220°C)
Baking sheet sprayed with vegetable spray

1. In a food processor, combine black beans, bread crumbs, dill, onions, carrots, cornmeal, egg, garlic and salt. Pulse on and off until well combined. With wet hands, scoop up 1/4 cup (50 mL) of mixture and form into a patty. Put on prepared baking sheet. Repeat procedure for remaining patties.
2. Bake 15 minutes, turning at the halfway point.
3. Meanwhile, make the sauce: In a small bowl, stir together sour cream, mayonnaise, lemon juice, garlic and dill.
4. Serve burgers hot with sauce on side.

Tips

+ Serve in a pita or tortilla with lettuce, tomatoes and onions.
+ Another simple topping can be made with 3 parts 2% yogurt and 1 part Dijon mustard.
+ Substitute black beans with another bean of your choice.

Make Ahead

+ Prepare mixture and sauce up to 1 day in advance. Reheat gently.

Nutritional Analysis (Per Serving)
+ Calories: 126
+ Protein: 7 g
+ Cholesterol: 27 mg
+ Sodium: 262 mg
+ Fat, total: 2 g
+ Carbohydrates: 20 g
+ Fiber: 5 g
+ Fat, saturated: 0.4 g

Bean and Sweet Potato Chili on Garlic Polenta

Chili

2 tsp	vegetable oil	10 mL
1½ tsp	minced garlic	7 mL
1½ cups	chopped leeks	375 mL
1 cup	chopped red bell peppers	250 mL
1	can (19 oz/540 mL) tomatoes, puréed	1
1½ cups	canned red kidney beans, rinsed and drained	375 mL
1¼ cups	chopped peeled sweet potatoes	300 mL
1 tbsp	fennel seeds	15 mL
2 tsp	chili powder	10 mL
1 tsp	dried basil	5 mL

Polenta

3¼ cups	Basic Vegetable Stock (see recipe, page 52)	800 mL
1 cup	cornmeal	250 mL
1 tsp	minced garlic	5 mL

Serves 6

1. In a large nonstick saucepan, heat oil over medium-high heat. Add garlic, leeks and red peppers; cook 4 minutes or until softened. Stir in tomatoes, beans, sweet potatoes, fennel seeds, chili powder and basil; bring to a boil. Reduce heat to medium-low, cover and cook 20 to 25 minutes or until sweet potatoes are tender.

2. Meanwhile, in a deep saucepan, bring vegetable stock to a boil. Reduce heat to low and gradually whisk in cornmeal and garlic. Cook 5 minutes, stirring frequently.

3. Pour polenta into a serving dish. Spoon chili over top. Serve immediately.

Tips

+ Use any cooked beans you have on hand.
+ Try fresh fennel instead of leeks.
+ Polenta is delicious, nutritious and takes minutes to make.
+ A great source of fiber.

Make Ahead

+ Prepare chili up to 2 days in advance. Cook polenta just before serving.

Nutritional Analysis (Per Serving)

+ Calories: 327
+ Protein: 11 g
+ Cholesterol: 0 mg
+ Sodium: 362 mg
+ Fat, total: 3 g
+ Carbohydrates: 65 g
+ Fiber: 10 g
+ Fat, saturated: 0.3 g

Zucchini, Mushroom and Bean Loaf with Tomato Sauce

1 tsp	vegetable oil	5 mL
2 tsp	minced garlic	10 mL
1 cup	chopped onions	250 mL
½ cup	finely chopped carrots	125 mL
2 cups	chopped zucchini	500 mL
1 cup	chopped mushrooms	250 mL
1½ cups	canned chickpeas, rinsed and drained	375 mL
1½ cups	canned white kidney beans, rinsed and drained	375 mL
⅓ cup	dry seasoned bread crumbs	75 mL
3 tbsp	chili sauce	45 mL
2 tbsp	grated Parmesan cheese	25 mL
2	eggs	2
1 tsp	dried basil	5 mL
¾ cup	prepared tomato pasta sauce	175 mL

Beans, including soy, white and navy, are high in fiber, calcium and protein and low in fat. Include more beans in your meals and snacks, in spreads, dips, soups and chili.

Serves 6 to 8
Preheat oven to 350°F (180°C)
9- by 5-inch (2 L) loaf pan sprayed with vegetable spray

1. In a nonstick frying pan, heat oil over medium-high heat. Add garlic, onions and carrots; cook 4 minutes. Stir in zucchini and mushrooms; cook 8 minutes or until softened.

2. In a food processor, combine zucchini mixture, chickpeas, white kidney beans, seasoned bread crumbs, chili sauce, Parmesan, eggs and basil. Pulse on and off until finely chopped and well combined. Press into prepared loaf pan.

3. Bake, uncovered, about 40 minutes or until tester inserted in center comes out clean. Heat tomato sauce and serve with sliced loaf.

Tips

✦ This vegetarian loaf tastes a lot like chicken. The combination of puréed beans provides a meaty texture.

✦ Replace bottled chili sauce with barbecue sauce or ketchup.

✦ This loaf is a good source of fiber.

Make Ahead

✦ Prepare up to 1 day in advance and serve cold or reheated.

Nutritional Analysis (Per Serving)
✦ Calories: 190 ✦ Protein: 11 g ✦ Cholesterol: 55 mg
✦ Sodium: 489 mg ✦ Fat, total: 4 g ✦ Carbohydrates: 30 g
✦ Fiber: 8 g ✦ Fat, saturated: 1 g

Black Bean, Corn and Leek Frittata

1½ tsp	vegetable oil	7 mL
2 tsp	minced garlic	10 mL
¾ cup	chopped leeks	175 mL
½ cup	chopped red bell peppers	125 mL
½ cup	canned or frozen corn kernels, drained	125 mL
½ cup	canned black beans, rinsed and drained	125 mL
⅓ cup	chopped fresh coriander	75 mL
2	eggs	2
3	egg whites	3
⅓ cup	2% milk	75 mL
¼ tsp	salt	1 mL
¼ tsp	freshly ground black pepper	1 mL
2 tbsp	grated Parmesan cheese	25 mL

For added fiber, make whole-grain foods, vegetables, fruit and legumes (beans, peas and lentils) part of your everyday meal plans.

Serves 4 to 6

1. In a nonstick saucepan sprayed with vegetable spray, heat oil over medium-high heat. Add garlic, leeks and red peppers; cook 4 minutes or until softened. Remove from heat; stir in corn, black beans and coriander.
2. In a bowl whisk together whole eggs, egg whites, milk, salt and pepper. Stir in cooled vegetable mixture.
3. Spray a 12-inch (30 cm) nonstick frying pan with vegetable spray. Heat over medium-low heat. Pour in frittata mixture. Cook 5 minutes, gently lifting sides of frittata to let uncooked egg mixture flow under frittata. Sprinkle with Parmesan. Cover and cook another 3 minutes or until frittata is set. Slip frittata onto serving platter.
4. Cut into wedges and serve immediately.

Tips

✦ Here's a great variation on the traditional omelet — but with less fat and cholesterol.

✦ Replace beans and vegetables with other varieties of your choice.

✦ Coriander can be replaced with dill, parsley and basil.

Make Ahead

✦ Combine entire mixture early in the day. Cook just before serving.

Nutritional Analysis (Per Serving)
✦ Calories: 101   ✦ Protein: 7 g   ✦ Cholesterol: 74 mg
✦ Sodium: 253 mg   ✦ Fat, total: 4 g   ✦ Carbohydrates: 10 g
✦ Fiber: 2 g   ✦ Fat, saturated: 1.1 g

Black Bean Quesadillas with Spinach Cheese Filling

2 tsp	vegetable oil	10 mL
2 tsp	minced garlic	10 mL
1 cup	chopped onions	250 mL
½ cup	well-squeezed, thawed frozen chopped spinach	125 mL
1 cup	canned black beans, rinsed and drained	250 mL
2 oz	goat cheese	50 g
⅓ cup	chopped fresh coriander	75 mL
⅓ cup	shredded part-skim mozzarella cheese (about 1 oz/25 g)	75 mL
⅓ cup	5% ricotta cheese	75 mL
6	small (6-inch/15 cm) flour tortillas	6
⅓ cup	salsa	75 mL

Serves 3
Preheat oven to 425°F (220°C)
Two baking sheets sprayed with vegetable spray

1. In a nonstick frying pan, heat oil over medium-high heat. Add garlic and onions; cook 6 minutes or until softened. Stir in spinach and remove from heat. Mash ½ cup (125 mL) of the black beans. Add mashed beans and remaining whole beans to spinach mixture.

2. In a bowl combine goat cheese, coriander, mozzarella and ricotta.

3. Lay 3 tortillas on baking sheets. Divide bean mixture among tortillas and spread to within ½ inch (1 cm) of edges. Spread cheese mixture over beans and top with salsa. Top with 3 remaining tortillas and press gently to stick.

4. Bake 5 minutes or until heated through.

Tips

✦ Feel free to replace beans, goat cheese and coriander with other choices you prefer.

✦ When using frozen spinach, use a sharp knife to cut about one-half package (10 oz/300 g); refreeze remaining portion.

Make Ahead

✦ Prepare entire mixture up to 1 day in advance. Bake just before serving.

Nutritional Analysis (Per Serving)
✦ Calories: 393 ✦ Protein: 20 g ✦ Cholesterol: 13 mg
✦ Sodium: 666 mg ✦ Fat, total: 13 g ✦ Carbohydrates: 49 g
✦ Fiber: 10 g ✦ Fat, saturated: 4 g

Gnocchi with Tomatoes, Olives and Goat Cheese

2 tsp	vegetable oil	10 mL
2 tsp	minced garlic	10 mL
3/4 cup	chopped onions	175 mL
1	can (19 oz/540 mL) tomatoes, crushed	1
1/3 cup	sliced stuffed green olives	75 mL
1 tsp	dried basil	5 mL
1/2 tsp	dried oregano	2 mL
1	bay leaf	1
2 oz	goat cheese	50 g
1 1/2 lb	potato gnocchi	750 g

Serves 4 to 6

1. In nonstick saucepan, heat oil over medium heat. Add garlic and onions and cook for 4 minutes or until softened. Add tomatoes, olives, basil, oregano and bay leaf; bring to a boil, reduce heat to medium-low and cook uncovered for 15 minutes, or until thickened, stirring occasionally. Add goat cheese and stir until it melts. Set aside.

2. In large pot of boiling water, cook gnocchi according to package directions; drain. Serve sauce over gnocchi.

Tips

+ Replace gnocchi with tortellini or ravioli.
+ This recipe can be halved.
+ Green olives add a distinct flavor, but can be replaced with black olives.
+ Goat cheese can be replaced with feta or, if a milder taste is desired, ricotta cheese.

Make Ahead

+ Sauce can be prepared early in the day and reheated. If too thick, add a little water.

Nutritional Analysis (Per Serving)
+ Calories: 317   + Protein: 9 g   + Cholesterol: 5 mg
+ Sodium: 504 mg   + Fat, total: 7 g   + Carbohydrates: 55 g
+ Fiber: 4 g   + Fat, saturated: 2 g

Vegetarian Shepherd's Pie with Peppered Potato Topping

2 tsp	vegetable oil	10 mL
2 tsp	minced garlic	10 mL
1 cup	chopped onions	250 mL
¾ cup	finely chopped carrots	175 mL
1½ cups	prepared tomato pasta sauce	375 mL
1 cup	canned red kidney beans, rinsed and drained	250 mL
1 cup	canned chickpeas, rinsed and drained	250 mL
½ cup	Basic Vegetable Stock (see recipe, page 52) or water	125 mL
1½ tsp	dried basil	7 mL
2	bay leaves	2
4 cups	diced potatoes	1 L
½ cup	2% milk	125 mL
⅓ cup	light sour cream	75 mL
¼ tsp	freshly ground black pepper	1 mL
¾ cup	shredded cheddar cheese	175 mL
3 tbsp	grated Parmesan cheese	45 mL

Serves 6 to 8
Preheat oven to 350°F (180°C)
13- by 9-inch (3 L) baking dish

1. In a saucepan heat oil over medium-high heat. Add garlic, onions and carrots; cook 4 minutes or until onion is softened. Stir in tomato sauce, kidney beans, chickpeas, stock, basil and bay leaves; reduce heat to medium-low, cover and cook 15 minutes or until vegetables are tender. Remove bay leaves. Transfer sauce to a food processor; pulse on and off just until chunky. Spread over bottom of baking dish.

2. Place potatoes in a saucepan; add cold water to cover. Bring to a boil, reduce heat and simmer 10 to 12 minutes or until tender. Drain; mash with milk, sour cream and pepper. Spoon on top of sauce in baking dish. Sprinkle with cheeses.

3. Bake, uncovered, 20 minutes or until hot.

Tips
+ This shepherd's pie rivals the beef version — creamy, thick and rich tasting. Beans provide the meat-like texture.

+ For a different twist, try using sweet potatoes in the topping.

+ Try other cheeses such as mozzarella or Swiss.

Make Ahead
+ Prepare up to 1 day in advance. Reheat gently.

+ Freeze for up to 3 weeks.

Nutritional Analysis (Per Serving)
+ Calories: 238   + Protein: 11 g   + Cholesterol: 10 mg
+ Sodium: 522 mg   + Fat, total: 7 g   + Carbohydrates: 36 g
+ Fiber: 5 g   + Fat, saturated: 2 g

Mediterranean Kasha Casserole with Sun-Dried Tomatoes

3 cups	Basic Vegetable Stock (see recipe, page 52)	750 mL
1 cup	whole-grain kasha	250 mL
2 tsp	vegetable oil	10 mL
2 tsp	minced garlic	10 mL
1 cup	chopped onions	250 mL
1½ cups	diced unpeeled eggplant	375 mL
1½ cups	diced unpeeled zucchini	375 mL
2 cups	chopped mushrooms	500 mL
1 cup	diced plum tomatoes	250 mL
1 cup	prepared tomato pasta sauce	250 mL
1 tsp	dried basil	5 mL
½ tsp	dried oregano	2 mL
½ cup	chopped softened sun-dried tomatoes	125 mL
⅓ cup	sliced black olives	75 mL
2 oz	feta cheese, crumbled (optional)	50 g

Originally from Russia, kasha is the name given to buckwheat seeds that have been hulled and, most often, either finely or coarsely ground. Despite its name, buckwheat isn't a type of wheat; in fact, it is not a cereal at all.

Serves 6 to 8

1. In a saucepan bring vegetable stock and kasha to a boil; reduce heat to low, cover and cook until liquid is absorbed, about 10 to 12 minutes.

2. Meanwhile, in a large nonstick saucepan sprayed with vegetable spray, heat oil over medium-high heat. Add garlic and onions; cook 2 minutes. Stir in eggplant and zucchini; cook 5 minutes, stirring often. Stir in mushrooms, tomatoes, tomato sauce, basil and oregano; cook 4 minutes, stirring occasionally. Remove from heat; stir in sun-dried tomatoes and olives.

3. Combine kasha with vegetable mixture. Serve sprinkled with feta cheese, if desired.

Tips

✦ Kasha is a nutritious and delicious grain. Use whole-grain kasha to prevent sticking.

✦ To soften sun-dried tomatoes, pour boiling water over them and soak 15 minutes or until soft. Drain and chop.

✦ You can either leave the cheese out or substitute one of your choice.

Make Ahead

✦ Prepare up to 2 days in advance. Reheat gently.

Nutritional Analysis (Per Serving)

✦ Calories: 143   ✦ Protein: 5 g   ✦ Cholesterol: 0 mg
✦ Sodium: 325 mg   ✦ Fat, total: 3 g   ✦ Carbohydrates: 28 g
✦ Fiber: 3 g   ✦ Fat, saturated: 0.4 g

Polenta with Chèvre and Roasted Vegetables

Polenta

3 cups	vegetable or chicken stock	750 mL
1 cup	cornmeal	250 mL
1	medium red bell pepper, cut into quarters	1
1	medium yellow pepper, cut into quarters	1
1	medium red onion, sliced	1
2	small zucchini (about 8 oz/250 g), cut in half lengthwise	2
1 tbsp	olive oil	15 mL
1	small head garlic, top 1/2 inch (1 cm) cut off	1
1 tbsp	balsamic vinegar	15 mL
2 oz	goat cheese (chèvre)	50 g

Great garlic: *It appears that garlic's sulfur compounds can help the liver detoxify carcinogens, stimulate immune function and kill certain cancer cells. The Iowa Women's Health Study followed 42,000 women for five years and found that those who ate 0.7 g garlic each day (less than 1 clove) had a 32% reduced risk of colon cancer compared with women who consumed no garlic. A Harvard study found that regular garlic consumption reduced the risk of colon cancer in men by 23%.*

Serves 4
Preheat oven to 425°F (220°C)
8-inch (2 L) square baking dish sprayed with vegetable spray
Large baking sheet lined with foil

1. In a deep saucepan over medium-high heat, bring stock to a boil. Reduce heat to low; gradually whisk in cornmeal. Cook, stirring, for 5 minutes. Pour into baking dish, smoothing top; chill.

2. In a bowl combine red pepper, yellow pepper, onion, zucchini and olive oil; transfer to prepared baking sheet. Wrap garlic loosely in foil; add to baking sheet. Roast vegetables in preheated oven, turning occasionally, for 45 minutes or until tender. Squeeze garlic out of skins; chop remaining vegetables. Transfer all to a bowl. Sprinkle with balsamic vinegar; toss to coat well.

3. Turn polenta onto cutting board; cut into 4 squares. In a large nonstick frying pan sprayed with vegetable spray, cook polenta over medium-high heat for 2 minutes or until golden. Turn; cook for 1 minute. Spoon polenta onto serving plates. Top with vegetable mixture; sprinkle with goat cheese. Serve.

Tip

✦ Chèvre is a white, tart-flavored cheese made from goat's milk. At least, it's supposed to be — some cheese sold as chèvre contains cow's milk, so read the label carefully! Depending on the producer, goat cheese can be drier or creamier in texture. Either way, at only 15% milk fat, it is a lower-fat cheese. And because it's so flavorful, a little goes a long way.

Nutritional Analysis (Per Serving)
✦ Calories: 253 ✦ Protein: 8 g ✦ Cholesterol: 8 mg
✦ Sodium: 155 mg ✦ Fat, total: 9 g ✦ Carbohydrates: 39 g
✦ Fiber: 6 g ✦ Fat, saturated: 3.1 g

Fish and Seafood

Salmon Fillets with Black Bean Sauce

1 lb	salmon fillets	500 g
1/4 cup	chopped green onions (about 2 medium)	50 mL

Sauce

1/2 cup	chicken stock	125 mL
5 tsp	brown sugar	25 mL
1 tbsp	black bean sauce	15 mL
2 tsp	rice wine vinegar	10 mL
2 tsp	soya sauce	10 mL
2 tsp	sesame oil	10 mL
1 1/4 tsp	cornstarch	6 mL
3/4 tsp	minced gingerroot	4 mL
1/2 tsp	minced garlic	2 mL

Whole black bean sauce is less salty tasting than the puréed version. If whole black bean sauce is not available, increase the sugar to taste.

Serves 4
Preheat oven to 425°F (220°C)
Baking dish sprayed with vegetable spray

1. Put salmon fillets in single layer in prepared baking dish.
2. *Sauce:* In saucepan whisk together stock, brown sugar, black bean sauce, vinegar, soya sauce, sesame oil, cornstarch, ginger and garlic; cook over medium heat, stirring, for 4 minutes or until sauce thickens slightly. Pour over fish and bake uncovered 10 minutes per inch (2.5 cm) thickness of fish, or until fish flakes easily when pierced with a fork. Serve sprinkled with green onions.

Make Ahead
✦ Prepare sauce up to 48 hours ahead and keep refrigerated. Stir again before using.

Nutritional Analysis (Per Serving)
✦ Calories: 196 ✦ Protein: 23 g ✦ Cholesterol: 56 mg
✦ Sodium: 417 mg ✦ Fat, total: 8 g ✦ Carbohydrates: 7 g
✦ Fiber: 0 g ✦ Fat, saturated: 2 g

Salmon over White-and-Black-Bean Salsa

1 lb	salmon steaks	500 g

Salsa

1 cup	canned black beans, drained	250 mL
1 cup	canned white navy beans, drained	250 mL
3/4 cup	chopped tomatoes	175 mL
1/2 cup	chopped green peppers	125 mL
1/4 cup	chopped red onions	50 mL
1/4 cup	chopped fresh coriander	50 mL
2 tbsp	balsamic vinegar	25 mL
2 tbsp	lemon juice	25 mL
1 tbsp	olive oil	15 mL
1 tsp	minced garlic	5 mL

If you're not using canned beans, 1 cup (250 mL) dry yields 3 cups (750 mL) cooked.

Serves 4
Start barbecue or preheat oven to 425°F (220°C)

1. *Salsa:* In bowl combine black beans, white beans, tomatoes, green peppers, red onions and coriander. In small bowl whisk together vinegar, lemon juice, olive oil and garlic; pour over bean mixture and toss to combine.
2. Barbecue fish or bake uncovered for approximately 10 minutes for each 1-inch (2.5 cm) thickness of fish, or until fish flakes with a fork. Serve fish over bean salsa.

Make Ahead
✦ Prepare bean mixture earlier in the day and keep refrigerated. Stir before serving.

Nutritional Analysis (Per Serving)
✦ Calories: 319 ✦ Protein: 32 g ✦ Cholesterol: 56 mg
✦ Sodium: 313 mg ✦ Fat, total: 9 g ✦ Carbohydrates: 29 g
✦ Fiber: 9 g ✦ Fat, saturated: 2 g

Polenta with Chèvre and Roasted Vegetables (page 238) ➤

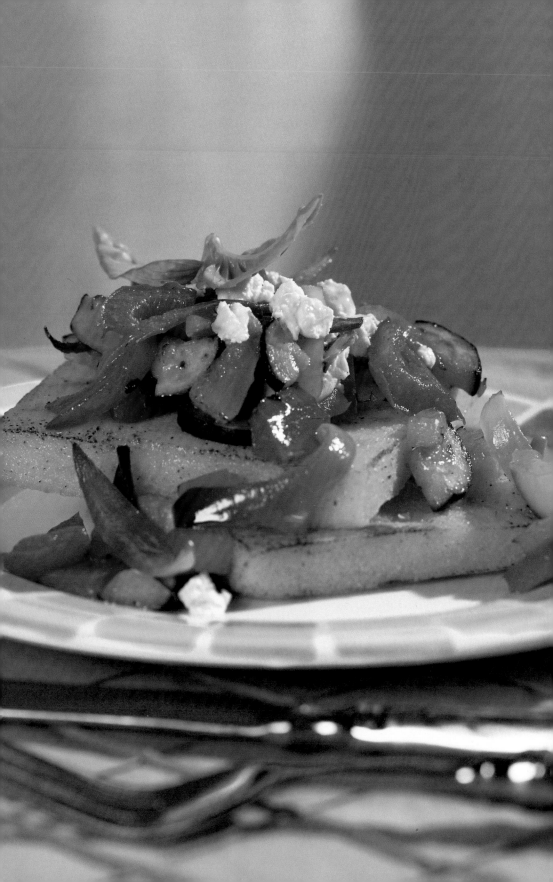

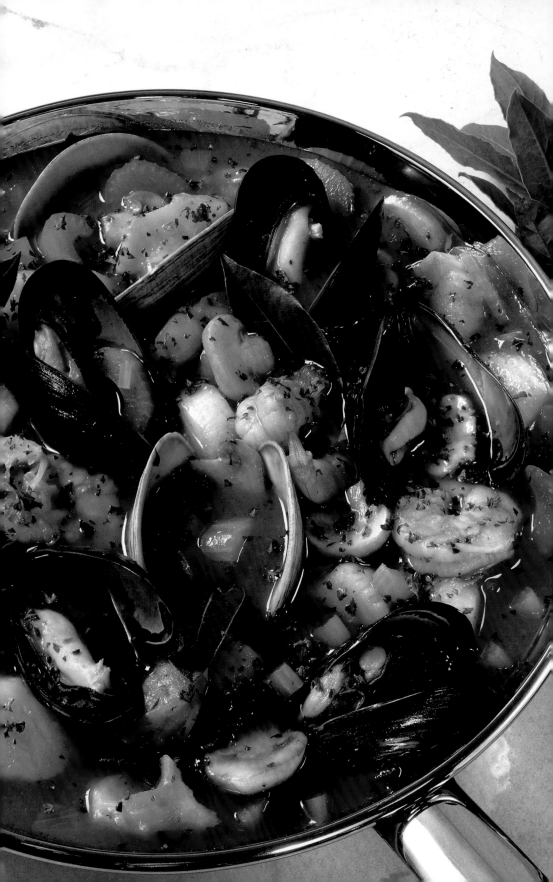

Salmon Burgers with Mango Salsa

1/3 cup	finely chopped green peppers	75 mL
1/4 cup	finely chopped fresh dill (or 1 tsp/5 mL dried)	50 mL
3 tbsp	chopped chives	45 mL
3 tbsp	bread crumbs	45 mL
1	egg	1
2 tsp	minced garlic	10 mL
1 lb	salmon, cut into chunks	500 g
Salsa		
3/4 cup	finely diced mangoes or peaches	175 mL
1/2 cup	finely diced red peppers	125 mL
1/4 cup	finely diced green peppers	50 mL
1/4 cup	finely diced red onions	50 mL
2 tbsp	chopped fresh coriander	25 mL
1 tbsp	lemon juice	15 mL
1 tsp	olive oil	5 mL
1/2 tsp	minced garlic	2 mL

Serves 4 or 5

1. Put peppers, dill, chives, bread crumbs, egg, garlic and salmon in food processor; process on and off until chunky. Do not purée. Form into 4 or 5 burgers.
2. *Salsa:* In bowl combine mango, red peppers, green peppers, red onions, coriander, lemon juice, olive oil and garlic; mix thoroughly.
3. In nonstick skillet sprayed with nonstick vegetable spray, or on the barbecue, cook patties over medium-high heat for 2 to 3 minutes; turn and cook another 1 minute or until just done at the center. Serve with salsa.

Make Ahead
+ Prepare burgers and salsa early in the day and refrigerate. Cook just before eating.

Nutritional Analysis (Per Serving)
+ Calories: 186   + Protein: 21 g   + Cholesterol: 88 mg
+ Sodium: 145 mg   + Fat: 6 g   + Carbohydrates: 4 g
+ Fiber: 0 g

Sole with Spinach and Cream Sauce

2 tsp	vegetable oil	10 mL
3/4 cup	chopped onions	175 mL
1 tsp	crushed garlic	5 mL
Half	package (10 oz/300 g) fresh spinach, cooked and drained	Half
	Salt and pepper	
1/3 cup	white wine	75 mL
1 tbsp	lemon juice	15 mL
1 lb	sole fillets	500 g
1 1/2 tsp	margarine	7 mL
1 tbsp	all-purpose flour	15 mL
1/3 cup	2% milk	75 mL
2 tbsp	grated Parmesan cheese	25 mL

The fish in this classic entrée can be substituted with trout, flounder, halibut or turbot.

Serves 4

1. In small skillet, heat oil; sauté onions and garlic for 3 minutes. Add spinach and cook for 2 minutes. Season with salt and pepper to taste. Spread over flat serving dish. Set aside.
2. In large skillet, bring wine, lemon juice and fish fillets to boil. Reduce heat, cover and simmer just until fish is barely opaque, approximately 3 minutes. With slotted spoon, carefully place fish over spinach mixture, reserving poaching liquid.
3. In small pan, melt margarine; stir in flour and cook for 1 minute. Add milk and reserved poaching liquid; simmer, stirring, until thickened. Stir in 1 tbsp (15 mL) cheese; pour over fish. Sprinkle with remaining cheese.

Nutritional Analysis (Per Serving)
+ Calories: 188   + Protein: 22 g   + Cholesterol: 56 mg
+ Sodium: 182 mg   + Fat: 6 g   + Carbohydrates: 7 g
+ Fiber: 1 g

◄ Seafood Tomato Stew (page 253)

Sole Fillets with Mushroom Stuffing

1 lb	fish fillets, cut into 4 serving-sized pieces	500 g
1/3 cup	shredded mozzarella cheese	75 mL
1 tbsp	margarine, melted	15 mL
1 tbsp	lemon juice	15 mL
2 tbsp	chicken stock or white wine	25 mL
2 tbsp	chopped fresh parsley	25 mL

Stuffing

1 tsp	margarine	5 mL
1/2 cup	chopped mushrooms	125 mL
1/3 cup	chopped onions	75 mL
1 tsp	crushed garlic	5 mL
2 tbsp	dry bread crumbs	25 mL
2 tbsp	chopped fresh dill (or 1/2 tsp/2 mL dried dillweed)	25 mL
1 tbsp	water	15 mL

When working with sole, be gentle. It breaks quite easily.

Serves 4
Preheat oven to 425°F (220°C)
Baking dish sprayed with nonstick vegetable spray

1. *Stuffing:* In small nonstick skillet, melt margarine; sauté mushrooms, onions and garlic for 5 minutes. Add crumbs, dill and water; mix well.
2. Divide stuffing among fillets; sprinkle with cheese. Roll up fillets and fasten with toothpicks. Place in single layer in baking dish.
3. Combine margarine, lemon juice and stock; pour over fish. Bake for approximately 10 minutes or until fish flakes easily when tested with fork. Garnish with parsley.

Make Ahead
- Prepare stuffing early in the day, but roll up in fillets just before baking.

Nutritional Analysis (Per Serving)
- Calories: 175
- Protein: 22 g
- Cholesterol: 58 mg
- Sodium: 233 mg
- Fat: 7 g
- Carbohydrates: 5 g
- Fiber: 1 g

Orange Roughy with Mandarins

1 lb	orange roughy	500 g
1 cup	orange juice	250 mL
1 tsp	grated orange rind	5 mL
2 tsp	cornstarch	10 mL
1 cup	drained canned mandarin orange segments	250 mL

Substitute sole or halibut for the orange roughy.

Serves 4
Preheat oven to 400°F (200°C)
Baking dish sprayed with nonstick vegetable spray

1. Divide fish into 4 serving-sized pieces. Place in single layer in baking dish; pour in 1/4 cup (50 mL) of the orange juice. Cover and bake for approximately 10 minutes or until fish flakes easily when tested with fork. Gently remove fish to serving platter.
2. Meanwhile, in small saucepan, combine orange rind, cornstarch and remaining 3/4 cup (175 mL) orange juice; cook just until thickened, stirring constantly. Add mandarins and heat through; pour over fish.

Nutritional Analysis (Per Serving)
- Calories: 212
- Protein: 22 g
- Cholesterol: 77 mg
- Sodium: 60 mg
- Fat: 6 g
- Carbohydrates: 16 g
- Fiber: 1 g

Lake Trout with Red Pepper Sauce

1 lb	lake or salmon trout fillets	500 g
1 tsp	vegetable oil	5 mL
	Salt and pepper	
Sauce		
1½ tsp	margarine	7 mL
1 tsp	crushed garlic	5 mL
¼ cup	chopped onion	50 mL
1	medium sweet red pepper, diced	1
½ cup	chicken stock	125 mL
1½ tsp	vegetable oil	7 mL

This fish can also be broiled and the sauce served alongside.

When using margarine, choose a soft (non-hydrogenated) version to limit consumption of trans fats.

Serves 4
Preheat oven to 425°F (220°C)
Baking dish sprayed with nonstick vegetable spray

1. Brush fish with oil; season with salt and pepper to taste and place in single layer in baking dish.
2. *Sauce:* In nonstick skillet, heat margarine; sauté garlic and onion for 2 minutes. Add red pepper and stock; simmer for 5 minutes.
3. Pour sauce into food processor; add oil and purée until smooth. Pour over fish. Bake for 12 to 15 minutes or just until fish flakes easily when tested with fork.

Make Ahead
+ Prepare and refrigerate sauce up to a day before.

Nutritional Analysis (Per Serving)
+ Calories: 204 + Protein: 25 g + Cholesterol: 42 mg
+ Sodium: 168 mg + Fat: 10 g + Carbohydrates: 2 g
+ Fiber: 0.5 g

Halibut with Lemon and Pecans

½ cup	bread crumbs	125 mL
1 tsp	dried parsley	5 mL
½ tsp	dried basil	2 mL
½ tsp	crushed garlic	2 mL
1½ tsp	grated Parmesan cheese	7 mL
1 lb	halibut, cut into 4 serving-sized pieces	500 g
1	egg white	1
2 tbsp	margarine	25 mL
2 tbsp	white wine	25 mL
4 tsp	lemon juice	20 mL
1 tbsp	chopped fresh parsley	15 mL
1	green onion, chopped	1
1 tbsp	chopped pecans, toasted	15 mL

If using a thin piece of fish, you can probably skip the baking time. The fish will cook through in the skillet.

Serves 4
Preheat oven to 400°F (200°C)
Baking dish sprayed with nonstick vegetable spray

1. In shallow dish, combine bread crumbs, dried parsley, basil, garlic and cheese. Dip fish pieces into egg white, then into bread crumb mixture.
2. In large nonstick skillet, melt 1 tbsp (15 mL) of the margarine; add fish and cook just until browned on both sides. Transfer fish to baking dish and bake for 5 to 10 minutes or until fish flakes easily when tested with fork. Remove to serving platter and keep warm.
3. To skillet, add remaining margarine, wine, lemon juice, parsley, onions and pecans; cook for 1 minute. Pour over fish.

Nutritional Analysis (Per Serving)
+ Calories: 231 + Protein: 24 g + Cholesterol: 61 mg
+ Sodium: 302 mg + Fat: 9 g + Carbohydrates: 10 g
+ Fiber: 1 g

Halibut with Chunky Tomato Sauce and Black Olives

1 tbsp	margarine	15 mL
1 tsp	crushed garlic	5 mL
1 cup	sliced mushrooms	250 mL
2/3 cup	chopped onions	150 mL
2	large tomatoes, diced	2
1 tsp	each dried basil and oregano (or 2 tbsp/25 mL each chopped fresh	5 mL
1/3 cup	sliced black olives	75 mL
1 lb	halibut, cut into 4 serving-sized pieces	500 g
1 tbsp	grated Parmesan cheese	15 mL

For those with a taste for spicy food, add a sprinkle of chili flakes or powder along with seasonings.

Serves 4
Preheat oven to 425°F (220°C)
Baking dish sprayed with nonstick vegetable spray

1. In large nonstick skillet, melt margarine; sauté garlic, mushrooms and onions until softened, approximately 3 minutes.
2. Add tomatoes, basil, oregano and olives; simmer for 3 minutes.
3. Place fish in baking dish large enough to arrange in single layer; pour sauce over top. Bake for 10 to 15 minutes or until fish flakes easily when tested with fork. Serve sprinkled with Parmesan cheese.

Nutritional Analysis (Per Serving)
- Calories: 184
- Protein: 23 g
- Cholesterol: 61 mg
- Sodium: 262 mg
- Fat: 6 g
- Carbohydrates: 8 g
- Fiber: 2 g

Halibut Burgers with Dijon Mustard Glaze

1 lb	halibut or seabass, cut into chunks	500 g
3 tbsp	seasoned bread crumbs	45 mL
1	egg	1
2 tsp	minced garlic	10 mL
1/3 cup	finely chopped red peppers	75 mL
1/4 cup	finely chopped fresh basil (or 1 tsp/5 mL dried)	50 mL
1 tsp	vegetable oil	5 mL
3 tbsp	2% yogurt	45 mL
1 tbsp	Dijon mustard	15 mL

Try different toppings, such as salsa or guacamole.

Serves 4 or 5

1. Put fish, bread crumbs, egg, garlic, red peppers and basil in food processor; pulse on and off until fish is chunky. Do not purée. Form into 4 or 5 burgers.
2. In nonstick skillet sprayed with vegetable spray, heat oil (or heat barbecue); cook patties over medium-high heat for about 3 or 4 minutes; turn and cook another 3 minutes until browned.
3. In small bowl whisk together yogurt and mustard. Serve burgers with mustard sauce drizzled on top.

Make Ahead
- Prepare mustard sauce up to a day before serving. Stir before serving.
- Prepare burgers early in the day. Cook just before serving.

Nutritional Analysis (Per Serving)
- Calories: 144
- Protein: 21 g
- Cholesterol: 82 mg
- Sodium: 145 mg
- Fat: 5 g
- Carbohydrates: 3 g
- Fiber: 0 g

Red Snapper with Dill Tomato Sauce

1 tbsp	vegetable oil	15 mL
1 tsp	crushed garlic	5 mL
½ cup	sliced sweet red pepper	125 mL
½ cup	sliced sweet green pepper	125 mL
½ cup	sliced onions	125 mL
½ cup	sliced mushrooms	125 mL
1 cup	puréed drained canned tomatoes	250 mL
½ tsp	dried oregano	2 mL
3 tbsp	chopped fresh dill (or 1 tsp/5 mL dried dillweed)	45 mL
1 lb	red snapper, divided into 4 portions	500 g
1 tbsp	grated Parmesan cheese	15 mL

Serves 4
Preheat oven to 425°F (220°C)
Baking dish sprayed with nonstick vegetable spray

1. In large nonstick skillet, heat oil; sauté garlic, red and green peppers, onions and mushrooms until softened, approximately 5 minutes.
2. Add tomatoes and oregano; simmer for 5 minutes. Add dill; cook for 1 more minute.
3. Place red snapper in single layer in baking dish; pour sauce over top. Bake for 18 to 25 minutes or until fish flakes easily when tested with fork. Sprinkle Parmesan over top.

Tip
✦ You can substitute perch, grouper or tilefish for red snapper.

Nutritional Analysis (Per Serving)
✦ Calories: 170 ✦ Protein: 23 g ✦ Cholesterol: 61 mg
✦ Sodium: 216 mg ✦ Fat: 5 g ✦ Carbohydrates: 7 g
✦ Fiber: 2 g

Cod with Almonds and Lemon Sauce

1 lb	cod, cut into 4 serving-sized pieces	500 g
2 tbsp	chopped fresh dill (or 1 tsp/5 mL dried dillweed)	25 mL
4 tsp	margarine, melted	20 mL
4 tsp	lemon juice	20 mL
1 tsp	crushed garlic	5 mL
2 tbsp	sliced almonds, toasted	25 mL

Pecans also suit this dish.

When using margarine, choose a soft (non-hydrogenated) version to limit consumption of trans fats.

Serves 4
Preheat oven to 425°F (220°C)
Baking dish sprayed with nonstick vegetable spray

1. Place fish in baking dish large enough to arrange in single layer. Combine dill, margarine, lemon juice and garlic; pour over fish.
2. Bake until fish flakes easily when tested with fork, approximately 10 minutes. Sprinkle with almonds.

Tips
✦ Any firm white fish can be substituted, such as haddock or halibut.
✦ Toast nuts in skillet on top of stove on high, or in 450°F (230°C) oven for 2 minutes or until golden.

Nutritional Analysis (Per Serving)
✦ Calories: 152 ✦ Protein: 22 g ✦ Cholesterol: 60 mg
✦ Sodium: 146 mg ✦ Fat: 6 g ✦ Carbohydrates: 1 g
✦ Fiber: 0 g

Swordfish with Mango Coriander Salsa

1½ lbs	swordfish steaks	750 g
1 tsp	vegetable oil	5 mL
Salsa		
1½ cups	finely diced mango or peach	375 mL
¾ cup	finely diced red peppers	175 mL
½ cup	finely diced green peppers	125 mL
½ cup	finely diced red onions	125 mL
¼ cup	chopped fresh coriander	50 mL
2 tbsp	lemon juice	25 mL
2 tsp	olive oil	10 mL
1 tsp	minced garlic	5 mL

This salsa can also be used over chicken or pork.

Serves 6
Start barbecue or preheat oven to 425°F (220°C)

1. Brush fish with 1 tsp (5 mL) of oil on both sides. Barbecue or bake fish for 10 minutes per inch (2.5 cm) thickness, or until it flakes easily when pierced with a fork.
2. Meanwhile, in bowl combine mango, red peppers, green peppers, red onions, coriander, lemon juice, olive oil and garlic; mix thoroughly. Serve over fish.

Tip
✦ Any firm fish can be substituted. Try tuna or shark.

Make Ahead
✦ Make salsa early in the day and refrigerate.

Nutritional Analysis (Per Serving)
✦ Calories: 197   ✦ Protein: 22 g   ✦ Cholesterol: 43 mg
✦ Sodium: 101 mg   ✦ Fat, total: 7 g   ✦ Carbohydrates: 11 g
✦ Fiber: 2 g   ✦ Fat, saturated: 2 g

Swordfish Gratin

1½ tsp	margarine	7 mL
1 cup	sliced mushrooms	250 mL
½ cup	sliced sweet green pepper	125 mL
½ cup	sliced onions	125 mL
1 tsp	crushed garlic	5 mL
½ tsp	dried basil	2 mL
½ tsp	dried oregano	2 mL
1 cup	tomato sauce	250 mL
1 lb	swordfish, cut into 4 serving-sized pieces	500 g
½ cup	shredded mozzarella cheese	125 mL

When using margarine, choose a soft (non-hydrogenated) version to limit consumption of trans fats.

Serves 4
Preheat oven to 425°F (220°C)

1. In nonstick skillet, melt margarine; sauté mushrooms, green pepper, onions and garlic for 5 minutes or until softened. Add basil, oregano and tomato sauce; simmer for 5 minutes. Pour half of mixture into baking dish. Place fish over top. Pour remaining sauce over top. Sprinkle with cheese.
2. Bake for 10 to 15 minutes or until fish flakes easily when tested with fork.

Tip
✦ Any other meaty fish can be substituted for the swordfish. Tuna, marlin or shark are good substitutes.

Nutritional Analysis (Per Serving)
✦ Calories: 217   ✦ Protein: 24 g   ✦ Cholesterol: 67 mg
✦ Sodium: 520 mg   ✦ Fat: 9 g   ✦ Carbohydrates: 8 g
✦ Fiber: 2 g

Pecan-Coated Swordfish with Lemon Sauce

1	egg	1
3 tbsp	2% milk	45 mL
1/2 cup	finely chopped pecans	125 mL
2 tbsp	seasoned bread crumbs	25 mL
1 lb	swordfish	500 g
3 tbsp	all-purpose flour	45 mL
2 tsp	vegetable oil	10 mL

Sauce

2/3 cup	chicken stock	150 mL
2 tbsp	lemon juice	25 mL
2 tbsp	sugar	25 mL
2 tsp	cornstarch	10 mL
1/2 tsp	grated lemon zest	2 mL
2 tbsp	chopped fresh parsley	25 mL

Serves 4
Preheat oven to 425°F (220°C)
Baking dish sprayed with vegetable spray

1. In shallow bowl whisk together egg and milk. Combine pecans and bread crumbs and put on a plate. Dust fish with flour, dip in egg wash and coat with pecan mixture.

2. Heat oil in large nonstick skillet sprayed with vegetable spray over medium heat; add fish and cook for 2 minutes per side or until both sides are golden. Place in prepared baking dish. Bake uncovered for 10 minutes per inch (2.5 cm) thickness of fish or until fish flakes easily when pierced with a fork.

3. While fish bakes, in saucepan whisk together stock, lemon juice, sugar, cornstarch and lemon zest; cook over medium heat for 3 or 4 minutes or until sauce thickens slightly. Pour sauce over fish and sprinkle with parsley.

Tips

✦ Try almonds or cashews instead of pecans.

✦ Tuna, shark or any firm white fish would be a good substitute for swordfish.

Make Ahead

✦ Prepare fish earlier in the day and refrigerate before baking.

✦ Prepare sauce earlier in the day. Add more stock before serving if sauce is too thick.

Nutritional Analysis (Per Serving)
✦ Calories: 341   ✦ Protein: 27 g   ✦ Cholesterol: 99 mg
✦ Sodium: 528 mg   ✦ Fat, total: 19 g   ✦ Carbohydrates: 17 g
✦ Fiber: 1 g   ✦ Fat, saturated: 3 g

Zucchini Stuffed with Crabmeat, Tomatoes and Dill

4	zucchini	4
2 tsp	margarine or butter	10 mL
1 tsp	minced garlic	5 mL
⅓ cup	chopped onions	75 mL
6 oz	chopped crabmeat	150 g
⅓ cup	chopped tomatoes	75 mL
3 tbsp	seasoned bread crumbs	45 mL
3 tbsp	chopped fresh dill (or 2 tsp/10 mL dried)	45 mL
2 tbsp	light sour cream	25 mL
2 tbsp	chopped green onions (about 1 medium)	25 mL
1 tbsp	grated Parmesan cheese	15 mL

When using margarine, choose a soft (non-hydrogenated) version to limit consumption of trans fats.

Serves 4
Preheat oven to 400°F (200°C)
Baking sheet

1. Trim ends of zucchini. Cook in boiling water, covered, for 5 minutes or until tender. Rinse with cold water and drain. Cut in half lengthwise; scoop out pulp, leaving shell intact. Chop pulp and squeeze out moisture. Set aside. Place shells on baking sheet.

2. In nonstick saucepan, heat margarine over medium heat; cook garlic and onions for 4 minutes or until softened. Add zucchini pulp and cook for 4 minutes more.

3. Place vegetable mixture in food processor along with crabmeat, tomatoes, bread crumbs, dill, sour cream and green onions. Pulse on and off just until finely chopped. Divide among shells. Sprinkle with Parmesan.

4. Bake for 10 minutes or until heated through.

Tips
+ Try yellow zucchini if available.
+ Diced, cooked shrimp can substitute for crabmeat. Imitation crab (surimi) can also be used.

Make Ahead
+ Shells can be filled up to a day ahead, covered and kept in refrigerator. Bake for 20 minutes to heat thoroughly.

Nutritional Analysis (Per Serving)
+ Calories: 113
+ Protein: 10 g
+ Cholesterol: 4 mg
+ Sodium: 756 mg
+ Fat, total: 3 g
+ Carbohydrates: 12 g
+ Fiber: 3 g
+ Fat, saturated: 0.9 g

Scallops in Black Bean Sauce
with Asparagus and Oyster Mushrooms

1 lb	scallops	500 g
1 tsp	vegetable oil	5 mL
2½ cups	asparagus cut into 1-inch (2.5 cm) pieces	625 mL
2 cups	sliced oyster mushrooms	500 mL
2	medium green onions, chopped	2

Sauce

¾ cup	chicken stock	175 mL
2 tbsp	black bean sauce	25 mL
2 tbsp	honey	25 mL
2 tsp	rice wine vinegar	10 mL
2 tsp	soya sauce	10 mL
2 tsp	sesame oil	10 mL
1 tbsp	cornstarch	15 mL
1 tsp	minced garlic	5 mL
1 tsp	minced gingerroot	5 mL

Black bean sauce is made from fermented soybeans and a lot of salt. Doesn't sound too appetizing, does it? And it isn't — at least, not on its own. But put it together with a liquid and sweetener, and this sauce is outstanding! Try it with vegetables, fish, chicken and meat. You can find bottled black bean sauce in the Asian section of your supermarket.

Serves 4

1. Heat a nonstick skillet sprayed with vegetable spray over high heat; add scallops and cook for 2 to 3 minutes, turning frequently, or until just cooked at center. Remove from heat and drain any excess liquid.

2. In small bowl, whisk together stock, black bean sauce, honey, vinegar, soya sauce, sesame oil, cornstarch, garlic and ginger; set aside.

3. Heat oil in nonstick pan over medium-high heat. Cook asparagus and mushrooms for 5 minutes or until tender-crisp. Drain any excess liquid. Stir sauce again and add to pan. Cook for 1 minute or until bubbly and thickened slightly. Return scallops to pan and cook for 30 seconds or until heated through. Serve over rice or pasta. Garnish with green onions.

Tips

✦ Whole black bean sauce is less salty than the puréed version.

✦ If puréed sauce is too salty, increase honey to taste.

✦ Regular mushrooms are acceptable as a substitute. They give off more liquid, so drain off excess.

✦ Any firm seafood can be used.

✦ Broccoli can be substituted for asparagus.

Make Ahead

✦ Prepare sauce up to 48 hours ahead. Keep refrigerated and stir again before using.

Nutritional Analysis (Per Serving)
✦ Calories: 222   ✦ Protein: 23 g   ✦ Cholesterol: 37 mg
✦ Sodium: 604 mg   ✦ Fat, total: 6 g   ✦ Carbohydrates: 20 g
✦ Fiber: 2 g   ✦ Fat, saturated: 0.7 g

Seafood Kebabs with Pineapple and Green Pepper in Apricot Glaze

1 lb	firm white fish, cut into 2-inch (5 cm) cubes	500 g
16	dried apricots	16
1	green pepper, cut into 16 chunks	1
16	pineapple chunks	16
Glaze		
1/3 cup	apricot jam	75 mL
2 tbsp	lemon juice	25 mL
1 tbsp	vegetable oil	15 mL
1 tbsp	water	15 mL
1 tbsp	chopped fresh coriander or parsley	15 mL
1 tsp	Dijon mustard	5 mL
1 tsp	minced garlic	5 mL
3/4 tsp	curry powder	4 mL

Serves 4

Barbecue or preheat oven to 425°F (220°C)

1. Alternately thread fish cubes, apricots, green pepper and pineapple chunks onto 4 long or 8 short barbecue skewers.

2. *Glaze:* In small bowl whisk together apricot jam, lemon juice, oil, water, coriander, mustard, garlic and curry. Brush kebabs with some of sauce; reserve remainder of sauce to serve with cooked kebabs.

3. Barbecue or bake kebabs for 5 to 8 minutes, turning once, or just until seafood is opaque.

Tips

✦ Swordfish, shrimps or scallops are a good choice for fish.

✦ Peach jam can substitute for the apricot jam.

✦ If fresh pineapple is unavailable, use canned.

Make Ahead

✦ Prepare kebabs and the glaze up to 24 hours ahead, keeping separate until just ready to cook.

Nutritional Analysis (Per Serving)

✦ Calories: 317   ✦ Protein: 23 g   ✦ Cholesterol: 54 mg
✦ Sodium: 118 mg   ✦ Fat, total: 5 g   ✦ Carbohydrates: 47 g
✦ Fiber: 3 g   ✦ Fat, saturated: 0.6 g

Mussels with Tomatoes, Basil and Garlic

2 lb	mussels	1 kg
1½ tsp	vegetable oil	7 mL
½ cup	finely diced onions	125 mL
2 tsp	crushed garlic	10 mL
1	can (14 oz/398 mL) tomatoes, drained and chopped	1
⅓ cup	dry white wine	75 mL
1 tbsp	chopped fresh basil (or ½ tsp/2 mL dried)	15 mL
1½ tsp	chopped fresh oregano (or ¼ tsp/1 mL dried)	7 mL

Serves 4

1. Scrub mussels under cold water; pull off hairy beards. Discard any that do not close when tapped. Set aside.

2. In large nonstick saucepan, heat oil; sauté onions and garlic for 2 minutes. Add tomatoes, wine, basil and oregano; cook for 3 minutes, stirring constantly.

3. Add mussels; cover and cook until mussels fully open, 4 to 5 minutes. Discard any that do not open. Arrange mussels in bowls; pour sauce over top.

Tips

✦ When buying mussels, look for shells that are tightly closed.

✦ Fresh juicy tomatoes are excellent when in season.

✦ Substitute clams for the mussels.

Nutritional Analysis (Per Serving)
✦ Calories: 108   ✦ Protein: 10 g   ✦ Cholesterol: 22 mg
✦ Sodium: 351 mg   ✦ Fat: 2 g   ✦ Carbohydrates: 8 g
✦ Fiber: 2 g

Scallops with Basil Tomato Sauce

1 tbsp	margarine	15 mL
3/4 cup	chopped onions	175 mL
1 tsp	crushed garlic	5 mL
3/4 cup	diced sweet green pepper	175 mL
3/4 cup	sliced mushrooms	175 mL
2 tsp	all-purpose flour	10 mL
1 cup	2% milk	250 mL
2 tbsp	tomato paste	25 mL
1 1/4 tsp	dried basil (or 2 tbsp/25 mL chopped fresh)	6 mL
1 lb	scallops, sliced in half if large	500 g
1 tbsp	grated Parmesan cheese	15 mL

When using margarine, choose a soft (non-hydrogenated) version to limit consumption of trans fats.

Serves 4

1. In large nonstick skillet, melt margarine; sauté onions, garlic, green pepper and mushrooms until softened, approximately 5 minutes. Stir in flour and cook for 1 minute, stirring.
2. Add milk, tomato paste and basil; cook, stirring continuously, until thickened, 2 to 3 minutes.
3. Add scallops; cook just until opaque, 2 to 3 minutes. Place on serving dish; sprinkle with Parmesan cheese.

Tip
- Shrimp or squid can be used in place of the scallops, or try a combination of the two.

Nutritional Analysis (Per Serving)
- Calories: 226
- Protein: 29 g
- Cholesterol: 41 mg
- Sodium: 459 mg
- Fat: 6 g
- Carbohydrates: 14 g
- Fiber: 2 g

Chinese Shrimp Sauté with Green Onions and Pecans

1 1/2 cups	chopped broccoli florets	375 mL
1 1/2 cups	snow peas, trimmed	375 mL
2/3 cup	chicken stock	150 mL
2 tbsp	hoisin sauce	25 mL
1 tbsp	cornstarch	15 mL
1 tsp	minced gingerroot (or 1/2 tsp/2 mL ground)	5 mL
1 tbsp	olive oil	15 mL
1 1/2 tsp	crushed garlic	7 mL
3/4 cup	chopped sweet red pepper	175 mL
1 lb	medium shrimp, peeled and deveined	500 g
1 tbsp	chopped pecans	15 mL
1	green onion, finely chopped	1

Serves 4

1. Blanch broccoli and snow peas in boiling water just until color brightens; drain and set aside.
2. Combine chicken stock, hoisin sauce, cornstarch and ginger until mixed. Set aside.
3. In large skillet, heat oil; sauté garlic and red pepper for 2 minutes. Add shrimp and hoisin mixture; sauté just until shrimp turns pink and sauce thickens. Add broccoli, snow peas and pecans; toss well. Sprinkle with green onions.

Tip
- The shrimp can be replaced with scallops or a combination of both.

Nutritional Analysis (Per Serving)
- Calories: 244
- Protein: 29 g
- Cholesterol: 221 mg
- Sodium: 779 mg
- Fat: 6 g
- Carbohydrates: 17 g
- Fiber: 4 g

Seafood Tomato Stew

1 tbsp	vegetable oil	15 mL
Half	medium onion, chopped	Half
Half	celery stalk, chopped	Half
1 tsp	crushed garlic	5 mL
¼ lb	mushrooms, sliced	125 g
2	cans (each 19 oz/540 mL) tomatoes, crushed	2
2 tbsp	tomato paste	25 mL
⅓ cup	white wine or fish stock	75 mL
1½ tsp	dried oregano	7 mL
1½ tsp	dried basil	7 mL
2	bay leaves	2
24	mussels	24
½ lb	shrimp, peeled and deveined	250 g
½ lb	scallops	250 g
½ lb	firm white fish (cod, halibut, haddock), cut into bite-sized pieces	250 g
	Chopped fresh parsley	

Serves 6

1. In large nonstick saucepan, heat oil; sauté onion, celery, garlic and mushrooms until softened, approximately 5 minutes.
2. Add tomatoes, tomato paste, wine, oregano, basil and bay leaves; cover and simmer for 25 minutes, stirring occasionally.
3. Scrub mussels under cold water; remove any beards. Discard any that do not close when tapped.
4. Add mussels, shrimp, scallops and fish to pot; cover and cook for 5 to 8 minutes or until mussels open, shrimp are pink and scallops and fish are opaque. Discard any mussels that do not open. Discard bay leaves. Serve immediately.

Tips

✦ Known as a *cioppino*, this seafood dish can be made with any combination of seafood. Other chopped vegetables can also be added.

✦ Serve with French or Italian bread.

Make Ahead

✦ Follow steps 1 to 3 early in day. Later, reheat the sauce, then add seafood and cook as directed.

Nutritional Analysis (Per Serving)
✦ Calories: 238 ✦ Protein: 33 g ✦ Cholesterol: 106 mg
✦ Sodium: 749 mg ✦ Fat: 6 g ✦ Carbohydrates: 14 g
✦ Fiber: 3 g

Seafood with Rice, Mushrooms and Tomatoes

1 lb	cooked seafood (any combination of shrimp, scallops, squid or firm white fish)	500 g
1 tbsp	vegetable oil	15 mL
1½ tsp	crushed garlic	7 mL
1 cup	chopped onions	250 mL
¾ cup	chopped sweet green or red pepper	175 mL
1 cup	sliced mushrooms	250 mL
1 cup	rice	250 mL
2½ cups	chicken stock	625 mL
1 cup	frozen peas	250 mL
1 cup	chopped tomatoes	250 mL
1½ tsp	each dried oregano and basil (or 2 tbsp/25 mL each chopped fresh)	7 mL
1 tbsp	grated Parmesan cheese	15 mL
	Chopped fresh parsley	

Serves 4 to 6

1. Cut seafood into bite-sized pieces and set aside.

2. In large nonstick saucepan, heat oil; sauté garlic, onions, green peppers and mushrooms until softened. Add rice and sauté, stirring, just until rice begins to turn brown, 3 to 5 minutes. Add stock; cover and simmer for 20 to 30 minutes or until rice is tender and most liquid is absorbed.

3. Add peas, tomatoes, oregano and basil; cook on medium heat for 3 minutes or until peas are cooked. Add seafood and cook until heated through. Place in serving dish. Sprinkle Parmesan and parsley over top.

Tip

✦ Try brown rice instead of plain rice to increase the fiber. Cook 10 minutes longer.

Make Ahead

✦ Prepare a couple of hours before serving and serve at room temperature.

Nutritional Analysis (Per Serving)
✦ Calories: 281   ✦ Protein: 21 g   ✦ Cholesterol: 88 mg
✦ Sodium: 823 mg   ✦ Fat: 5 g   ✦ Carbohydrates: 37 g
✦ Fiber: 3 g

Shrimp Risotto with Artichoke Hearts and Parmesan

3 cups	seafood or chicken stock	750 mL
½ cup	chopped onions	125 mL
2 tsp	minced garlic	10 mL
1 cup	Arborio rice (risotto rice)	250 mL
1 tsp	dried basil	5 mL
Half	can (14 oz/398 mL) artichoke hearts, drained and chopped	Half
8 oz	raw shrimp, shelled and chopped	250 g
¼ cup	chopped green onions	50 mL
¼ cup	grated low-fat Parmesan cheese	50 mL
¼ tsp	freshly ground black pepper	1 mL

Bring on the shellfish: *If you have high blood cholesterol, don't worry about enjoying shrimp! Yes, they are fairly high in cholesterol. But for most people, cholesterol in foods has little or no effect on blood cholesterol. What counts the most is saturated fat (found in animal foods and processed foods with hydrogenated oils), which your body uses as a building block for blood cholesterol. And seafood contains very little saturated fat. In fact, a 3-oz (90 g) serving of shrimp has less than 1 g fat. The same goes for lobster!*

Serves 4

1. In a saucepan over medium-high heat, bring stock to a boil; reduce heat to low. In another nonstick saucepan sprayed with vegetable spray, cook onions and garlic over medium-high heat for 3 minutes or until softened. Add rice and basil; cook for 1 minute.

2. Using a ladle, add ½ cup (125 mL) stock to rice; stir to keep rice from sticking to pan. When liquid is absorbed, add another ½ cup (125 mL) stock. Reduce heat if necessary to maintain a slow, steady simmer. Repeat this process, ladling in hot stock and stirring constantly, for 15 minutes, reducing amount of stock added to ¼ cup (50 mL) near end of cooking time.

3. Add artichokes and shrimp; cook, adding more stock as necessary, for 3 minutes or until shrimp turn pink and rice is tender but firm. Add green onions, Parmesan cheese and pepper. Serve immediately.

Tip

✦ If you haven't got the time or ingredients necessary to make seafood stock from scratch, you can buy it canned or in powdered form (1 tsp [5 mL] in 1 cup [250 mL] boiling water yields 1 cup [250 mL] stock). Keep in mind, however, that these stocks are often loaded with sodium. To cut back on the sodium, try using only ½ tsp (2 mL) powder — or try the seafood stock on page 53, which has no added salt at all!

Nutritional Analysis (Per Serving)
- ✦ Calories: 174
- ✦ Protein: 19 g
- ✦ Cholesterol: 93 mg
- ✦ Sodium: 300 mg
- ✦ Fat, total: 3 g
- ✦ Carbohydrates: 15 g
- ✦ Fiber: 1 g
- ✦ Fat, saturated: 1.4 g

Jumbo Shells Stuffed with Crabmeat, Cheese and Dill

18	jumbo pasta shells	18
6 oz	crabmeat or surimi (dried imitation crab)	175 g
1³/₄ cups	5% ricotta cheese	425 mL
²/₃ cup	shredded low-fat mozzarella cheese	150 mL
2	green onions, sliced	2
3 tbsp	low-fat milk	45 mL
1	large egg	1
¹/₄ cup	chopped fresh dill (or 1 tsp/5 mL dried)	50 mL
¹/₄ tsp	freshly ground black pepper	1 mL
1 cup	tomato pasta sauce	250 mL
3 tbsp	low-fat milk	45 mL

Serves 6
Preheat oven to 350°F (180°C)
13- by 9-inch (3 L) baking dish

1. In a large pot of boiling water, cook shells for 14 minutes or until tender; drain. Rinse under cold running water; drain. Set aside.

2. In a bowl combine crabmeat, ricotta cheese, mozzarella cheese, green onions, milk, egg, dill and pepper. Stuff approximately 2¹/₂ tbsp (35 mL) mixture into each pasta shell.

3. In a bowl combine tomato sauce and milk; spread half over bottom of baking dish. Add stuffed shells; pour remaining sauce over top. Bake, covered with foil, for 20 minutes or until heated through.

Tips

✦ When many of us were growing up, if you'd gone to the store and asked for "tomato pasta sauce" they wouldn't have had a clue what you were talking about. Back then it was just plain old "spaghetti sauce." Well, it's basically the same stuff. Don't use canned tomato sauce, however; it's too salty and has a slightly bitter aftertaste. Better choices for this recipe are commercially prepared sauce in a jar or, if you have the time, your own homemade sauce.

✦ If you don't have jumbo shells you can substitute 12 manicotti or cannelloni pasta shells.

✦ Try replacing the crab meat with diced cooked chicken.

Nutritional Analysis (Per Serving)
✦ Calories: 295 ✦ Protein: 21 g ✦ Cholesterol: 75 mg
✦ Sodium: 328 mg ✦ Fat, total: 10 g ✦ Carbohydrates: 30 g
✦ Fiber: 328 g ✦ Fat, saturated: 5.4 g

Fish with Tomato, Basil and Cheese Topping

1 cup	chopped tomatoes	250 mL
½ cup	grated mozzarella cheese	125 mL
¼ cup	sliced black olives	50 mL
¼ cup	chopped green onions (about 2 medium)	50 mL
2 oz	goat cheese	50 g
1 tsp	minced garlic	5 mL
1½ tsp	dried basil	7 mL
1 lb	fish fillets	500 g

Fatty fish, including salmon, sardines, tuna, mackerel and rainbow trout, are high in omega-3 fatty acids, which are thought to play a role in preventing heart disease. Include fish in your diet 2 to 3 times a week.

Serves 4
Preheat oven to 425°F (220°C)
Baking dish sprayed with vegetable spray

1. In bowl, combine tomatoes, mozzarella, black olives, green onions, goat cheese, garlic and basil; mix well.
2. Place fish in prepared pan; top with tomato mixture. Bake uncovered approximately 15 minutes for each 1-inch (2.5 cm) thickness of fish fillet, or until fish flakes easily with a fork.

Tips
+ This dish suits any type of fish.
+ If goat cheese is too intense for you, try ricotta or feta.
+ Baking time is increased due to the added sauce, according to fish guidelines.

Make Ahead
+ Tomato mixture can be prepared earlier in the day and refrigerated.

Nutritional Analysis (Per Serving)
+ Calories: 195
+ Protein: 27 g
+ Cholesterol: 63 mg
+ Sodium: 287 mg
+ Fat, total: 7 g
+ Carbohydrates: 5 g
+ Fiber: 1 g
+ Fat, saturated: 2 g

Crunchy Fish with Cucumber Dill Relish

Relish

2 cups	finely chopped cucumbers	500 mL
1/3 cup	chopped fresh dill	75 mL
1/3 cup	2% yogurt	75 mL
1/4 cup	finely diced green onions (about 2 medium)	50 mL
1/4 cup	finely diced green peppers	50 mL
3 tbsp	light mayonnaise	45 mL
1 tsp	minced garlic	5 mL

Crunchy Fish

2 cups	corn flakes	500 mL
1 tbsp	grated Parmesan cheese	15 mL
1 tsp	minced garlic	5 mL
1/2 tsp	dried basil	2 mL
1	egg	1
3 tbsp	2% milk	45 mL
3 tbsp	all-purpose flour	45 mL
1 lb	firm white fish fillets	500 g
1 tbsp	margarine or butter	15 mL

When using margarine, choose a soft (non-hydrogenated) version to limit consumption of trans fats.

Serves 4

1. *Relish:* In bowl, combine cucumbers, dill, yogurt, green onions, green peppers, mayonnaise and garlic; mix to combine and set aside.
2. Put corn flakes, Parmesan, garlic and basil in food processor; process until fine and put on a plate. In shallow bowl whisk together egg and milk. Dust fish with flour.
3. Dip fish fillets in egg wash, then coat with crumb mixture. In large nonstick skillet sprayed with vegetable spray, melt margarine over medium heat. Add fillets and cook for 5 minutes or until browned, turn and cook for 2 minutes longer, or until fish is browned and flakes easily when pierced with a fork. Serve topped with cucumber dill relish.

Tips

+ Try to make the relish as close to the time of serving as possible; otherwise the cucumber will make the sauce too watery.
+ Use cod, snapper or haddock.
+ Use 1 1/2 tsp (7 mL) dried dillweed if fresh dill is unavailable.
+ The flatter the fish, the faster it cooks.

Make Ahead

+ Prepare fish early in the day and keep refrigerated until ready to bake.

Nutritional Analysis (Per Serving)

+ Calories: 274
+ Protein: 27 g
+ Cholesterol: 112 mg
+ Sodium: 429 mg
+ Fat, total: 9 g
+ Carbohydrates: 20 g
+ Fiber: 1 g
+ Fat, saturated: 2 g

Fish Fillets with Corn and Red Pepper Salsa

1 lb	fish fillets	500 g
Salsa		
1	large red pepper	1
1½ cups	corn kernels	375 mL
⅓ cup	chopped red onions	75 mL
¼ cup	chopped fresh coriander	50 mL
2 tbsp	fresh lime or lemon juice	25 mL
3 tsp	olive oil	15 mL
2 tsp	minced garlic	7 mL

Hold the tartar, please! *Yikes! Bet you didn't realize that a small 2-tbsp (30 mL) portion of tartar sauce packs 170 calories and 18 g fat! But when you consider its mayonnaise base (consisting of vegetable oil and egg yolks), these numbers are no surprise. Want a better alternative? Try the corn and red pepper salsa in this recipe.*

Serves 4
Preheat broiler
Baking dish sprayed with vegetable spray

1. *Salsa:* Broil red pepper for 15 to 20 minutes, turning occasionally, until charred on all sides. Remove pepper and set oven at 425°F (220°C). When pepper is cool, remove skin, seeds and stem. Chop and put in small bowl along with corn, onions, coriander, lime juice, 2 tsp (10 mL) of olive oil and 1 tsp (5 mL) of the garlic; mix well.

2. Put fish in single layer in prepared baking dish and brush with remaining 1 tsp (5 mL) garlic and 1 tsp (5 mL) oil. Bake uncovered for 10 minutes per inch (2.5 cm) thickness of fish or until fish flakes easily when pierced with a fork. Serve with salsa.

Tips

+ After broiling pepper, put in small bowl and cover tightly with plastic wrap; this allows the skin to be removed easily.

+ The fresh pepper can be replaced with 4 oz (125 g) sweet pepper packed in water in a jar.

+ Roasted corn gives an exceptional flavor in this recipe. Either barbecue or broil until just cooked and charred, along with pepper. Remove kernels with a sharp knife.

Make Ahead

+ Prepare salsa earlier in the day and refrigerate.

Nutritional Analysis (Per Serving)
+ Calories: 211
+ Protein: 24 g
+ Cholesterol: 54 mg
+ Sodium: 320 mg
+ Fat, total: 5 g
+ Carbohydrates: 19 g
+ Fiber: 2 g
+ Fat, saturated: 1 g

Fish with Sun-Dried Tomato Pesto, Feta and Black Olives

1½ lbs	fish fillets	750 g
1 oz	feta cheese, crumbled	25 g
2 tbsp	chopped black olives	25 mL
Sauce		
¼ cup	well-packed, chopped sun-dried tomatoes	50 mL
2 tbsp	chopped fresh basil or parsley	25 mL
1½ tbsp	olive oil	20 mL
1½ tbsp	grated Parmesan cheese	20 mL
1 tbsp	toasted pine nuts	15 mL
1 tsp	minced garlic	5 mL
⅓ cup	chicken stock	75 mL

Serves 6
Preheat oven to 425°F (220°C)
Baking dish sprayed with vegetable spray

1. *Sauce:* Put sun-dried tomatoes, basil, olive oil, Parmesan, pine nuts and garlic in food processor; process until finely chopped. With machine running, gradually add stock through feed tube; process until smooth.

2. Put fish in single layer in prepared baking dish; spread sun-dried pesto on top. Sprinkle with feta and olives. Bake uncovered for 15 minutes per inch (2.5 cm) thickness of fish or until fish flakes easily when pierced with a fork.

Tips

✦ Use dry sun-dried tomatoes in this recipe, not the kind packed in oil. Pour boiling water over top, soak for 15 minutes or until softened, then chop.

✦ Any type of fish works well with this dish.

✦ Normally, fish is baked for 10 minutes per inch (2.5 cm) of thickness. However, when a thick sauce is used, 5 minutes must be added to the baking time.

Make Ahead

✦ Prepare sauce up to 48 hours in advance and keep refrigerated.

✦ This sauce can also be frozen for up to 6 weeks.

Nutritional Analysis (Per Serving)
✦ Calories: 172   ✦ Protein: 24 g   ✦ Cholesterol: 60 mg
✦ Sodium: 295 mg   ✦ Fat, total: 7 g   ✦ Carbohydrates: 2 g
✦ Fiber: 0 g   ✦ Fat, saturated: 2 g

Baked Whole Fish Stuffed with Vegetables and Dilled Rice

1 tbsp	vegetable oil	15 mL
1½ tsp	crushed garlic	7 mL
½ cup	chopped onion	125 mL
½ cup	chopped sweet green or red pepper	125 mL
⅓ cup	chopped celery	75 mL
½ cup	sliced mushrooms	125 mL
1¼ cups	cooked rice	300 mL
½ cup	chicken stock	125 mL
2 tbsp	chopped fresh dill (or 1 tsp/5 mL dried dillweed)	25 mL
2 tbsp	chopped fresh parsley	25 mL
1 tbsp	grated Parmesan cheese	15 mL
	Salt and pepper	
1	whole trout, pickerel or salmon (2 to 3 lb/1 to 1.5 kg), cleaned, boned if possible	1
4	slices lemon	4

Serves 4
Preheat oven to 400°F (200°C)

1. In large nonstick skillet, heat oil; sauté garlic, onion, green pepper and celery until softened, approximately 5 minutes. Add mushrooms and cook for 3 minutes.

2. Add rice, stock, dill, parsley, cheese, and salt and pepper to taste; cook for 1 minute, mixing to combine, or until stock is evaporated.

3. Place fish on large sheet of lightly oiled foil. Stuff with rice mixture; place lemon slices over top. Fold foil to enclose fish completely; place on baking sheet and bake for approximately 30 minutes, or 10 minutes per inch (2.5 cm) of thickness, or until fish flakes easily when tested with fork.

Tip
✦ This stuffing can also be used as a filling between fish fillets. Use whatever vegetables are on hand.

Make Ahead
✦ Make filling early in the day, but do not stuff fish until just before baking.

Nutritional Analysis (Per Serving)
✦ Calories: 412 ✦ Protein: 59 g ✦ Cholesterol: 157 mg
✦ Sodium: 618 mg ✦ Fat: 8 g ✦ Carbohydrates: 22 g
✦ Fiber: 2 g

Peppers with Barley Stuffing and Tuna-Caper Dressing

3 cups	vegetable or chicken stock	750 mL
¾ cup	pearl barley	175 mL
4	medium red, yellow or green bell peppers, top 1 inch (2.5 cm) cut off, ribs and seeds removed	4

Dressing

Half	can (6 oz/175 g) water-packed tuna, drained	Half
¼ cup	water	50 mL
1 tbsp	light mayonnaise	15 mL
1 tbsp	olive oil	15 mL
2 tsp	fresh lemon juice	10 mL
2 tsp	drained capers	10 mL
1 tsp	minced garlic	5 mL
½ cup	diced ripe plum tomatoes	125 mL
⅓ cup	diced red onions	75 mL
¼ cup	chopped green onions	50 mL
3 tbsp	diced black olives	45 mL

Canned tuna isn't expensive, so don't try to save money by purchasing anything other than white, water-packed tuna. Cheaper varieties of "light" tuna don't taste as good, and, when packed in oil, they certainly aren't light! In fact, oil-packed tuna contains double the calories and 6 times the fat.

Serves 4

1. In a saucepan over medium-high heat, bring stock to a boil. Add barley; reduce heat to medium-low. Cook, covered, for 45 minutes or until barley is tender; drain any excess liquid.

2. In a large pot of boiling water, cook peppers for 5 minutes; drain. Set aside to cool.

3. In a food processor or blender, combine tuna, water, mayonnaise, olive oil, lemon juice, capers and garlic; purée.

4. In a bowl combine barley, tomatoes, red onions, green onions and black olives. Pour dressing over; toss to coat well. Spoon mixture into peppers; top with reserved pepper tops. Serve.

Tips

✦ This tuna dressing makes a wonderful sauce over cooked beef, especially steak. I also use it for a dip with vegetables or as a sauce over pasta. It will keep in the refrigerator for up to 5 days.

✦ This is a perfect dish for entertaining, either as an appetizer or as a side dish. Use a variety of colored bell peppers and be sure to save the lids of the peppers for a dramatic garnish. Also garnish with sliced basil.

Nutritional Analysis (Per Serving)
✦ Calories: 307   ✦ Protein: 17 g   ✦ Cholesterol: 19 mg
✦ Sodium: 445 mg   ✦ Fat, total: 10 g   ✦ Carbohydrates: 41 g
✦ Fiber: 8 g   ✦ Fat, saturated: 1.3 g

Poultry

❖ ❖

Chicken with Rice, Green Olives and Tomato Sauce

4	chicken legs	4
1/3 cup	all-purpose flour	75 mL
2 tsp	vegetable oil	10 mL
2 tsp	minced garlic	10 mL
1 1/2 cups	chopped onions	375 mL
1 1/2 cups	chopped green peppers	375 mL
1 cup	white rice	250 mL
1	can (19 oz/540 mL) tomatoes, puréed	1
1 1/2 cups	chicken stock	375 mL
1/2 cup	sliced stuffed green olives	125 mL
2 tsp	drained capers	10 mL
2 tsp	dried basil	10 mL
1 1/2 tsp	dried oregano	7 mL
1	bay leaf	1

Serves 4
Preheat oven to 400°F (200°C)
9- by 13-inch baking dish (3.5 L) sprayed with vegetable spray

1. In large nonstick skillet sprayed with vegetable spray, heat 1 tsp (5 mL) of the oil over high heat. Dust chicken with flour. Cook for 8 minutes, turning often, or until browned on all sides. Put in prepared baking dish.

2. In nonstick skillet, heat remaining 1 tsp (5 mL) oil over medium heat. Add garlic, onions and green peppers; cook for 4 minutes or until softened. Stir in rice, tomatoes, stock, olives, capers, basil, oregano and bay leaf; bring to a boil and pour over chicken. Cover tightly with aluminum foil and bake for 30 minutes, or until juices run clear when leg is pierced at thickest point and rice is tender. Remove skin before eating.

Tips

✦ Bone-in chicken breasts or a combination of breasts and legs can be used in this recipe. Bone-in breast will cook in less time than legs.

✦ A combination of wild and white rice can be used.

Nutritional Analysis (Per Serving)
✦ Calories: 522 ✦ Protein: 34 g ✦ Cholesterol: 92 mg
✦ Sodium: 964 mg ✦ Fat, total: 10 g ✦ Carbohydrates: 76 g
✦ Fiber: 8 g ✦ Fat, saturated: 2 g

Chicken Fagioli (Bean Tomato Sauce)

4	chicken legs	4
1/4 cup	all-purpose flour	50 mL
2 tsp	vegetable oil	10 mL
2 tsp	minced garlic	10 mL
1/2 cup	chopped onions	125 mL
1/3 cup	chopped carrots	75 mL
1/3 cup	chopped celery	75 mL
1 1/2 cups	red kidney beans, drained	375 mL
1 cup	puréed canned tomatoes	250 mL
3/4 cup	chicken stock	175 mL
1 1/2 tsp	dried basil	7 mL
1 tsp	dried oregano	5 mL

Serves 4

1. In large nonstick skillet sprayed with vegetable spray, heat 1 tsp (5 mL) of the oil over high heat. Dust chicken with flour and cook for 8 minutes, turning often, or until browned on all sides. Set aside and wipe skillet clean.

2. Reduce heat to medium. Add remaining 1 tsp (5 mL) oil to skillet. Add garlic, onions, carrots and celery; cook for 5 minutes or until softened. Mash 1/2 cup (125 mL) of the kidney beans; add mashed and whole beans, tomatoes, stock, basil and oregano to skillet. Bring to a boil, reduce heat to medium-low, add browned chicken pieces, cover and cook for 30 minutes or until juices run clear when legs are pierced at thickest point. Stir occasionally. Remove skin before eating.

Tips

✦ Use bone-in chicken breasts instead of legs; reduce browning time to 4 minutes and reduce cooking time to 20 minutes.

✦ White kidney beans or a combination of red and white can be used.

✦ A great dish to reheat.

Nutritional Analysis (Per Serving)
✦ Calories: 316   ✦ Protein: 33 g   ✦ Cholesterol: 92 mg
✦ Sodium: 538 mg   ✦ Fat, total: 7 g ✦ Carbohydrates: 31 g
✦ Fiber: 8 g   ✦ Fat, saturated: 1 g

Chicken with Black Bean Sauce and Sautéed Mushrooms

2 tsp	vegetable oil	10 mL
4	chicken legs	4
1/3 cup	all-purpose flour	75 mL
2 1/2 cups	sliced mushrooms	625 mL

Sauce

1 cup	chicken stock	250 mL
3 tbsp	honey	45 mL
3 tbsp	black bean sauce	45 mL
1 tbsp	soya sauce	15 mL
1 tbsp	rice wine vinegar	15 mL
1 tbsp	sesame oil	15 mL
1 tbsp	cornstarch	15 mL
2 tsp	minced garlic	10 mL
1 tsp	minced gingerroot	5 mL
1/2 cup	chopped green onions (about 4 medium)	125 mL

Serves 4
Preheat oven to 400°F (200°C)
Baking dish

1. In large nonstick skillet sprayed with vegetable spray, heat oil over high heat. Dust chicken pieces with flour; cook for 8 minutes, turning often, or until well browned on all sides. Transfer to baking dish. Bake for 30 to 40 minutes or until juices run clear when pierced at thickest point. Pour off fat and place on serving platter and keep covered.

2. In a nonstick skillet sprayed with vegetable spray, sauté mushrooms until just cooked (approximately 4 minutes). Drain any excess liquid and set aside.

3. Meanwhile, in saucepan whisk together stock, honey, black bean sauce, soya sauce, vinegar, sesame oil, cornstarch, garlic and ginger until smooth; cook over medium heat for 5 minutes, or until slightly thickened. Add mushrooms and pour over baked chicken. Garnish with green onions. Remove skin before eating.

Tips

◆ Try using oyster mushrooms instead of regular button mushrooms.

◆ Of the two kinds of bottled black bean sauce available — whole black bean sauce and puréed black bean garlic sauce — the whole bean sauce is lower in sodium.

Make Ahead

◆ Prepare sauce and mushrooms earlier in the day. Add more stock if sauce is too thick.

Nutritional Analysis (Per Serving)
◆ Calories: 344   ◆ Protein: 28 g   ◆ Cholesterol: 92 mg
◆ Sodium: 708 mg   ◆ Fat, total: 12 g   ◆ Carbohydrates: 30 g
◆ Fiber: 2 g   ◆ Fat, saturated: 2 g

Chicken with Roasted Pepper and Prosciutto

1	small red pepper	1
1 lb	skinless, boneless chicken breasts (about 4)	500 g
1 oz	sliced prosciutto (4 thin slices)	25 g
2 oz	mozzarella cheese, cut into 4 equal-sized pieces	50 g
1	egg white	1
2 tbsp	water	25 mL
2/3 cup	seasoned bread crumbs	150 mL
2 tsp	vegetable oil	10 mL

Serve chicken breasts whole, or slice crosswise into medallions and fan out on the plate for a pretty presentation.

Serves 4
Preheat oven to broil
Baking sheet sprayed with vegetable spray

1. Broil red pepper for 15 to 20 minutes, turning often until charred on all sides. Preheat oven to 425°F (220°C). Put pepper in bowl and cover tightly with plastic wrap. When cool enough to handle, remove stem, skin and seeds, and cut into thin strips.

2. Pound chicken breasts between sheets of waxed paper to 1/4-inch (5 mm) thickness. Divide prosciutto slices among flattened chicken breasts. Place a piece of cheese at the short end of each breast, and place roasted pepper strips on top of the cheese. Starting at the filling end, carefully roll the breasts up tightly. Use a toothpick to hold chicken breast together.

3. In small bowl, whisk together egg white and water. Put bread crumbs on a plate. Dip each chicken roll in egg white mixture, then in bread crumbs. Heat oil in nonstick skillet sprayed with vegetable spray. Cook over high heat for 3 minutes, turning often, or until browned on all sides. Transfer to prepared baking sheet and bake for 10 to 15 minutes. Remove toothpicks before serving.

Tips

✦ Use 4 oz (125 g) of bottled roasted red peppers rather than roasting your own.

✦ If prosciutto is unavailable, use thin slices of smoked ham.

✦ If a more intense flavor is desired, use a stronger tasting cheese.

Nutritional Analysis (Per Serving)
✦ Calories: 269   ✦ Protein: 34 g   ✦ Cholesterol: 78 mg
✦ Sodium: 717 mg   ✦ Fat, total: 7 g   ✦ Carbohydrates: 14 g
✦ Fiber: 0 g   ✦ Fat, saturated: 2 g

Chicken Cacciatore with Thick Tomato Sauce

4	chicken drumsticks, skinned	4
4	chicken thighs, skinned	4
	All-purpose flour for dusting	
1 tbsp	vegetable oil	15 mL
2 tsp	crushed garlic	10 mL
1 cup	chopped onion	250 mL
1/2 cup	chopped sweet green pepper	125 mL
1 cup	sliced mushrooms	250 mL
1	can (19 oz/540 mL) tomatoes, crushed	1
2 tbsp	tomato paste	25 mL
1 tsp	dried basil	5 mL
1 tsp	dried oregano	5 mL
1/4 cup	red wine	50 mL
1 tbsp	grated Parmesan cheese	15 mL
1/4 cup	chopped fresh parsley	50 mL

Serves 4

1. Dust chicken with flour. In large nonstick skillet, heat oil; sauté chicken just until browned on all sides. Remove and set aside.

2. To skillet, add garlic, onion, green pepper and mushrooms; sauté for 5 minutes or until softened. Add tomatoes, tomato paste, basil, oregano and wine; stir to mix well.

3. Return chicken to skillet; cover and simmer for 20 to 30 minutes or until juices run clear when chicken is pierced, stirring occasionally and turning pieces over. Serve sprinkled with cheese and parsley.

Tip

✦ You can use vegetables such as zucchini or eggplant to replace the peppers and mushrooms.

Nutritional Analysis (Per Serving)
✦ Calories: 192   ✦ Protein: 17 g   ✦ Cholesterol: 4 mg
✦ Sodium: 341 mg   ✦ Fat: 7 g   ✦ Carbohydrates: 13 g
✦ Fiber: 3 g

Chicken and Eggplant Parmesan

4	crosswise slices of eggplant, skin on, approximately ½ inch (1 cm) thick	4
1	whole egg	1
1	egg white	1
1 tbsp	water or milk	15 mL
⅔ cup	seasoned bread crumbs	150 mL
3 tbsp	chopped fresh parsley (or 2 tsp/10 mL dried)	45 mL
1 tbsp	grated Parmesan cheese	15 mL
1 lb	skinless, boneless chicken breasts (about 4)	500 g
2 tsp	vegetable oil	10 mL
1 tsp	minced garlic	5 mL
½ cup	tomato pasta sauce	125 mL
½ cup	grated mozzarella cheese	125 mL

> *Choose lean meat, fish and poultry with skins removed over high-fat deli meats, bacon and sausages.*

Serves 4
Preheat oven to 425°F (220°C)
Baking sheet sprayed with vegetable spray

1. In small bowl, whisk together whole egg, egg white and water. On plate stir together bread crumbs, parsley and Parmesan. Dip eggplant slices in egg wash, then coat with bread-crumb mixture. Place on prepared pan and bake for 20 minutes, or until tender, turning once.

2. Meanwhile, pound chicken breasts between sheets of waxed paper to ¼-inch (5 mm) thickness. Dip chicken in remaining egg wash, then coat with remaining bread-crumb mixture. Heat oil and garlic in nonstick skillet sprayed with vegetable spray and cook for 4 minutes, or until golden brown, turning once.

3. Spread 1 tbsp (15 mL) of tomato sauce on each eggplant slice. Place one chicken breast on top of each eggplant slice. Spread another 1 tbsp (15 mL) of tomato sauce on top of each chicken piece. Sprinkle with cheese and bake for 5 minutes or until cheese melts.

Tips

✦ Turkey, veal or pork scallopini can replace chicken.

✦ A stronger cheese, such as Swiss, can replace mozzarella.

✦ A great dish to reheat the next day.

Nutritional Analysis (Per Serving)
✦ Calories: 317   ✦ Protein: 36 g   ✦ Cholesterol: 130 mg
✦ Sodium: 612 mg   ✦ Fat, total: 10 g   ✦ Carbohydrates: 20 g
✦ Fiber: 2 g   ✦ Fat, saturated: 3 g

Chicken Tetrazzini

8 oz	spaghetti	250 g
4 tsp	margarine	20 mL
1½ tsp	crushed garlic	7 mL
1 cup	chopped onion	250 mL
1 cup	chopped sweet red pepper	250 mL
1 cup	sliced mushrooms	250 mL
3 tbsp	all-purpose flour	45 mL
1½ cups	chicken stock	375 mL
1 cup	2% milk	250 mL
3 tbsp	white wine	45 mL
1½ tsp	Dijon mustard	7 mL
4 oz	cooked boneless skinless chicken pieces	125 g
½ cup	shredded cheddar cheese	125 mL
1 tbsp	grated Parmesan cheese	15 mL
	Chopped fresh parsley	

When using margarine, choose a soft (non-hydrogenated) version to limit consumption of trans fats.

Serves 4 to 6
Preheat broiler

1. In saucepan of boiling water, cook spaghetti according to package directions or until firm to the bite; drain.

2. Meanwhile, in nonstick saucepan, melt margarine; sauté garlic, onion, red pepper and mushrooms until softened, approximately 5 minutes. Add flour and cook, stirring, for 1 minute.

3. Add stock, milk, wine and mustard; cook, stirring, for 3 minutes or until thickened. Add chicken.

4. Add sauce to spaghetti and toss to mix well; place in baking dish. Sprinkle cheddar and Parmesan cheeses over top; bake until top is golden, approximately 5 minutes. Garnish with parsley.

Tips

✦ Try this dish with macaroni or penne instead of spaghetti.

✦ Substitute fresh tuna or swordfish for the chicken.

✦ Mozzarella cheese can replace the cheddar.

✦ Substitute the chicken with 4 oz (125 g) of cooked seafood for a change.

Nutritional Analysis (Per Serving)
✦ Calories: 318 ✦ Protein: 17 g ✦ Cholesterol: 29 mg
✦ Sodium: 505 mg ✦ Fat: 9 g ✦ Carbohydrates: 40 g
✦ Fiber: 2 g

Sautéed Chicken with Tropical Fruit Sauce

Sauce

3/4 cup	canned pineapple bits, drained	175 mL
1/2 cup	orange or pineapple juice	125 mL
1/2 cup	chicken stock	125 mL
1/4 cup	chopped dried apricots	50 mL
2 tbsp	brown sugar	25 mL
1 tbsp	soya sauce	15 mL
1 tbsp	cornstarch	15 mL
1 tsp	minced garlic	5 mL
1 tsp	grated orange zest	5 mL
1	egg white	1
2 tbsp	water	25 mL
3/4 cup	seasoned bread crumbs	175 mL
1 1/2 lb	skinless, boneless chicken breasts (approximately 6)	750 g
1 tsp	vegetable oil	5 mL

Serves 6

1. In small saucepan, combine pineapple, juice, stock, apricots, brown sugar, soya sauce, cornstarch, garlic and zest until smooth and well blended; cook over medium heat for 5 minutes, or until slightly thickened. Reduce heat to low and keep warm.

2. In shallow bowl, whisk together egg white and water. Put bread crumbs on a plate. Between sheets of waxed paper pound breasts to 1/4-inch (5 mm) thickness.

3. Dip chicken in egg wash, then in bread crumbs. In large nonstick skillet sprayed with vegetable spray, heat oil over medium-high heat. Cook for 2 minutes per side, or until just done at center. Serve with sauce.

Tips

✦ Dates can replace the apricots.

✦ If fresh pineapple is available, add to sauce when you've finished cooking.

✦ Veal or turkey scallopini can replace chicken.

Make Ahead

✦ Sauce can be made up to a day ahead. Reheat gently, adding more stock if too thick.

Nutritional Analysis (Per Serving)
✦ Calories: 253   ✦ Protein: 29 g   ✦ Cholesterol: 66 mg
✦ Sodium: 668 mg   ✦ Fat, total: 3 g   ✦ Carbohydrates: 27 g
✦ Fiber: 1 g   ✦ Fat, saturated: 0.6 g

Chinese Lemon Chicken on a Bed of Red Peppers and Snow Peas

1 tsp	vegetable oil	5 mL
1½ cups	thinly sliced red peppers	375 mL
1½ cups	sugar snap peas or halved snow peas	375 mL
1 lb	skinless, boneless chicken breasts (about 4)	500 g
¼ cup	all-purpose flour	50 mL
2 tsp	vegetable oil	10 mL
Sauce		
1 cup	chicken stock	250 mL
3 tbsp	lemon juice	45 mL
2 tbsp	granulated sugar	25 mL
1 tbsp	vegetable oil	15 mL
4 tsp	cornstarch	20 mL
1 tsp	sesame oil	5 mL
1 tsp	grated lemon zest	5 mL
½ tsp	minced garlic	2 mL
2 tbsp	chopped fresh parsley	25 mL

Serves 4

1. In a large nonstick skillet sprayed with vegetable spray, heat 1 tsp (5 mL) oil over medium heat and sauté red peppers and peas just until tender-crisp (approximately 3 minutes). Place in serving dish.

2. Between sheets of waxed paper, pound chicken breasts to ¼-inch (5 mm) thickness. Dust with flour. In large nonstick skillet sprayed with vegetable spray, heat oil; sauté chicken until browned on both sides and just cooked (approximately 6 to 8 minutes).

3. In saucepan combine stock, lemon juice, sugar, oil, cornstarch, sesame oil, lemon zest and garlic; cook over medium heat for 2 to 3 minutes or until thickened. Pour some sauce over chicken. Sprinkle with parsley. Serve individual servings with remaining sauce.

Tips

+ This is a beautiful looking dish. If you substitute any vegetables, try to keep contrasting colors.

+ Replace chicken with turkey, veal or pork scallopini.

Make Ahead

+ Prepare sauce earlier in the day. Add a little water if too thick before serving.

Nutritional Analysis (Per Serving)
+ Calories: 290 + Protein: 29 g + Cholesterol: 66 mg
+ Sodium: 313 mg + Fat, total: 10 g + Carbohydrates: 20 g
+ Fiber: 2 g + Fat, saturated: 1 g

Chinese Chicken with Garlic Ginger Sauce

3 lb	whole chicken	1.5 kg
Sauce		
⅓ cup	chicken stock	75 mL
¼ cup	chopped green onions (about 2 medium)	50 mL
3 tbsp	vegetable oil	45 mL
4 tsp	soya sauce	20 mL
1 tsp	minced garlic	5 mL
1 tsp	minced gingerroot	5 mL

To get more mono- and polyunsaturated fat in your diet, use olive, canola, safflower, corn, soybean or sunflower oils for cooking.

Serves 6

1. Remove neck and giblets from chicken and discard. Place chicken in large saucepan and add water to cover. Cover saucepan and bring to a boil over high heat. Reduce heat to low and simmer, covered, for 45 minutes, or until juices run clear from chicken leg when pierced.

2. Meanwhile, whisk together stock, green onions, oil, soya sauce, garlic and ginger in a small bowl.

3. Remove chicken from pot and let cool slightly. Remove skin; cut into serving pieces. Serve with dipping sauce.

Tips

✦ This is delicious served cold.

✦ This is a simple-looking chicken dish, but unbelievably tasty. Great for leftovers.

✦ Increase garlic and ginger to taste.

Make Ahead

✦ Prepare up to a day ahead and serve at room temperature.

Nutritional Analysis (Per Serving)
✦ Calories: 156 ✦ Protein: 17 g ✦ Cholesterol: 53 mg
✦ Sodium: 337 mg ✦ Fat, total: 9 g ✦ Carbohydrates: 1 g
✦ Fiber: 0 g ✦ Fat, saturated: 1 g

Teriyaki Chicken Stir-Fry with Asparagus and Red Peppers

Sauce

1/2 cup	chicken stock or water	125 mL
1/4 cup	rice wine vinegar	50 mL
4 tbsp	honey	60 mL
3 tbsp	soya sauce	45 mL
1 tbsp	sesame oil	15 mL
2 tsp	minced garlic	10 mL
2 tsp	minced ginger	10 mL
2 1/2 tsp	cornstarch	12 mL
12 oz	penne	375 g
12 oz	boneless skinless chicken breast, cut into thin strips	375 g
2 tsp	vegetable oil	10 mL
1 1/2 cups	sliced red peppers	375 mL
1 1/2 cups	asparagus cut into 1-inch (2.5 cm) pieces	375 mL

Serves 6

1. In small bowl, combine stock, vinegar, honey, soya sauce, sesame oil, garlic, ginger and cornstarch; mix well.

2. In large pot of boiling water, cook penne until tender but firm. Drain and place in serving bowl. Meanwhile, in wok or skillet sprayed with vegetable spray, stir-fry chicken for 2 1/2 minutes or until just cooked at center. Drain any excess liquid and remove chicken from wok.

3. Add oil to wok and stir-fry red peppers and asparagus for 4 minutes or until tender-crisp; stir sauce again and add to wok along with chicken. Cook for 1 minute or until slightly thickened. Toss with drained pasta.

Tips

✦ Replace asparagus with broccoli, snow peas or sugar snap peas.

✦ Chicken can be replaced with pork, beef steak or seafood.

Make Ahead

✦ Prepare sauce up to a day ahead. Stir before using.

Nutritional Analysis (Per Serving)

✦ Calories: 373   ✦ Protein: 22 g   ✦ Cholesterol: 33 mg
✦ Sodium: 642 mg   ✦ Fat, total: 6 g   ✦ Carbohydrates: 59 g
✦ Fiber: 2 g   ✦ Fat, saturated: 1 g

Chicken with Teriyaki Vegetables

4	boneless skinless chicken breasts	4
1 tsp	vegetable oil	5 mL
1 tsp	crushed garlic	5 mL
1	large sweet red pepper, sliced thinly	1
1 cup	snow peas, trimmed	250 mL
Marinade		
3 tbsp	sherry	45 mL
3 tbsp	brown sugar	45 mL
2 tbsp	water	25 mL
2 tbsp	soya sauce	25 mL
2 tbsp	vegetable oil	25 mL
1½ tsp	minced gingerroot	7 mL

Serves 4
Preheat oven to 425°F (220°C)
Baking dish sprayed with nonstick vegetable spray

1. *Marinade:* In medium bowl, combine sherry, sugar, water, soya sauce, oil and ginger. Set aside.
2. Place chicken between 2 sheets of waxed paper; pound until thin and flattened. Add to bowl and marinate for 30 minutes.
3. Remove chicken and place in baking dish. Pour marinade into saucepan; cook for 3 to 4 minutes or until thickened and syrupy. Set 2 tbsp (25 mL) aside; brush remainder over chicken. Cover and bake for 10 to 15 minutes or until no longer pink inside.
4. Meanwhile, in large nonstick skillet, heat oil; sauté garlic, red pepper and snow peas for 2 minutes. Add reserved marinade; cook for 2 minutes, stirring constantly. Serve over chicken.

Tip
✦ Chicken quarters or breasts with the bone in can also be used. Bake for 20 to 30 minutes or until no longer pink inside.

Nutritional Analysis (Per Serving)
✦ Calories: 221 ✦ Protein: 26 g ✦ Cholesterol: 62 mg
✦ Sodium: 318 mg ✦ Fat: 7 g ✦ Carbohydrates: 9 g
✦ Fiber: 1 g

Chicken Breasts Stuffed with Spinach and Cheese with Tomato Garlic Sauce

4	boneless skinless chicken breasts	4
1½ tsp	vegetable oil	7 mL
½ tsp	crushed garlic	2 mL
1	medium green onion, finely chopped	1
¼ cup	drained cooked chopped spinach	50 mL
¼ cup	diced mushrooms	50 mL
¼ cup	shredded mozzarella cheese	50 mL
¼ cup	chicken stock	50 mL
Sauce		
1½ tsp	margarine	7 mL
1 tsp	crushed garlic	5 mL
1½ cups	diced tomatoes	375 mL
⅓ cup	chicken stock	75 mL
1 tbsp	chopped fresh parsley	15 mL

When using margarine, choose a soft (non-hydrogenated) version to limit consumption of trans fats.

Serves 4
Preheat oven to 400°F (200°C)
Baking dish sprayed with nonstick vegetable spray

1. Place chicken between 2 sheets of waxed paper; pound until flattened. Set aside.

2. In nonstick skillet, heat oil; sauté garlic, onion, spinach and mushrooms until softened. Spoon evenly over breasts; sprinkle with cheese. Roll up and fasten with toothpicks.

3. Place chicken in baking dish; pour in stock. Cover and bake for 10 minutes or until chicken is no longer pink. Remove chicken to serving dish and keep warm.

4. *Sauce:* Meanwhile, in small saucepan, melt margarine; sauté garlic for 1 minute. Stir in tomatoes and chicken stock; cook for 3 minutes or until heated through. Add parsley and serve over chicken.

Tips

✦ Be sure not to overcook the chicken or it will become dry.

✦ If using fresh spinach, use 1½ cups (375 mL). Cook, drain well and chop.

Nutritional Analysis (Per Serving)
✦ Calories: 216   ✦ Protein: 30 g   ✦ Cholesterol: 70 mg
✦ Sodium: 247 mg   ✦ Fat: 8 g   ✦ Carbohydrates: 4 g
✦ Fiber: 1 g

Maple Chicken with Peppers and Mustard over Rotini

6 oz	skinless boneless chicken breast	175 g
8 oz	rotini	250 g
1/3 cup	pure maple syrup	75 mL
1/3 cup	chicken stock	75 mL
3 tbsp	balsamic vinegar	45 mL
2 tbsp	olive oil	25 mL
1 tbsp	Dijon mustard	15 mL
2 tsp	cornstarch	10 mL
1 tsp	minced garlic	5 mL
1 cup	thinly sliced red bell peppers	250 mL
1/3 cup	chopped green onions	75 mL

B vitamins and heart disease: *Several studies have shown that a diet lacking in B vitamins may increase the risk of heart disease by causing a high blood level of homocysteine, an amino acid that we normally convert to other harmless amino acids with the help of three B vitamins: folate, B_6 and B_{12}. When homocysteine levels are high, the result can be damaged blood vessel walls and a build-up of cholesterol. Good sources of folate include spinach, lentils, and enriched pasta. One serving of this pasta dish provides 25% of your daily folate needs (0.4 mg). For more on B vitamins, see page 210.*

Serves 4

1. In a nonstick saucepan sprayed with vegetable spray or on a preheated grill, cook chicken over medium-high heat, turning once, for 12 minutes or until cooked through. Cut chicken into cubes; set aside.

2. In a large pot of boiling water, cook rotini for 8 to 10 minutes or until tender but firm; drain. Meanwhile, in another saucepan over medium-high heat, combine maple syrup, chicken stock, balsamic vinegar, olive oil, Dijon mustard, cornstarch and garlic; whisk well. Cook, stirring constantly, for 3 minutes or until thickened and bubbly. Add red peppers; reduce heat to medium-low. Cook, covered, for 2 minutes or until peppers are tender.

3. In a large serving bowl, combine pasta, chicken, green onions and sauce; toss to coat well. Serve immediately.

Tip

✦ Be sure that you buy only pure maple syrup for this recipe. That means 100% maple syrup — not maple flavored syrup or the kind that contains some (usually no more than 15%) maple syrup. These artificial syrups contain mostly water, sugar and corn syrup; pure maple syrup is distilled from maple sap, and is twice as sweet as sugar.

Nutritional Analysis (Per Serving)

✦ Calories: 396 ✦ Protein: 17 g ✦ Cholesterol: 24 mg
✦ Sodium: 116 mg ✦ Fat, total: 8 g ✦ Carbohydrates: 64 g
✦ Fiber: 3 g ✦ Fat, saturated: 1.3 g

Chicken with Red Pepper and Onions

4	chicken breasts or legs	4
	All-purpose flour for dusting	

Sauce

1 tbsp	margarine	15 mL
1½ tsp	crushed garlic	7 mL
¾ cup	diced onion	175 mL
1½ cups	diced sweet red pepper	375 mL
1 tbsp	all-purpose flour	15 mL
1⅓ cups	chicken stock	325 mL
	Parsley sprigs	

Cut down on foods that have been fried or deep-fried and those that contain hydrogenated vegetable oils.

When using margarine, choose a soft (non-hydrogenated) version to limit consumption of trans fats.

Serves 4
Preheat oven to 400°F (200°C)
Baking dish sprayed with nonstick vegetable spray

1. Dust chicken with flour. In large nonstick skillet sprayed with nonstick vegetable spray, brown chicken on both sides, approximately 10 minutes. Place in baking dish; cover and bake for 20 to 30 minutes or until no longer pink inside and juices run clear when chicken is pierced.

2. *Sauce:* Meanwhile, in small saucepan, melt margarine; sauté garlic, onion and red pepper for 5 minutes or until softened. Add flour and cook, stirring, for 1 minute. Add stock and cook, stirring, just until thickened, approximately 3 minutes.

3. Place chicken on serving dish; pour sauce over top. Garnish with parsley. Remove skin before eating.

Tip

✦ This red pepper sauce can also be puréed.

Nutritional Analysis (Per Serving)
✦ Calories: 250 ✦ Protein: 35 g ✦ Cholesterol: 84 mg
✦ Sodium: 383 mg ✦ Fat: 8 g ✦ Carbohydrates: 13 g
✦ Fiber: 0 g

Chicken, Red Pepper and Snow Pea Stir-Fry

8 oz	boneless skinless chicken breasts, cubed	250 g
	All-purpose flour for dusting	
1 tbsp	vegetable oil	15 mL
1 tsp	sesame oil	5 mL
1 tsp	crushed garlic	5 mL
1 cup	thinly sliced sweet red pepper	250 mL
1 cup	sliced water chestnuts	250 mL
1 cup	snow peas, cut in half	250 mL
¼ cup	cashews, coarsely chopped	50 mL
1	large green onion, chopped	1

Sauce

½ cup	chicken stock	125 mL
1 tbsp	soya sauce	15 mL
1 tbsp	hoisin sauce	15 mL
2 tsp	cornstarch	10 mL
1 tsp	minced gingerroot	5 mL

Serves 4

1. *Sauce:* In small bowl, mix together stock, soya sauce, hoisin sauce, cornstarch and ginger; set aside.
2. Dust chicken cubes with flour. In nonstick skillet, heat vegetable and sesame oils; sauté garlic, chicken, red pepper, water chestnuts and snow peas over high heat just until vegetables are tender-crisp, approximately 2 minutes.
3. Add sauce to skillet; cook for 2 minutes or just until chicken is no longer pink inside and sauce has thickened. Garnish with cashews and green onions.

Tips

✦ You can substitute other vegetables, such as asparagus, broccoli or bean sprouts, for the snow peas.

✦ Tender beef or veal can replace the chicken.

Nutritional Analysis (Per Serving)
✦ Calories: 248   ✦ Protein: 17 g   ✦ Cholesterol: 31 mg
✦ Sodium: 614 mg ✦ Fat: 10 g   ✦ Carbohydrates: 21 g
✦ Fiber: 3 g

Chicken with Paprika in Vegetable Cream Sauce

4	chicken breasts or legs	4
	All-purpose flour for dusting	
1 tbsp	vegetable oil	15 mL
2 tsp	crushed garlic	10 mL
³/₄ cup	chopped onion	175 mL
³/₄ cup	chopped sweet red or green pepper	175 mL
³/₄ cup	sliced mushrooms	175 mL
1 cup	chicken stock	250 mL
2 tsp	paprika	10 mL
2 tsp	all-purpose flour	10 mL
¹/₄ cup	light sour cream	50 mL

Serves 4

1. Dust chicken with flour. In large nonstick skillet sprayed with nonstick vegetable spray, sauté chicken until browned on both sides, approximately 10 minutes. Remove and set aside.

2. In same skillet, heat oil; sauté garlic, onion, red pepper and mushrooms until softened, approximately 5 minutes. Add chicken stock.

3. Return chicken to pan; sprinkle chicken with paprika. Cover and simmer for 20 to 30 minutes or until chicken is no longer pink inside and juices run clear when chicken is pierced. Remove chicken to serving platter.

4. Mix flour with sour cream until well combined; add to skillet and cook on low heat, stirring, until thickened, 3 to 4 minutes. Pour over chicken. Remove skin before eating.

Tip

✦ For an extravagant change, try fresh wild mushrooms, such as oyster mushrooms.

Nutritional Analysis (Per Serving)
✦ Calories: 215 ✦ Protein: 31 g ✦ Cholesterol: 72 mg
✦ Sodium: 279 mg ✦ Fat: 5 g ✦ Carbohydrates: 15 g
✦ Fiber: 2 g

Chicken with Red Wine Sauce and Chopped Dates

4	chicken breasts or legs	4
	All-purpose flour for dusting	
1 tbsp	vegetable oil	15 mL
1	medium onion, chopped	1
2 tsp	crushed garlic	10 mL
2	large carrots, sliced	2
1/2 lb	mushrooms, sliced	250 g
1 1/4 cups	chicken stock	300 mL
2/3 cup	dry red wine	150 mL
2 tbsp	tomato paste	25 mL
1 tsp	dried oregano	5 mL
1 tsp	dried basil	5 mL
1/2 tsp	dried rosemary	2 mL
1/2 cup	chopped dates	125 mL
	Parsley sprigs	

Serves 4
Preheat oven to 400°F (200°C)

1. Dust chicken with flour. In large nonstick skillet sprayed with nonstick vegetable spray, sauté chicken until browned on both sides, approximately 10 minutes. Place in baking dish.

2. In same skillet, heat oil; sauté onion, garlic, carrots and mushrooms until softened, 5 to 8 minutes. Add stock, wine, tomato paste, oregano, basil and rosemary; cover and simmer for 10 minutes, stirring occasionally. Stir in dates.

3. Pour sauce over chicken. Bake for 30 minutes, basting occasionally, or until chicken is no longer pink inside and juices run clear when chicken is pierced. Garnish with parsley. Remove skin before eating.

Tips

✦ Instead of dates, try chopped prunes for a change.

✦ Store dry herbs in tightly closed containers away from heat, light and moisture.

Nutritional Analysis (Per Serving)
✦ Calories: 310　✦ Protein: 31 g　✦ Cholesterol: 66 mg
✦ Sodium: 393 mg　✦ Fat: 5 g　✦ Carbohydrates: 36 g
✦ Fiber: 5 g

Chicken with Leeks, Sweet Potatoes and Dates

4	chicken breasts or legs	4
	All-purpose flour for dusting	
1 tbsp	margarine	15 mL
2 tsp	crushed garlic	10 mL
2 cups	chopped leeks	500 mL
2 cups	chopped peeled sweet potatoes	500 mL
1½ cups	chicken stock	375 mL
⅓ cup	white wine	75 mL
½ tsp	cinnamon	2 mL
½ tsp	ground ginger	2 mL
½ cup	chopped dates	125 mL

When using margarine, choose a soft (non-hydrogenated) version to limit consumption of trans fats.

Serves 4
Preheat oven to 400°F (200°C)

1. Dust chicken with flour. In nonstick skillet sprayed with nonstick vegetable spray, brown chicken on both sides, approximately 10 minutes. Place in baking dish.

2. In same skillet, melt margarine; sauté garlic, leeks and potatoes until softened, approximately 10 minutes, stirring constantly. Add chicken stock, wine, cinnamon and ginger; cover and simmer for 10 minutes. Stir in dates.

3. Pour sauce over chicken; bake for 20 to 30 minutes, basting occasionally, or until chicken is no longer pink inside and juices run clear when chicken is pierced. Remove skin before eating.

Tips

✦ If leeks are unavailable, use the same measurement of sliced onions.

✦ Dried apricots or raisins can replace the dates, or use a combination.

✦ If using a food processor to chop the dates, grease the blade with vegetable oil first to avoid sticking.

Nutritional Analysis (Per Serving)
✦ Calories: 400   ✦ Protein: 34 g   ✦ Cholesterol: 84 mg
✦ Sodium: 427 mg   ✦ Fat: 8 g   ✦ Carbohydrates: 48 g
✦ Fiber: 5 g

Chicken Breasts Wrapped in Phyllo with Basil and Tomatoes

4	boneless skinless chicken breasts	4
1½ tsp	margarine	7 mL
½ tsp	crushed garlic	2 mL
½ cup	chopped onion	125 mL
½ cup	chopped mushrooms	125 mL
¼ cup	chopped tomatoes	50 mL
¼ tsp	dried basil (or 2 tbsp/25 mL chopped fresh)	1 mL
4	sheets phyllo	4
4 tsp	margarine, melted	20 mL
½ cup	tomato sauce, warmed	125 mL

> *When using margarine, choose a soft (non-hydrogenated) version to limit consumption of trans fats.*

Serves 4
Preheat oven to 400°F (200°C)
Baking sheet sprayed with nonstick vegetable spray

1. Place chicken between 2 sheets of waxed paper; pound until thin and flattened. Set aside.

2. In small nonstick skillet, melt margarine; sauté garlic, onion and mushrooms until softened, approximately 3 minutes. Add tomatoes and basil; cook for 1 minute. Spoon evenly over breasts. Roll up carefully and fasten with toothpicks.

3. Layer phyllo sheets; cut into 4 to make 16 squares. Place 2 squares on flat surface; brush with some margarine. Place 2 more squares over top. Place rolled breast over top and enclose with phyllo. Brush with margarine; place on baking sheet. Repeat with 3 other breasts.

4. Bake for 15 to 20 minutes or just until phyllo is golden and chicken is no longer pink. Serve with warmed tomato sauce.

Tip

✦ When testing doneness, carefully place tip of knife into chicken, trying not to break phyllo package.

Make Ahead

✦ Prepare filling ahead of time; assemble and bake right before eating.

Nutritional Analysis (Per Serving)
✦ Calories: 274   ✦ Protein: 28 g   ✦ Cholesterol: 66 mg
✦ Sodium: 391 mg ✦ Fat: 8 g   ✦ Carbohydrates: 18 g
✦ Fiber: 2 g

Crunchy Cheese Chicken Fingers

1 lb	skinless boneless chicken breasts, cut into 1-inch (2 cm) strips	500 g
1½ cups	Cheerios breakfast cereal	375 mL
2 tbsp	grated Parmesan cheese	25 mL
½ tsp	chili powder	2 mL
½ tsp	dried basil	2 mL
½ tsp	dried oregano	2 mL
1 tsp	minced garlic	5 mL
1	egg	1
2 tbsp	milk or water	25 mL

Serves 4
Preheat oven to 400°F (200°C)
Baking sheet sprayed with vegetable spray

1. Put Cheerios, Parmesan, chili powder, basil, oregano and garlic in food processor; process until Cheerios are fine crumbs. Place on plate.
2. In small bowl, whisk together egg and milk. Dip each chicken strip in egg wash, then roll in crumbs; place on prepared baking sheet. Bake for 10 to 15 minutes until browned and chicken is cooked through.

Tips

+ For a change — and less fat — substitute firm fish fillets (such as haddock, halibut or cod) for chicken.
+ Try other dried spices of your choice.
+ Bread crumbs or bran- or cornflakes can replace Cheerios.

Nutritional Analysis (Per Serving)
+ Calories: 190   + Protein: 33 g   + Cholesterol: 145 mg
+ Sodium: 325 mg   + Fat: 4 g   + Carbohydrates: 11 g
+ Fiber: 1 g

Baked Chicken with Tomatoes, Raisins and Almonds

1 tbsp	vegetable oil	15 mL
4	chicken breasts or legs	4
2 tsp	crushed garlic	10 mL
¾ cup	chopped red onion	175 mL
¾ cup	chopped sweet green pepper	175 mL
⅓ cup	chopped carrots	75 mL
2 tsp	curry powder	10 mL
1	can (19 oz/540 mL) tomatoes, crushed or puréed	1
⅓ cup	sliced pitted black olives	75 mL
⅓ cup	raisins	75 mL
2 tbsp	sliced almonds, toasted	25 mL

Serves 4
Preheat oven to 400°F (200°C)

1. In large nonstick skillet, heat half the oil; brown chicken on both sides, approximately 10 minutes. Remove chicken to baking dish. Pour off extra fat.

2. To skillet, add remaining oil, garlic, onion, green pepper and carrots; sauté until softened, approximately 5 minutes.

3. Stir in curry powder, tomatoes, olives and raisins; reduce heat, cover and simmer for 15 minutes, stirring occasionally.

4. Pour sauce over chicken; cover and bake for 30 minutes or until chicken is no longer pink inside and juices run clear when chicken is pierced. Sprinkle with almonds. Remove skin before eating.

Tips

✦ Adjust the amount of curry powder to your taste.

✦ For maximum freshness and flavor, store curry powder in airtight containers for no more than 2 months.

✦ Toast nuts either in 400°F (200°C) oven or in a skillet on top of stove for 3 to 5 minutes.

Nutritional Analysis (Per Serving)
✦ Calories: 260 ✦ Protein: 30 g ✦ Cholesterol: 66 mg
✦ Sodium: 410 mg ✦ Fat: 5 g ✦ Carbohydrates: 29 g
✦ Fiber: 4 g

Roasted Chicken with Pineapple, Carrots and Ginger

4	chicken breasts or legs	4
1 tbsp	margarine	15 mL
1 cup	chopped sweet green pepper	250 mL
1/2 cup	chopped onion	125 mL
1 cup	chopped carrot	250 mL
1 1/2 tsp	crushed garlic	7 mL
2 tsp	minced gingerroot	10 mL
1/2 cup	pineapple juice	125 mL
1 tbsp	cornstarch	15 mL
4 tsp	soya sauce	20 mL
2 tbsp	brown sugar	25 mL
1/2 cup	chicken stock	125 mL
1 cup	pineapple chunks	250 mL

When using margarine, choose a soft (non-hydrogenated) version to limit consumption of trans fats.

Serves 4
Preheat oven to 400°F (200°C)

1. In large nonstick skillet sprayed with nonstick vegetable spray, sauté chicken until browned on both sides, approximately 10 minutes. Place chicken in baking dish.

2. Pour off fat in skillet; add margarine. Add green pepper, onion, carrot, garlic and ginger; cook until vegetables are softened, approximately 5 minutes.

3. Meanwhile, combine pineapple juice, cornstarch, soya sauce, brown sugar and stock until well mixed. Pour into skillet along with pineapple chunks; cook for 3 to 4 minutes or until thickened.

4. Pour sauce over chicken; bake for 30 to 40 minutes or until juices run clear when chicken is pierced. Remove skin before eating.

Tips

+ Try red pepper in place of the green pepper for a more dramatic appearance.
+ Also try a sprinkle of cinnamon and nutmeg.
+ If using canned pineapple, use juice from can.

Nutritional Analysis (Per Serving)
+ Calories: 325   + Protein: 31 g   + Cholesterol: 90 mg
+ Sodium: 576 mg   + Fat: 9 g   + Carbohydrates: 26 g
+ Fiber: 3 g

Roasted Chicken with Asian Glaze and Fruit Sauce

1	whole chicken (2½ to 3 lb/ 1.25 to 1.5 kg)	1

Glaze

1 tsp	crushed garlic	5 mL
1 tsp	minced gingerroot (or ¼ tsp/1 mL ground ginger)	5 mL
¼ cup	honey	50 mL
¼ cup	sweet dessert wine (plum wine)	50 mL
Pinch	chili flakes	Pinch
1 tbsp	margarine, melted	15 mL
Pinch	dried coriander and/or cumin	Pinch
	Salt and pepper	
½ cup	chicken stock	125 mL

Sauce

1 tbsp	cornstarch	15 mL
½ cup	chicken stock	125 mL
¼ cup	chopped dates	50 mL
¼ cup	chopped dried apricots	50 mL

When using margarine, choose a soft (non-hydrogenated) version to limit consumption of trans fats.

Serves 4
Preheat oven to 400°F (200°C)

1. Place chicken in roasting pan.
2. *Glaze:* In small bowl, mix together garlic, ginger, honey, wine, chili flakes, margarine, coriander, salt and pepper to taste and stock; set half aside for sauce. Brush some of the remaining mixture over chicken. Bake for 50 to 60 minutes or until meat thermometer registers 185°(85°C), basting with more honey mixture every 15 minutes.
3. Cut chicken into 4 quarters; place on serving dish and keep warm.
4. *Sauce:* Pour reserved honey mixture into small saucepan; stir in cornstarch, mixing well. Add chicken stock along with dates and apricots; cook over medium heat, stirring, for 2 minutes or until thickened. Pour over chicken. Remove skin before eating.

Tips

✦ This glaze can also be used over Cornish hens or game birds.

✦ Substitute dried prunes or raisins for the dates or apricots for a change.

Nutritional Analysis (Per Serving)

✦ Calories: 367 ✦ Protein: 36 g ✦ Cholesterol: 100 mg
✦ Sodium: 378 mg ✦ Fat: 9 g ✦ Carbohydrates: 35 g
✦ Fiber: 1 g

Roasted Chicken Stuffed with Apples and Raisins

1	whole chicken (2½ to 3 lb/ 1.25 to 1.5 kg)	1

Stuffing

1½ tsp	margarine	7 mL
½ cup	diced onions	125 mL
⅓ cup	diced carrots	75 mL
1 cup	diced peeled apple	250 mL
¼ cup	raisins	50 mL
4 tsp	brown sugar	20 mL
½ tsp	cinnamon	2 mL
1 cup	cooked rice (preferably brown)	250 mL

Basting Sauce

2 tbsp	brown sugar	25 mL
½ cup	orange juice	125 mL
2 tsp	grated orange rind	10 mL
½ tsp	ground ginger	2 mL

When using margarine, choose a soft (non-hydrogenated) version to limit consumption of trans fats.

Serves 4
Preheat oven to 375°F (190°C)

1. *Stuffing:* In nonstick skillet, melt margarine; sauté onions and carrots until onions are softened. Add apple, raisins, sugar and cinnamon; cook, stirring, for 3 minutes. Stir in rice.

2. *Basting Sauce:* Meanwhile, in small saucepan, combine sugar, orange juice, orange rind and ginger; heat thoroughly.

3. Spoon stuffing into chicken and truss chicken. Place in roasting pan and pour sauce over chicken. Roast for about 1¼ hours or until meat thermometer registers 185°F (85°C), basting often with sauce. Tent chicken with foil if browning too fast. Serve with pan juices. Remove skin before eating.

Tips

✦ Stuff birds just prior to cooking to avoid contaminating with harmful bacteria.

✦ Dry dates or apricots can replace the raisins.

Make Ahead

✦ Stuffing can be made and refrigerated up to the day before.

Nutritional Analysis (Per Serving)
✦ Calories: 355   ✦ Protein: 35 g   ✦ Cholesterol: 104 mg
✦ Sodium: 261 mg   ✦ Fat: 8 g   ✦ Carbohydrates: 40 g
✦ Fiber: 2 g

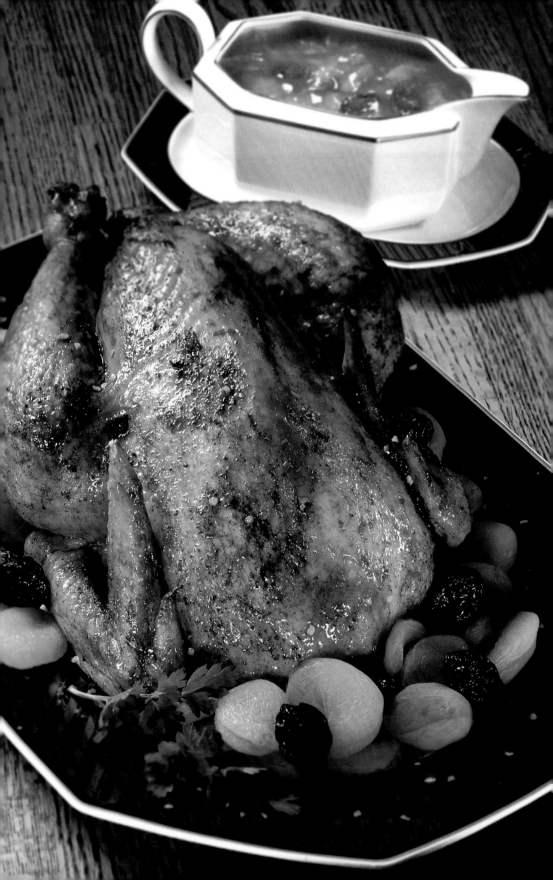

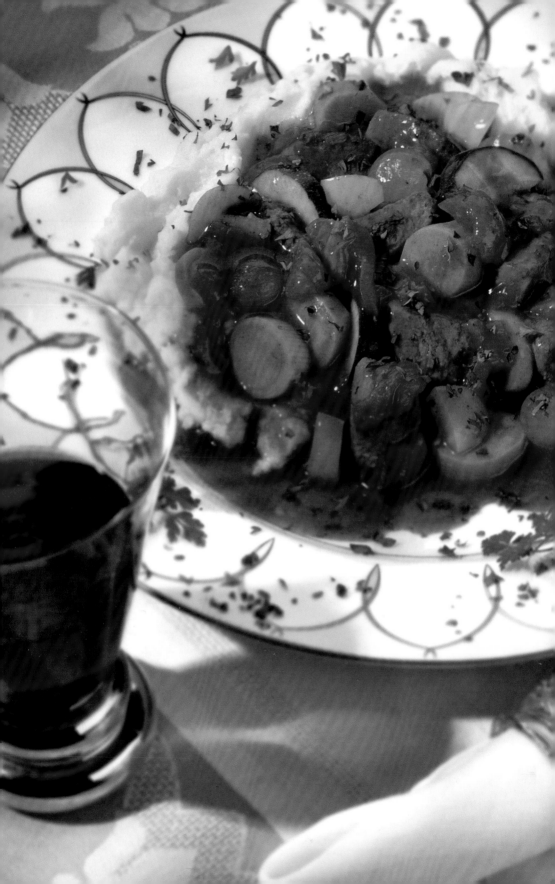

Sweet-and-Sour Chicken Meatballs over Rice

Meatballs

12 oz	ground chicken	375 g
1/4 cup	finely chopped onions	50 mL
2 tbsp	ketchup	25 mL
2 tbsp	bread crumbs	25 mL
1	egg	1
2 tsp	olive oil	10 mL
2 tsp	minced garlic	10 mL
1/3 cup	chopped onions	75 mL
2 cups	tomato juice	500 mL
2 cups	pineapple juice	500 mL
1/2 cup	chili sauce	125 mL
2 cups	white rice	500 mL

Asian chili sauce is a fiery concoction of chili peppers, garlic, sugar and rice vinegar. It's really hot! So if you've got a sensitive palate, use it sparingly. This sauce also makes a good substitute in recipes that call for hot chili peppers.

Serves 8

1. In bowl, combine chicken, onions, ketchup, bread crumbs and egg; mix well. Form each 1 tbsp (15 mL) into a meatball and place on plate; set aside.
2. In large saucepan, heat oil over medium heat. Add garlic and onions and cook just until softened, approximately 3 minutes. Add tomato and pineapple juices, chili sauce and meatballs. Cover and simmer uncovered for 30 to 40 minutes just until meatballs are tender.
3. Meanwhile, bring 4 cups (1 L) of water to a boil. Stir in rice, reduce heat, cover and simmer for 20 minutes or until liquid is absorbed. Remove from heat and let stand for 5 minutes, covered. Serve meatballs and sauce over rice.

Tips

✦ If your kids don't like rice, serve this dish over 1 lb (500 g) of spaghetti.

✦ You can omit onions.

✦ If children like pineapple, add 1 cup (250 mL) pineapple cubes (canned or fresh) at the end of the cooking time.

Make Ahead

✦ Make up to 2 days ahead and reheat. Can be frozen for up to 6 weeks. Great for leftovers.

Nutritional Analysis (Per Serving)

✦ Calories: 351   ✦ Protein: 15 g   ✦ Cholesterol: 54 mg
✦ Sodium: 558 mg   ✦ Fat, total: 6 g   ✦ Carbohydrates: 58 g
✦ Fiber: 2 g   ✦ Fat, saturated: 2 g

Chicken Kebabs with Ginger Lemon Marinade

8 oz	boneless skinless chicken breasts, cut into 2-inch (5 cm) cubes	250 g
16	squares sweet green pepper	16
16	pineapple chunks (fresh or canned)	16
16	cherry tomatoes	16

Ginger Lemon Marinade

3 tbsp	lemon juice	45 mL
2 tbsp	water	25 mL
1 tbsp	vegetable oil	15 mL
2 tsp	sesame oil	10 mL
1½ tsp	red wine vinegar	7 mL
4 tsp	brown sugar	20 mL
1 tsp	minced gingerroot (or ¼ tsp/1 mL ground)	5 mL
½ tsp	ground coriander	2 mL
½ tsp	ground fennel seeds (optional)	2 mL

Serves 4

1. *Ginger Lemon Marinade:* In small bowl, combine lemon juice, water, vegetable oil, sesame oil, vinegar, brown sugar, ginger, coriander and fennel seeds (if using); mix well. Add chicken and mix well; marinate for 20 minutes.

2. Alternately thread chicken cubes, green pepper, pineapple and tomatoes onto 4 long or 8 short barbecue skewers. Barbecue for 15 to 20 minutes or just until chicken is no longer pink inside, brushing often with marinade and rotating every 5 minutes.

Tips

♦ This tart yet sweet marinade complements veal and firm white fish, too.

♦ For a change, try a combination of red and yellow peppers along with the green pepper.

Nutritional Analysis (Per Serving)
♦ Calories: 110   ♦ Protein: 13 g   ♦ Cholesterol: 31 mg
♦ Sodium: 35 mg   ♦ Fat: 2 g   ♦ Carbohydrates: 10 g
♦ Fiber: 2 g

Chicken Bean Chili

1½ tsp	vegetable oil	7 mL
1 cup	diced carrots	250 mL
1 cup	chopped onions	250 mL
1 tsp	crushed garlic	5 mL
1	can (19 oz/540 mL) tomatoes, crushed	1
2 cups	chicken stock	500 mL
2 tsp	chili powder	10 mL
1½ tsp	dried basil	7 mL
1 tsp	dried oregano	5 mL
2 tbsp	tomato paste	25 mL
¾ cup	canned white kidney beans, drained	175 mL
¾ cup	canned black beans, drained	175 mL
¾ cup	corn niblets	175 mL
8 oz	skinless boneless chicken breast	250 g

Serves 4 to 6

1. In large nonstick saucepan, heat oil; sauté carrots, onions and garlic until softened, approximately 5 minutes.
2. Add tomatoes, stock, chili powder, basil, oregano, tomato paste, beans and corn. Simmer uncovered for 30 to 40 minutes, stirring occasionally.
3. Meanwhile, in small nonstick skillet sprayed with vegetable spray, sauté chicken until just cooked, approximately 3 minutes. Set aside.
4. When chili mixture is cooked, add sautéed chicken. Mix well and serve chili alone in bowl, wrapped in tortillas, or on top of a baked potato sprinkled with cheese.

Tips

✦ Serve over baked potatoes, in tortillas or tacos or over rice or pasta.

✦ Diced pork, beef or turkey can replace chicken.

✦ Other varieties of canned beans can be used.

Make Ahead

✦ Make and refrigerate up to a day ahead. Reheat gently, adding more stock if too thick.

Nutritional Analysis (Per Serving)
✦ Calories: 220　✦ Protein: 15 g　✦ Cholesterol: 17 mg
✦ Sodium: 575 mg　✦ Fat: 5 g　✦ Carbohydrates: 30 g
✦ Fiber: 5 g

Chicken Mushroom Ratatouille Chili

12 oz	skinless, boneless chicken breast, diced	375 g
2 tsp	vegetable oil	10 mL
2 tsp	minced garlic	10 mL
1 cup	chopped onions	250 mL
1/2 cup	chopped carrots	125 mL
1 2/3 cups	chopped green peppers	400 mL
1 2/3 cups	chopped, peeled eggplant	400 mL
1 1/2 cups	chopped mushrooms	375 mL
2 tbsp	tomato paste	25 mL
1	can (19 oz/540 mL) tomatoes, puréed	1
2 cups	chicken stock	500 mL
1 1/3 cups	chopped, peeled potatoes	325 mL
1 cup	canned red kidney beans, drained	250 mL
1 tbsp	chili powder	15 mL
1 1/2 tsp	dried basil	7 mL
2	bay leaves	2

Serves 4 to 6

1. In small nonstick skillet sprayed with vegetable spray, sauté chicken until no longer pink, approximately 3 minutes. Set aside.
2. In large nonstick saucepan sprayed with vegetable spray, heat oil over medium heat. Add garlic, onions, carrots, green peppers and eggplant; cook for 5 minutes or until softened. Add mushrooms and cook for 2 minutes longer.
3. Add tomato paste, tomatoes, stock, potatoes, beans, chili powder, basil and bay leaves; bring to a boil. Cover, reduce heat to low and simmer for 40 minutes, stirring occasionally. Add cooked chicken before serving.

Tips

✦ A great combination of ratatouille and chili in one dish.

✦ Other vegetables can be substituted.

✦ Other beans can also be used.

Make Ahead

✦ Prepare up to a day ahead and reheat gently, adding extra chicken stock if too thick.

✦ Great as leftovers.

Nutritional Analysis (Per Serving)
✦ Calories: 248 ✦ Protein: 18 g ✦ Cholesterol: 39 mg
✦ Sodium: 496 mg ✦ Fat: 7 g ✦ Carbohydrates: 31 g
✦ Fiber: 8 g

Turkey Ratatouille Chile

2 tsp	vegetable oil	10 mL	
2 tsp	minced garlic	10 mL	
1 cup	chopped onions	250 mL	
1²/₃ cups	chopped zucchini	400 mL	
1²/₃ cups	chopped peeled eggplant	400 mL	
1½ cups	chopped mushrooms	375 mL	
12 oz	ground turkey	375 g	
2 tbsp	tomato paste	25 mL	
1	can (19 oz/540 mL) tomatoes, puréed	1	
2 cups	chicken stock	500 mL	
1¹/₃ cups	peeled chopped potatoes	325 mL	
1 cup	canned red kidney beans, drained	250 mL	
1 tbsp	chili powder	15 mL	
1½ tsp	dried basil	7 mL	
1	bay leaf	1	

Serves 4 to 6

1. In large nonstick saucepan sprayed with vegetable spray, heat oil over medium heat. Add garlic, onions, zucchini and eggplant; cook for 5 minutes or until softened. Add mushrooms and cook 2 minutes longer. Remove vegetables from skillet and set aside. Add turkey to skillet and cook for 3 minutes, stirring to break it up, or until no longer pink. Drain fat and add cooked vegetables to skillet.

2. Add tomato paste, tomatoes, stock, potatoes, beans, chili powder, basil and bay leaf; bring to a boil. Cover, reduce heat to low and simmer for 40 minutes, stirring occasionally.

Tips

✦ A great combination of ratatouille and chili in one dish.

✦ Great as a family meal. Serve with French bread.

✦ Ground pork, veal or chicken can replace the turkey.

Make Ahead

✦ Prepare up to a day ahead and reheat gently, adding extra chicken stock if too thick.

Nutritional Analysis (Per Serving)
✦ Calories: 248 ✦ Protein: 18 g ✦ Cholesterol: 39 mg
✦ Sodium: 496 mg ✦ Fat, total: 7 g ✦ Carbohydrates: 31 g
✦ Fiber: 8 g ✦ Fat, saturated: 2 g

Spinach and Cheese Stuffed Turkey Breasts

4	skinless boneless turkey scallopini	4
1½ tsp	vegetable oil	7 mL
1 tsp	crushed garlic	5 mL
¼ cup	finely chopped red onions	50 mL
¼ cup	drained cooked chopped spinach	50 mL
¼ cup	diced red peppers	50 mL
¼ cup	shredded Swiss cheese	50 mL
¼ cup	chicken stock	50 mL
Sauce		
1½ tsp	margarine or butter	7 mL
1 tsp	crushed garlic	5 mL
1½ cups	diced plum tomatoes	375 mL
⅓ cup	chicken stock	75 mL
3 tbsp	chopped fresh basil	45 mL

When using margarine, choose a soft (non-hydrogenated) version to limit consumption of trans fats.

Serves 4
Preheat oven to 400°F (200°C)
Baking dish sprayed with nonstick vegetable spray

1. Place turkey between 2 sheets of waxed paper; pound until flattened. Set aside.
2. In nonstick skillet, heat oil; sauté garlic, onions, spinach and red peppers until softened, approximately 3 minutes. Spoon evenly over breasts; sprinkle with cheese. Roll up and fasten with toothpicks.
3. Place turkey in baking dish; pour in ¼ cup (50 mL) stock. Cover and bake for 12 to 15 minutes or until turkey is no longer pink. Remove turkey to serving dish and keep warm.
4. *Sauce:* Meanwhile, in small saucepan, melt margarine; sauté garlic for 1 minute. Stir in tomatoes and chicken stock; cook for 3 minutes or until heated through. Add basil and serve over turkey.

Tips
✦ Substitute boneless chicken breasts, or use veal or pork scallopini.
✦ If using fresh spinach, use 1½ cups (375 mL). Cook, drain well and chop.
✦ A milder cheese can replace Swiss.

Make Ahead
✦ Prepare sauce early in the day. Reheat gently.

Nutritional Analysis (Per Serving)
✦ Calories: 225   ✦ Protein: 30 g   ✦ Cholesterol: 80 mg
✦ Sodium: 247 mg ✦ Fat: 10 g   ✦ Carbohydrates: 4 g
✦ Fiber: 1 g

Meat

Flank Steak in Hoisin Marinade with Sautéed Mushrooms

Marinade

¼ cup	soya sauce	50 mL
¼ cup	hoisin sauce	50 mL
¼ cup	rice wine vinegar	50 mL
2 tbsp	brown sugar	25 mL
2 tbsp	vegetable oil	25 mL
1 tsp	minced gingerroot	5 mL
1 tsp	minced garlic	5 mL
1½ lb	flank steak	750 g
1 tsp	vegetable oil	5 mL
1 tsp	minced garlic	5 mL
3 cups	sliced mushrooms	750 mL
¾ cup	chopped green onions	175 mL

Serves 6
Preheat broiler or start barbecue

1. In small bowl whisk together soya sauce, hoisin sauce, vinegar, brown sugar, oil, ginger and garlic. Pour over steak and let marinate in refrigerator at least 2 hours or overnight. Bring to room temperature before cooking.

2. In large nonstick skillet, heat oil over medium-high heat. Add garlic and mushrooms and cook for 3 minutes or until softened. Add green onions and cook for 1 minute longer.

3. Barbecue or broil steak, basting with some of the marinade, until cooked to desired "doneness" (approximately 15 minutes). Bring remaining marinade to a boil and simmer for 3 minutes. Serve steak with mushrooms and sauce. Cut the steak across the grain thinly to ensure tenderness.

Tip

✦ Wild mushrooms such as oyster or portobello are a highlight to this dish.

✦ The longer a flank steak marinates, the tenderer the meat will be.

Make Ahead

✦ Prepare sauce up to 3 days ahead and keep refrigerated.

Nutritional Analysis (Per Serving)
✦ Calories: 266 ✦ Protein: 26 g ✦ Cholesterol: 44 mg
✦ Sodium: 768 mg ✦ Fat, total: 13 g ✦ Carbohydrates: 11 g
✦ Fiber: 1 g ✦ Fat, saturated: 4 g

Beef Cabbage Rolls with Orzo in Tomato Sauce

1	head green savoy cabbage, core removed	1
½ cup	orzo or any small shaped pasta	125 mL
1 cup	chopped mushrooms	250 mL
⅓ cup	chopped onions	75 mL
1 tsp	minced garlic	5 mL
8 oz	lean ground beef	250 g
3 tbsp	barbecue sauce	45 mL
½ tsp	dried basil	2 mL
1	large egg white	1

Sauce

1	can (28 oz/796 mL) tomatoes, with juice	1
3 tbsp	packed brown sugar	45 mL
1 tsp	dried basil	5 mL
½ cup	water	125 mL
1 tbsp	lemon juice	15 mL
⅓ cup	raisins	75 mL

Cruciferous crunch: *Studies suggest that eating more cabbage — as well as other cruciferous vegetables (cauliflower, broccoli, Brussels sprouts) — can decrease the risk of colon cancer. It may also protect from stomach, lung and breast cancer. Why? Well, for one thing they're loaded with fiber and vitamin C. In fact, one serving of these cabbage rolls gives you 3½ times the daily requirement for vitamin C. Cabbage is also full of natural compounds called indoles and monoterpenes. These phytochemicals may inhibit tumor growth and help the body detoxify cancer-causing substances.*

Serves 4

1. In a large pot of boiling water, cook whole cabbage for 20 to 25 minutes; drain. When cool enough to handle, separate leaves carefully. Set aside.

2. In a pot of boiling water, cook orzo for 8 to 10 minutes or until tender but firm; drain. Rinse under cold running water; drain. Set aside.

3. In a nonstick frying pan sprayed with vegetable spray, cook mushrooms, onions and garlic over medium-high heat for 7 minutes or until slightly browned; transfer to a bowl. Add orzo, ground beef, barbecue sauce, basil and egg white; mix well.

4. Place about ⅓ cup (75 mL) beef-orzo mixture in center of 1 cabbage leaf. Fold in sides; roll up. Repeat with remaining filling.

5. In a food processor, combine tomatoes, brown sugar, basil, water and lemon juice; purée. Add raisins; pour mixture into a large nonstick saucepan over medium-high heat. Bring to a boil; reduce heat to low. Add cabbage rolls; cook, covered, for 1 hour 15 minutes, turning rolls over at halfway point.

Tip

✦ Savoy cabbage has a distinctively loose, full head of crinkled leaves; it's mild in flavor and doesn't lose its color or texture after being simmered. It's not always available, however, so you may have to make do with ordinary green cabbage.

Nutritional Analysis (Per Serving)
- ✦ Calories: 395
- ✦ Protein: 22 g
- ✦ Cholesterol: 35 mg
- ✦ Sodium: 331 mg
- ✦ Fat, total: 10 g
- ✦ Carbohydrates: 53 g
- ✦ Fiber: 9 g
- ✦ Fat, saturated: 3.9 g

Grilled Flank Steak with Asian Fruit Sauce over Fettuccine

Marinade

½ cup	apricot jam	125 mL
½ cup	beef or chicken stock	125 mL
3 tbsp	orange juice concentrate	45 mL
2 tbsp	light soya sauce	25 mL
1½ tbsp	rice wine vinegar	20 mL
2 tsp	sesame oil	10 mL
2 tsp	minced garlic	10 mL
1½ tsp	minced gingerroot	7 mL
12 oz	flank steak	375 g
1 tbsp	cornstarch	15 mL
¾ cup	diced dried apricots	175 mL
¾ cup	diced canned pineapple, drained	175 mL
1 lb	fettuccine	500 g
1 cup	sliced green onions	250 mL

Flank steak is a boneless cut of beef that comes from — you guessed it! — the cow's flank, or lower hind quarters. It's very lean and, left on its own, pretty tough. But once marinated, flank steak is wonderful! Like all lean meat, it must be cooked quickly at a high temperature to keep it from drying out. And for maximum tenderness, be sure to cut thinly across the grain.

Serves 6

Preheat grill or cast-iron grill pan, greased, to medium-high heat
Shallow glass baking dish

1. In baking dish, combine apricot jam, stock, orange juice concentrate, soya sauce, vinegar, sesame oil, garlic and ginger. Place steak in marinade, turning to coat well. Let stand, covered, for 1 hour at room temperature or overnight in refrigerator, turning occasionally. Bring to room temperature before cooking.

2. Remove steak from marinade, reserving liquid. On preheated grill or in grill pan, cook flank steak for 5 to 7 minutes per side or according to taste. Meanwhile, in a saucepan over medium-high heat, bring marinade to a boil. Reduce heat to medium; simmer for 5 minutes. In a bowl combine cornstarch and 1 tbsp (15 mL) cold water; add to simmering marinade. Cook for 1 minute or until thickened. Add apricots and pineapple; cook for 2 minutes or until heated through. Remove from heat.

3. In a large pot of boiling water, cook fettuccine for 8 to 10 minutes or until tender but firm; drain. Meanwhile, let flank steak rest, covered with foil, for 5 minutes; slice thinly across grain. In a bowl combine sauce and pasta; toss well. Spoon onto a serving platter; arrange flank steak over pasta. Sprinkle with green onions; serve immediately.

Nutritional Analysis (Per Serving)

- Calories: 544
- Sodium: 180 mg
- Fiber: 3 g
- Protein: 27 g
- Fat, total: 8 g
- Fat, saturated: 2.3 g
- Cholesterol: 29 mg
- Carbohydrates: 89 g

Chinese Beef with Crisp Vegetables

1 tbsp	vegetable oil	15 mL
2 tsp	crushed garlic	10 mL
8 oz	lean beef, thinly sliced	250 g
1½ cups	chopped broccoli	375 mL
1½ cups	thinly sliced sweet red pepper	375 mL
1½ cups	snow peas	375 mL

Sauce

1 tbsp	cornstarch	15 mL
¾ cup	beef stock	175 mL
2 tbsp	soya sauce	25 mL
3 tbsp	brown sugar	45 mL
2 tbsp	sherry or rice vinegar	25 mL
1½ tsp	minced gingerroot (or ¼ tsp/1 mL ground)	7 mL

To increase the nutrient value of a meal, add extra vegetables and fruits — they provide important antioxidants and phytochemicals.

Serves 4

1. *Sauce:* In small bowl, combine cornstarch, beef stock, soya sauce, sugar, sherry and ginger; mix well and set aside.

2. In large nonstick skillet, heat oil; sauté garlic and beef just until beef is browned but not cooked through. Remove beef and set aside.

3. To skillet, add broccoli, red pepper and snow peas; sauté for 2 minutes. Return beef to pan. Stir sauce and add to pan; cook just until beef is cooked and sauce has thickened, approximately 2 minutes, stirring constantly.

Tips

✦ For a variation of this great-tasting, sweet stir-fry, try chicken or pork and other vegetables.

✦ Stir-fries make a wonderful meal because they use very little fat. Since they must be made quickly, it helps to have all ingredients measured and prepared before you start to cook.

Make Ahead

✦ Prepare sauce early in the day.

Nutritional Analysis (Per Serving)
✦ Calories: 199   ✦ Protein: 16 g   ✦ Cholesterol: 31 mg
✦ Sodium: 674 mg   ✦ Fat: 5 g   ✦ Carbohydrates: 22 g
✦ Fiber: 3 g

Steak Kebabs with Honey Garlic Marinade

2 tbsp	soya sauce	25 mL
2 tbsp	sherry or rice vinegar	25 mL
4 tsp	honey	20 mL
2 tsp	crushed garlic	10 mL
1½ tsp	sesame oil	7 mL
4 tsp	vegetable oil	20 mL
1 tbsp	water	15 mL
¾ lb	lean steak, cut into cubes	375 g
16	pieces (1 inch/2.5 cm) sweet green pepper	16
16	pieces (1 inch/2.5 cm) onion	16
16	small mushrooms	16
16	snow peas	16

Serves 4

1. In bowl, combine soya sauce, sherry, honey, garlic, sesame and vegetable oils and water. Add steak and marinate for 30 minutes, or longer in refrigerator.

2. Remove beef from marinade. Place marinade in small saucepan and cook for 3 to 5 minutes or until thick and syrupy.

3. Thread beef, green pepper, onion, mushrooms and snow peas alternately onto 8 metal skewers. Place on greased grill and barbecue for 10 to 15 minutes, turning often and brushing with marinade, or until cooked as desired. Serve with any remaining marinade.

Tips

✦ The longer you marinate the meat, the better the flavor will be.

✦ For a variation, change the kind of vegetables used.

✦ Pineapple is a delicious substitute for any of the vegetables.

Make Ahead

✦ Prepare steak up to a day before and allow it to sit in marinade, turning occasionally. Assemble kebabs and barbecue just prior to serving.

Nutritional Analysis (Per Serving)
✦ Calories: 228   ✦ Protein: 20 g   ✦ Cholesterol: 47 mg
✦ Sodium: 553 mg   ✦ Fat: 9 g   ✦ Carbohydrates: 16 g
✦ Fiber: 2 g

Where there's smoke... When you cook meat on an outdoor grill — whether charcoal, gas or electric — fat drips onto the coals and creates smoke. And while that smoke provides the grilled flavor, it also contains potentially cancer-causing substances called benzopyrenes which are deposited on the surface of the meat. A University of Chicago study found that a well-done charcoal-broiled steak contained as many benzopyrenes as the smoke from several hundred cigarettes. Until more is known about grilled food and cancer, North American cancer societies recommend eating barbecued foods in moderation. As well, here's what you can do to reduce the amount of smoke and benzopyrenes in barbecued food:

• *Grill lean cuts of meat, such as flank steak, sirloin, pork tenderloin, center-cut pork chops, poultry breast.*

• *Trim visible fat before cooking.*

• *Don't char meat; keep a water bottle handy for coals that flare up.*

• *Baste foods frequently during grilling (with a low-fat marinade!).*

Veal Chops with Creamy Mushroom Sauce

4	veal chops (6 oz/175 g each)	4
	All-purpose flour for dusting	
2 tbsp	margarine	25 mL
2 tsp	crushed garlic	10 mL
1½ cups	sliced mushrooms	375 mL
2 tbsp	all-purpose flour	25 mL
¼ cup	Marsala wine or sweet red wine	50 mL
¾ cup	2% milk	175 mL
⅓ cup	chicken stock	75 mL

When using margarine, choose a soft (non-hydrogenated) version to limit consumption of trans fats.

Serves 4
Preheat oven to 425°F (220°C)

1. Dust chops with flour.
2. In large nonstick skillet, melt 1 tbsp (15 mL) of the margarine; sauté garlic for 1 minute. Add veal and sauté until browned on both sides, approximately 5 minutes. Place in baking dish; cover and bake just until tender, approximately 10 minutes.
3. Meanwhile, add remaining margarine and mushrooms to skillet; cook, stirring occasionally, until softened and liquid is absorbed. Add flour and cook for 1 minute. Add wine, milk and stock; simmer until thickened, stirring continuously, approximately 2 minutes. Place veal on serving dish and pour sauce over top.

Tips

✦ Marsala wine gives this dish a subtle sweetness.

✦ Avoid overcooking the veal as it toughens.

✦ Substitute pork chops or lamb chops for a change.

Nutritional Analysis (Per Serving)
✦ Calories: 239   ✦ Protein: 18 g   ✦ Cholesterol: 65 mg
✦ Sodium: 202 mg   ✦ Fat: 10 g   ✦ Carbohydrates: 14 g
✦ Fiber: 1 g

Veal Scallopini with Goat Cheese and Tomato Sauce

1 lb	veal cutlets, pounded until thin	500 g
1	egg white	1
½ cup	dry bread crumbs	125 mL
1 tbsp	vegetable oil	15 mL
2 tsp	crushed garlic	10 mL
1 cup	tomato sauce	250 mL
2 oz	goat cheese, crumbled	50 g
	Chopped fresh parsley	

Serves 4
Preheat oven to 450°F (230°C)

1. Dip veal in egg white, then in bread crumbs until coated.

2. In large nonstick skillet sprayed with nonstick vegetable spray, heat oil; sauté garlic for 1 minute. Add veal and cook just until tender and browned on both sides. Remove from heat.

3. Place tomato sauce in baking dish. Top with veal and sprinkle with goat cheese. Bake, uncovered, for 5 minutes or until heated through. Garnish with parsley.

Tips

✦ Feta cheese or shredded mozzarella can be substituted for the goat cheese in this interesting version of veal parmigiana.

✦ Boneless chicken or pork cutlets can replace the veal.

Nutritional Analysis (Per Serving)
✦ Calories: 253   ✦ Protein: 23 g   ✦ Cholesterol: 87 mg
✦ Sodium: 697 mg ✦ Fat: 11 g   ✦ Carbohydrates: 14 g
✦ Fiber: 1 g

Veal Stew in Chunky Tomato Sauce

1 lb	boneless stewing veal, cut into 1-inch (2.5 cm) cubes	500 g
	All-purpose flour for dusting	
1 tbsp	vegetable oil	15 mL
2 tsp	crushed garlic	10 mL
1 cup	chopped onions	250 mL
1/2 cup	chopped sweet green pepper	125 mL
1 cup	chopped carrots	250 mL
1 1/2 cups	sliced mushrooms	375 mL
1 1/2 cups	beef stock	375 mL
1	bay leaf	1
1 tsp	dried oregano	5 mL
1 1/2 tsp	dried basil (or 2 tbsp/25 mL chopped fresh)	7 mL
1 cup	chopped peeled potato	250 mL
1 cup	tomato sauce	250 mL
2 tbsp	tomato paste	25 mL
1/4 cup	red wine	50 mL

Serves 4

1. Dust veal cubes in flour.
2. In large nonstick Dutch oven, heat oil; sauté veal for 2 minutes. Remove veal and set aside.
3. To pan, add garlic, onions, green pepper, carrots and mushrooms; sauté until softened, approximately 5 minutes.
4. Add stock, bay leaf, oregano, basil, potato, tomato sauce, tomato paste and wine. Return veal to pan; cover and simmer for 1 hour or until veal is tender, stirring occasionally. Discard bay leaf.

Tips

✦ For a different version, try beef or lamb and other vegetables.

✦ The longer the veal stews, the more tender the meat.

Make Ahead

✦ Prepare up to a day before and refrigerate, or freeze for longer storage. Reheat gently on a low heat.

Nutritional Analysis (Per Serving)
✦ Calories: 289 ✦ Protein: 24 g ✦ Cholesterol: 72 mg
✦ Sodium: 753 mg ✦ Fat: 8 g ✦ Carbohydrates: 30 g
✦ Fiber: 5 g

Veal with Pineapple Lime Sauce and Pecans

1 lb	veal scallopini	500 g
2 tsp	oil	10 mL
3 tbsp	flour	45 mL
Sauce		
¼ cup	chopped green onions (about 2 medium)	50 mL
2 tbsp	chopped pecans	25 mL
¼ cup	pineapple juice concentrate	50 mL
¼ cup	water	50 mL
1 tbsp	honey	15 mL
1 tbsp	fresh lime juice	15 mL
1 tsp	grated lime zest	5 mL

Serves 4

1. Between sheets of waxed paper pound veal to ¼-inch (5 mm) thickness. In large nonstick skillet sprayed with vegetable spray, heat oil over medium-high heat. Dredge veal in flour and cook for 2 minutes per side or until just done at center. Place on a serving dish and cover.

2. Add green onions and pecans to skillet. Cook for 2 minutes. Add pineapple juice concentrate, water, honey, lime juice and lime zest. Bring to a boil for 1 minute, or until slightly syrupy and thickened. Serve sauce over veal.

Tips

✦ Use chicken, pork or turkey scallopini to replace veal.

✦ Use frozen juice concentrate and replace remainder in freezer. Orange juice can also be used.

✦ If limes are unavailable, use lemons.

Make Ahead

✦ Prepare sauce earlier in the day and reheat gently before serving. Add more water if too thick.

Nutritional Analysis (Per Serving)
✦ Calories: 217   ✦ Protein: 24 g   ✦ Cholesterol: 84 mg
✦ Sodium: 71 mg   ✦ Fat, total: 6 g   ✦ Carbohydrates: 16 g
✦ Fiber: 1 g   ✦ Fat, saturated: 1 g

Mixed Meat Burgers with Cheese and Mushroom Pockets

8 oz	lean ground beef	250 g
8 oz	lean ground veal or chicken	250 g
2 tsp	crushed garlic	10 mL
1/4 cup	finely chopped red onions	50 mL
2 tbsp	barbecue sauce	25 mL
1	egg	1
2 tbsp	seasoned bread crumbs	25 mL

Stuffing

1 tsp	vegetable oil	5 mL
1/2 cup	finely chopped mushrooms	125 mL
1/4 cup	shredded mozzarella cheese	50 mL

Serves 4 to 5
Start barbecue or preheat oven to 450°F (230°C)

1. In bowl, mix together both meats, garlic, red onions, barbecue sauce, egg and bread crumbs until well combined. Form into 4 or 5 hamburgers.

2. *Stuffing:* In small nonstick skillet, heat oil and sauté mushrooms until softened. Make pocket in each hamburger and evenly stuff with mushrooms and cheese. Press meat mixture around opening to seal.

3. Place on greased grill and barbecue, or place on rack on baking sheet and bake for 10 to 15 minutes or until no longer pink inside, turning patties once.

Tips

✦ Other combinations of ground meat can be used.

✦ Substitute another cheese for the mozzarella.

✦ Try wild mushrooms, such as oyster mushrooms.

Make Ahead

✦ Make patties in advance and freeze. Thaw and barbecue just prior to serving.

Nutritional Analysis (Per Serving)
✦ Calories: 231 ✦ Protein: 21 g ✦ Cholesterol: 102 mg
✦ Sodium: 200 mg ✦ Fat: 12 g ✦ Carbohydrates: 5 g
✦ Fiber: 1 g

Spicy Meatball and Pasta Stew

Meatballs

8 oz	lean ground beef	250 g
1	egg	1
2 tbsp	ketchup or chili sauce	25 mL
2 tbsp	seasoned bread crumbs	25 mL
1 tsp	minced garlic	5 mL
½ tsp	chili powder	2 mL

Stew

2 tsp	vegetable oil	10 mL
1 tsp	minced garlic	5 mL
1¼ cups	chopped onions	300 mL
¾ cup	chopped carrots	175 mL
3½ cups	beef stock	875 mL
1	can (19 oz/540 mL) tomatoes, crushed	1
¾ cup	canned chickpeas, drained	175 mL
1 tbsp	tomato paste	15 mL
2 tsp	granulated sugar	10 mL
2 tsp	chili powder	10 mL
1 tsp	dried oregano	5 mL
1¼ tsp	dried basil	6 mL
⅔ cup	small shell pasta	150 mL

Serves 8

1. In large bowl, combine ground beef, egg, ketchup, bread crumbs, garlic and chili powder; mix well. Form each ½ tbsp (7 mL) into a meatball and place on a baking sheet; cover and set aside.

2. In large nonstick saucepan, heat oil over medium heat. Add garlic, onions and carrots and cook for 5 minutes or until onions are softened. Stir in stock, tomatoes, chickpeas, tomato paste, sugar, chili powder, oregano and basil; bring to a boil, reduce heat to medium-low, cover and let cook for 20 minutes. Bring to a boil again and stir in pasta and meatballs; let simmer for 10 minutes or until pasta is tender but firm, and meatballs are cooked.

Tips

✦ Ground chicken, turkey or veal can replace the beef.

✦ Chickpeas can be replaced with kidney beans.

Make Ahead

✦ Prepare up to a day ahead, adding more stock if too thick.

✦ Great for leftovers.

Nutritional Analysis (Per Serving)

✦ Calories: 189　✦ Protein: 10 g　✦ Cholesterol: 43 mg
✦ Sodium: 904 mg　✦ Fat, total: 7 g　✦ Carbohydrates: 22 g
✦ Fiber: 3 g　✦ Fat, saturated: 2 g

Chili Bean Stew

1½ tsp	vegetable oil	7 mL
1 tsp	crushed garlic	5 mL
1 cup	chopped onion	250 mL
8 oz	lean ground beef	250 g
1	can (19 oz/540 mL) tomatoes, crushed	1
2 cups	beef stock	500 mL
1½ cups	diced peeled potatoes	375 mL
¾ cup	drained canned red kidney beans	175 mL
¾ cup	corn niblets	175 mL
2 tbsp	tomato paste	25 mL
1½ tsp	chili powder	7 mL
1½ tsp	each dried oregano and basil	7 mL
⅓ cup	small shell pasta	75 mL

Serves 4 to 6

1. In large nonstick saucepan, heat oil; sauté garlic and onion until softened, approximately 5 minutes.
2. Add beef and cook, stirring to break up chunks, until no longer pink; pour off any fat.
3. Add tomatoes, stock, potatoes, kidney beans, corn, tomato paste, chili powder, oregano and basil. Cover and reduce heat; simmer for 40 minutes, stirring occasionally.
4. Add pasta; cook until firm to the bite, approximately 10 minutes.

Tip

✦ Ground chicken or veal can substitute for beef, and other cooked beans can be used instead of kidney beans.

Make Ahead

✦ Make and refrigerate up to a day before. Reheat gently, adding more stock if too thick.

Nutritional Analysis (Per Serving)
✦ Calories: 232   ✦ Protein: 15 g   ✦ Cholesterol: 22 mg
✦ Sodium: 580 mg   ✦ Fat: 6 g   ✦ Carbohydrates: 30 g
✦ Fiber: 5 g

Pork Stir-Fry with Sweet-and-Sour Sauce, Snow Peas and Red Peppers

Sauce

1 cup	chicken stock	250 mL
1/3 cup	brown sugar	75 mL
1/3 cup	ketchup	75 mL
2 tbsp	rice wine vinegar	25 mL
1 tbsp	soya sauce	15 mL
2 tsp	sesame oil	10 mL
4 tsp	cornstarch	20 mL
2 tsp	minced garlic	10 mL
1½ tsp	minced gingerroot	7 mL
12 oz	pork loin, cut into thin strips	375 g
1 tsp	vegetable oil	5 mL
1½ cups	snow peas or sugar snap peas	375 mL
1¼ cups	red pepper strips	300 mL
3/4 cup	green pepper strips	175 mL
1/2 cup	chopped green onions (about 4 medium)	125 mL

Chinese-food lovers beware!
If you love sweet-and-sour dishes, you'll really enjoy this recipe — particularly because it contains only 6 g fat per serving. By comparison, a typical serving of sweet-and-sour pork (batter dipped, deep fried, then stir-fried) has 71 g fat — that's more fat than the average women should consume in an entire day!

Serves 4

1. In small bowl combine stock, brown sugar, ketchup, vinegar, soya sauce, sesame oil, cornstarch, garlic and ginger; set aside.
2. In nonstick wok or skillet sprayed with vegetable spray, cook the pork strips over high heat for 2 minutes, stirring constantly, or until just done at center; remove from wok.
3. Add oil to wok. Cook snow peas, red and green peppers for 3 minutes, stirring constantly, or until tender-crisp. Stir sauce again and add to wok along with pork. Cook for 45 seconds or until thickened. Garnish with green onions.

Tips
- Use beef steak or boneless chicken breast instead of pork.
- Serve over pasta or rice.

Make Ahead
- Prepare sauce up to a day before.

Nutritional Analysis (Per Serving)
- Calories: 266
- Protein: 21 g
- Cholesterol: 46 mg
- Sodium: 802 mg
- Fat, total: 6 g
- Carbohydrates: 34 g
- Fiber: 3 g
- Fat, saturated: 1 g

Pork Tenderloin Roast with Dried Fruit

1½ lb	pork tenderloin	750 g
¼ cup	brown sugar	50 mL
¼ cup	orange marmalade	50 mL
¼ cup	beef stock	50 mL
¼ cup	red wine	50 mL
¼ cup	chopped dates	50 mL
¼ cup	chopped dried apricots	50 mL
¼ cup	raisins	50 mL

A great way to bring out the best flavor in pork. The dried fruits go well with the meat and increase the fiber content.

Serves 4 or 5
Preheat oven to 375°F (190°C)

1. Place meat in roasting pan. In small saucepan, heat sugar and marmalade; brush over pork.

2. Add stock, wine, dates, apricots and raisins to roasting pan.

3. Bake, covered, for 35 to 45 minutes or until no longer pink and meat thermometer registers 160° to 170°F (70° to 75°C), basting every 10 minutes with pan juices.

4. To serve, slice meat thinly and spoon sauce and fruit over meat.

Nutritional Analysis (Per Serving)
- Calories: 379
- Protein: 40 g
- Cholesterol: 126 mg
- Sodium: 138 mg
- Fat: 6 g
- Carbohydrates: 38 g
- Fiber: 1 g

Roasted Leg of Lamb with Crunchy Garlic Topping

1 tbsp	margarine	15 mL
2 tsp	crushed garlic	10 mL
⅓ cup	finely chopped onion	75 mL
½ cup	dry bread crumbs	125 mL
¼ cup	crushed bran cereal*	50 mL
¼ cup	chopped fresh parsley	50 mL
⅓ cup	chicken stock	75 mL
1	leg of lamb (2½ to 3 lb/1.25 to 1.5 kg), deboned	1
⅓ cup	red wine	75 mL
⅓ cup	beef stock	75 mL

* Use a wheat bran breakfast cereal

If you suspect the lamb will be tough, marinate it in milk, turning occasionally, for at least 3 hours before baking.

When using margarine, choose a soft (non-hydrogenated) version to limit consumption of trans fats.

Serves 6 to 8
Preheat oven to 375°F (190°C)

1. In large nonstick skillet, melt margarine; sauté garlic and onion until softened. Add bread crumbs, cereal, parsley and chicken stock; mix until well combined. If too dry, add more chicken stock.

2. Place lamb in roasting pan and pat bread crumb mixture over top. Pour wine and beef stock into pan. Cover and bake for 20 minutes. Uncover and bake for 15 to 20 minutes or until meat thermometer registers 140°F (60°C) for rare or until desired doneness. Serve with pan juices.

Nutritional Analysis (Per Serving)
- Calories: 227
- Protein: 25 g
- Cholesterol: 77 mg
- Sodium: 197 mg
- Fat: 9 g
- Carbohydrates: 6 g
- Fiber: 1 g

Lamb Vegetable Stew
over Garlic Mashed Potatoes

3 tsp	vegetable oil	15 mL
12 oz	leg of lamb, visible fat removed, cut into 1-inch (2.5 cm) cubes	375 g
3 tbsp	flour	45 mL
1 cup	pearl onions	250 mL
2 tsp	minced garlic	10 mL
1½ cups	sliced mushrooms	375 mL
1½ cups	chopped leeks	375 mL
1 cup	sliced carrots	250 mL
1 cup	chopped green or yellow peppers	250 mL
¾ cup	sliced zucchini	175 mL
¼ cup	tomato paste	50 mL
⅓ cup	red or white wine	75 mL
2 cups	chopped tomatoes	500 mL
2 cups	beef or chicken stock	500 mL
2 tsp	dried rosemary	10 mL
1	bay leaf	1

Mashed Potatoes

1½ lb	potatoes, peeled and quartered	750 g
1 tbsp	margarine or butter	15 mL
1 tbsp	minced garlic	15 mL
1 cup	chopped onion	250 mL
½ cup	chicken stock	125 mL
⅓ cup	light sour cream	75 mL
¼ tsp	ground black pepper	1 mL

Substitute stewing beef for lamb.

When using margarine, choose a soft (non-hydrogenated) version to limit consumption of trans fats.

Serves 4 to 6

1. In large nonstick saucepan, heat 2 tsp (10 mL) of the oil over medium-high heat. Dust the lamb cubes in the flour and add to the saucepan. Cook for 5 minutes or until well browned on all sides. Remove lamb from saucepan.

2. Blanch the pearl onions in a pot of boiling water for 1 minute; refresh in cold water and drain. Peel and set aside.

3. In same saucepan, heat remaining 1 tsp (5 mL) oil over medium heat; add garlic, mushrooms, leeks, carrots, green peppers, zucchini and pearl onions. Cook for 8 to 10 minutes or until softened and browned, stirring occasionally. Stir in tomato paste and wine. Return lamb to saucepan along with tomatoes, beef stock, rosemary and bay leaf. Bring to a boil, cover, reduce heat to medium-low, and simmer for 25 minutes or until carrots and meat are tender.

4. Meanwhile, put potatoes in a saucepan with water to cover; bring to a boil and cook for 15 minutes or until tender when pierced with the tip of a knife. In nonstick skillet, melt margarine over medium heat; add garlic and onions and cook for 4 minutes or until softened. Drain cooked potatoes and mash with chicken stock and sour cream. Stir in onion mixture and pepper. Place potato mixture on large serving platter and pour stew over top.

Make Ahead

✦ Prepare mashed potatoes recipe up to a day ahead. Reheat gently before serving.

✦ Prepare stew early in the day and gently reheat before serving.

Nutritional Analysis (Per Serving)

✦ Calories: 343   ✦ Protein: 19 g   ✦ Cholesterol: 40 mg
✦ Sodium: 504 mg   ✦ Fat, total: 8 g   ✦ Carbohydrates: 51 g
✦ Fiber: 7 g   ✦ Fat, saturated: 3 g

Curried Lamb Casserole with Sweet Potatoes

³⁄₄ lb	lamb, cut into ³⁄₄-inch (2 cm) cubes	375 g
	All-purpose flour for dusting	
1 tbsp	vegetable oil	15 mL
2 tsp	crushed garlic	10 mL
1 cup	chopped onion	250 mL
1 cup	finely chopped carrots	250 mL
¹⁄₂ cup	finely chopped sweet green pepper	125 mL
1 cup	cubed peeled sweet potatoes	250 mL
1¹⁄₂ cups	sliced mushrooms	375 mL
2¹⁄₂ cups	beef stock	625 mL
¹⁄₃ cup	red wine	75 mL
3 tbsp	tomato paste	45 mL
2 tsp	curry powder	10 mL

Serves 4

1. Dust lamb with flour.
2. In large nonstick Dutch oven, heat oil, sauté lamb for 2 minutes or just until seared all over. Remove lamb and set aside.
3. To skillet, add garlic, onion, carrots, green pepper and sweet potatoes; cook, stirring often, for 8 to 10 minutes or until tender. Add mushrooms and cook until softened, approximately 3 minutes.
4. Add stock, wine, tomato paste and curry powder. Return lamb to pan; cover and simmer for 1¹⁄₂ hours, stirring occasionally.

Tips

+ Other vegetables can be used in this recipe.
+ Adjust the curry powder to your taste.
+ Serve over rice, linguine or couscous.

Make Ahead

+ Make and refrigerate up to a day ahead and reheat on low heat. This dish can also be frozen.

Nutritional Analysis (Per Serving)
+ Calories: 296   + Protein: 22 g   + Cholesterol: 47 mg
+ Sodium: 556 mg   + Fat: 8 g   + Carbohydrates: 30 g
+ Fiber: 5 g

Leg of Lamb with Pesto and Wild Rice

Stuffing

1 tsp	vegetable oil	5 mL
2 tsp	minced garlic	10 mL
1 cup	chopped onions	250 mL
1 cup	chopped red or green peppers	250 mL
3/4 cup	wild rice	175 mL
3/4 cup	white rice	175 mL
3 cups	beef or chicken stock	750 mL
1/3 cup	store-bought pesto	75 mL
3 lb	boneless leg of lamb with a pocket	1.5 kg
1 tsp	vegetable oil	5 mL
1 tsp	minced garlic	5 mL
2/3 cup	beef stock	150 mL
1/2 cup	red or white wine	125 mL

Serves 8
Preheat oven to 375°F (190°C)

1. In saucepan, heat oil over medium heat. Add garlic and onions and cook for 3 minutes or until softened. Add red peppers and cook for 2 minutes longer. Add rices and cook, stirring, for 3 minutes. Add stock; bring to a boil, cover, reduce heat to medium-low and simmer covered for 20 to 25 minutes or until rice is tender and liquid absorbed. Stir in pesto. Set aside to cool.

2. Stuff leg of lamb with some of the cooled rice mixture; put leftover stuffing in a casserole dish and cover. Rub lamb with oil and garlic and place on rack in roasting pan. Truss lamb with string. Pour stock and wine under lamb. Bake covered for 20 minutes, basting with pan juices every 10 minutes. Uncover lamb and bake another 20 to 25 minutes, basting every 10 minutes. Add extra stock if liquids evaporate. Put casserole dish with leftover stuffing in the oven for the last 20 minutes. Serve meat with juices.

Tips

+ Lamb can be butterflied and filled, then gently folded over and tied with a string.
+ Store-bought pesto saves time, but is higher in calories and fat.

Make Ahead

+ If using your own pesto, prepare up to 2 days before and keep refrigerated. Can also be frozen for up to 4 weeks.

Nutritional Analysis (Per Serving)
+ Calories: 406
+ Protein: 38 g
+ Cholesterol: 105 mg
+ Sodium: 643 mg
+ Fat, total: 13 g
+ Carbohydrates: 30 g
+ Fiber: 2 g
+ Fat, saturated: 4 g

Acorn Squash with Rice, Pineapple and Molasses (page 327) ➤
Overleaf: Baked French Wedge Potatoes (page 333)
Opposite overleaf: Sweet Potato, Apple and Raisin Casserole (page 334)

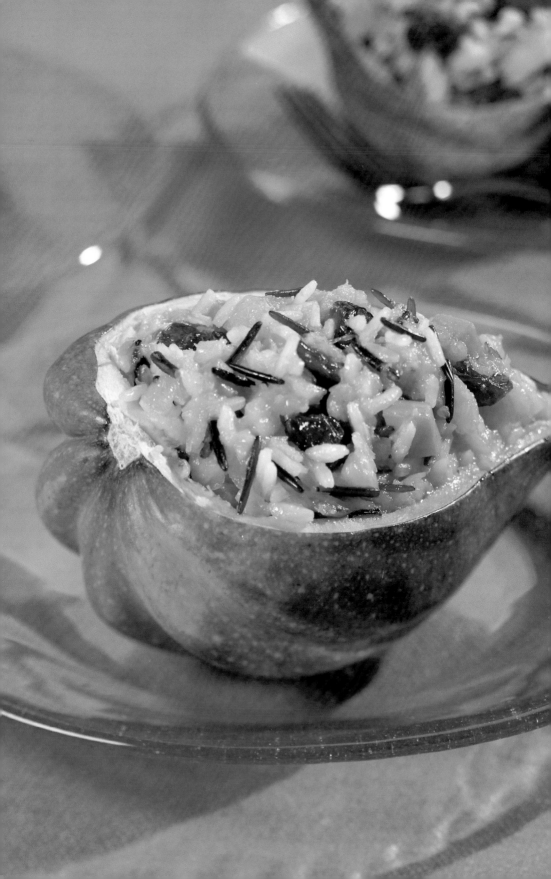

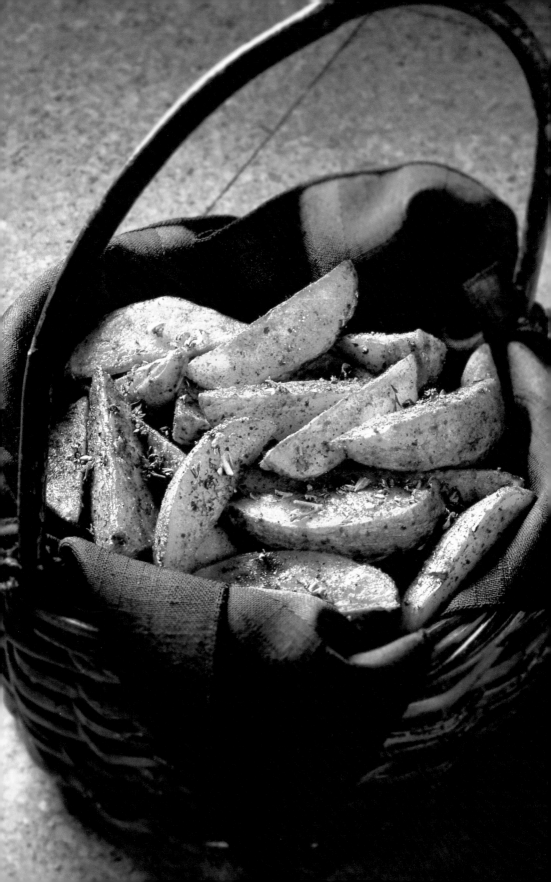

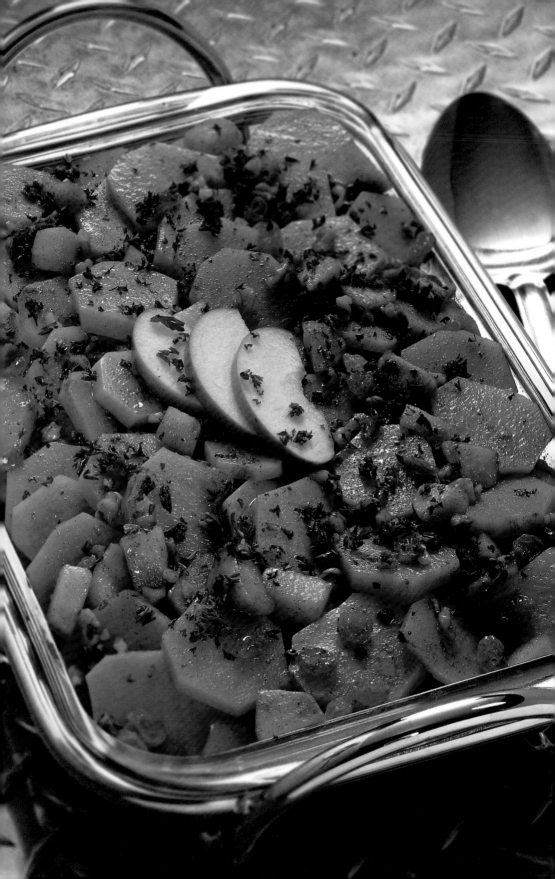

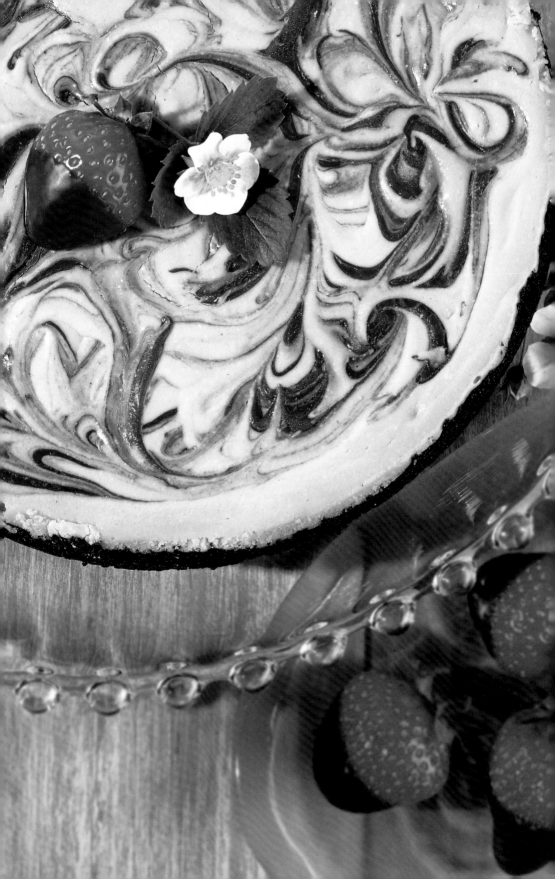

Vegetables

◄ Marble Mocha Cheesecake (page 344)

Potato Cheese Casserole

4	medium potatoes, peeled and thinly sliced	4
1½ tsp	margarine	7 mL
1 cup	chopped onions	250 mL
1 tsp	crushed garlic	5 mL
2 tbsp	all-purpose flour	25 mL
1¾ cups	2% warm milk	425 mL
3 tbsp	chopped fresh dill (or 1 tsp/5 mL dried dillweed)	45 mL
	Salt and pepper	
½ cup	shredded cheddar cheese	125 mL

Substitute another cheese of your choice, such as Swiss or mozzarella.

When using margarine, choose a soft (non-hydrogenated) version to limit consumption of trans fats.

Serves 4 to 5
Preheat oven to 375°F (190°C)

1. In saucepan of boiling water, cook potatoes just until fork-tender, approximately 10 minutes; drain. Arrange in baking dish just large enough to lay in single layer of overlapping slices.
2. In medium nonstick saucepan, melt margarine; sauté onions and garlic for 5 minutes or until softened. Add flour and cook, stirring, for 1 minute. Slowly stir in milk, simmer until thickened, stirring constantly, 3 to 4 minutes. Add dill; season with salt and pepper to taste.
3. Pour sauce over potatoes; sprinkle with cheese. Cover and bake for approximately 1 hour or until potatoes are tender.

Nutritional Analysis (Per Serving)
- Calories: 207
- Protein: 8 g
- Cholesterol: 18 mg
- Sodium: 134 mg
- Fat: 6 g
- Carbohydrates: 29 g
- Fiber: 2 g

Cheese and Red Pepper Stuffed Potatoes

2	large baking potatoes	2
⅓ cup	2% cottage cheese	75 mL
¼ cup	2% yogurt	50 mL
2 tbsp	2% milk	25 mL
1 tsp	vegetable oil	5 mL
1½ tsp	crushed garlic	7 mL
¼ cup	finely diced onion	50 mL
¼ cup	finely diced sweet red pepper	50 mL
2 tbsp	chopped fresh dill (or 1 tsp/5 mL dried dillweed)	25 mL
	Salt and pepper	
2 tbsp	grated Parmesan cheese	25 mL

Use ricotta instead of cottage cheese for a creamier consistency. There will, however, be slightly more calories per serving.

Serves 4
Preheat oven to 425°F (220°C)

1. Pierce potatoes with fork; bake or microwave just until tender. Cool and slice lengthwise in half; carefully scoop out pulp, leaving shell intact. Place pulp in mixing bowl or food processor.
2. Add cottage cheese, yogurt and milk; mix well. (Or process using on/off motion; do not purée.) Set aside.
3. In nonstick skillet, heat oil; sauté garlic, onion and red pepper until tender. Add dill, and salt and pepper to taste; add to potato mixture and mix well. Do not purée.
4. Stuff into potato shells; sprinkle with Parmesan. Place on baking sheet and bake for 10 minutes or until hot.

Nutritional Analysis (Per Serving)
- Calories: 170
- Protein: 7 g
- Cholesterol: 5 mg
- Sodium: 147 mg
- Fat: 3 g
- Carbohydrates: 30 g
- Fiber: 2 g

Potato Parmesan with Tomato Sauce and Cheese

3	large potatoes, scrubbed but not peeled (about 1 lb/500 g)	3
1	egg	1
1	egg white	1
3 tbsp	2% milk or water	45 mL
1/2 cup	dry seasoned bread crumbs	125 mL
2 tbsp	chopped fresh dill (or 1/2 tsp/2 mL dried)	25 mL
1 tbsp	grated Parmesan cheese	15 mL
3/4 cup	prepared tomato pasta sauce	175 mL
1/2 cup	shredded part-skim mozzarella cheese (about 2 oz/50 g)	125 mL

Serves 4 to 6
Preheat oven to 350°F (180°C)
Baking sheet sprayed with vegetable spray

1. In a saucepan add cold water to cover to potatoes. Bring to a boil; cook 20 to 25 minutes or just until barely tender when pierced with a fork. Drain. When cool enough to handle, cut into 1/2-inch (1 cm) round slices (or rinse with cold water if in a hurry).

2. In small bowl, whisk together whole egg, egg white and milk.

3. On a plate stir together bread crumbs, dill and Parmesan.

4. Dip potato slices in egg wash, coat with crumb mixture and place on prepared baking sheet. Repeat with all potato slices.

5. Bake 15 minutes, turning at the halfway point, or until golden and tender when pierced with a fork. Top each slice with some tomato sauce and sprinkle with mozzarella; bake 5 minutes longer.

Tips
✦ Yukon gold potatoes are great in this recipe.
✦ Fresh parsley or basil can replace dill.
✦ Try this with eggplant or zucchini. Boil just until tender.

Make Ahead
✦ Cook potatoes up to 2 days in advance.
✦ Prepare entire recipe 1 day in advance; bake just before serving.

Nutritional Analysis (Per Serving)
✦ Calories: 174 ✦ Protein: 8 g ✦ Cholesterol: 42 mg
✦ Sodium: 433 mg ✦ Fat, total: 5 g ✦ Carbohydrates: 26 g
✦ Fiber: 2 g ✦ Fat, saturated: 2 g

Greek Baked Stuffed Potatoes with Tomato, Olives and Cheese

3	medium baking potatoes	3
2 tsp	vegetable oil	10 mL
1½ tsp	minced garlic	7 mL
⅔ cup	chopped green peppers	150 mL
½ cup	chopped red onions	125 mL
1½ tsp	dried oregano	7 mL
⅔ cup	chopped fresh tomatoes	150 mL
⅓ cup	sliced black olives	75 mL
¼ cup	chopped green onions (about 2 medium)	50 mL
¼ cup	2% yogurt	50 mL
¼ cup	2% milk	50 mL
1½ oz	feta cheese, crumbled	40 g

Deciphering the "% MF" mystery:
Look at the label on any dairy product and you'll see a number followed by "% MF." Ever wonder what it means? It's the percentage of milk fat (that's the "MF") present in a given volume of milk or weight of cheese. For example, 31% MF on a package of cheddar cheese means there are 31 g fat in 100 g cheese, or 9 g fat in a 1 oz (30 g) serving. By comparison, feta cheese, at 22% MF, has only 6 g fat per 1 oz (30 g) serving.

Serves 6
Preheat oven to 425°F (220°C)

1. Bake the potatoes for 45 minutes to 1 hour, or until easily pierced with the tip of a sharp knife.

2. Meanwhile, in a nonstick skillet, heat oil over medium heat. Add garlic, green peppers, red onions and oregano and cook for 7 minutes or until softened, stirring occasionally. Stir in tomatoes, black olives and green onions and cook 1 minute more. Remove from heat.

3. When potatoes are cool enough to handle, cut in half lengthwise and scoop out flesh, leaving shells intact. Place shells on baking sheet. Mash potato and add yogurt, milk and 1 oz (25 g) of the feta. Stir in vegetable mixture. Divide among potato skin shells, sprinkle with remaining feta and bake for 15 minutes, or until heated through.

Tips

✦ Use plum tomatoes if available — they have less liquid. Or you can remove the seeds from regular tomatoes.

✦ If in a hurry, microwave potatoes. Each potato cooks in approximately 8 minutes at high power.

✦ Goat cheese or another sharp cheese can replace feta.

Make Ahead

✦ Prepare filling and stuff potatoes early in the day. Bake an extra 5 minutes or until hot.

Nutritional Analysis (Per Serving)
- ✦ Calories: 143
- ✦ Protein: 4 g
- ✦ Cholesterol: 8 mg
- ✦ Sodium: 349 mg
- ✦ Fat, total: 6 g
- ✦ Carbohydrates: 19 g
- ✦ Fiber: 2 g
- ✦ Fat, saturated: 2 g

Three-Mushroom Tomato Potato Stew

1 cup	sliced dried mushrooms	250 mL
2 tsp	vegetable oil	10 mL
1½ cups	chopped onions	375 mL
2 tsp	minced garlic	10 mL
1 cup	chopped carrots	250 mL
4 cups	thinly sliced oyster mushrooms	1 L
3 cups	thinly sliced button mushrooms	750 mL
2 cups	Basic Vegetable Stock (see recipe, page 52)	500 mL
1	can (19 oz/540 mL) tomatoes	1
¾ cup	chopped peeled sweet potatoes	175 mL
¾ cup	chopped peeled potatoes	175 mL
2 tbsp	tomato paste	25 mL
2	bay leaves	2
1 tsp	dried basil	5 mL
1 tsp	dried thyme	5 mL
¼ tsp	coarsely ground black pepper	1 mL

Okay, so you've just returned from the market with a bag of mushrooms. Kind of dirty, aren't they? Maybe you should give them a good wash before putting them in the refrigerator. Don't! Keep them as they are, in a paper bag, and refrigerate until ready to use. Then, before cooking, wipe the mushrooms with a damp cloth or, if you must, give them a quick rinse. Otherwise, water will penetrate the mushrooms and change their wonderful texture.

Serves 4

1. In a small bowl, add 2 cups (500 mL) boiling water to cover dried mushrooms. Soak 15 minutes. Drain, reserving soaking liquid; measure out 1 cup (250 mL).

2. In a large nonstick saucepan sprayed with vegetable spray, heat oil over medium-high heat. Add onions, garlic and carrots; cook, stirring occasionally, 5 minutes or until softened and browned. Stir in fresh mushrooms; cook 8 minutes longer, stirring occasionally, or until all liquid is absorbed.

3. Stir in dried mushrooms, reserved 1 cup (250 mL) mushroom liquid, stock, tomatoes, sweet potatoes, potatoes, tomato paste, bay leaves, basil, thyme and pepper. Bring to a boil, reduce heat to medium-low, cover, and cook 20 minutes or until potatoes are tender.

Tips

+ If using whole dried mushrooms, slice after soaking.

+ Use any combination of wild mushrooms. If not available, use common mushrooms.

+ Serve over pasta, rice, couscous or any other type of cooked grain.

+ If dried mushrooms are unavailable, substitute 2 cups (500 mL) sliced button mushrooms and add 1 cup (250 mL) more stock.

Make Ahead

+ Prepare up to 1 day in advance. Reheat gently, adding more stock if too thick.

Nutritional Analysis (Per Serving)

+ Calories: 187   + Protein: 7 g   + Cholesterol: 0 mg
+ Sodium: 254 mg   + Fat, total: 4 g   + Carbohydrates: 37 g
+ Fiber: 7 g   + Fat, saturated: 0.4 g

Sweet Potato and Carrot Casserole with Molasses and Pecans

1 lb	sweet potatoes, peeled and cut into ½-inch (1 cm) cubes	500 g
1 lb	carrots, peeled and thinly sliced	500 g
1¼ cups	canned pineapple chunks, drained	300 mL
½ cup	raisins	125 mL
⅓ cup	packed brown sugar	75 mL
2 tbsp	orange juice	25 mL
1 tbsp	margarine or butter	15 mL
1 tbsp	molasses	15 mL
1½ tsp	cinnamon	7 mL
3 tbsp	chopped pecans	45 mL

When using margarine, choose a soft (non-hydrogenated) version to limit consumption of trans fats.

Serves 6
Preheat oven to 350°F (180°C)
8-inch (2 L) square baking dish sprayed with vegetable spray

1. In a saucepan of boiling water, cook sweet potatoes and carrots for approximately 7 minutes or until tender. Drain. Toss sweet potatoes and carrots together along with pineapple and raisins; put in prepared baking dish.

2. In saucepan, heat brown sugar, orange juice, margarine, molasses and cinnamon over medium heat, stirring, for 1 minute, or until melted and smooth. Pour syrup over vegetables and sprinkle pecans on top. Bake for 15 minutes or until heated through.

Tips
+ Use chunked fresh pineapple instead of canned.
+ Dates are a great substitute for raisins.
+ Pecans can be replaced with almonds, walnuts or cashews.

Make Ahead
+ Prepare entire dish early in the day and bake just before serving.

Nutritional Analysis (Per Serving)
+ Calories: 288 + Protein: 3 g + Cholesterol: 0 mg
+ Sodium: 67 mg + Fat, total: 5 g + Carbohydrates: 62 g
+ Fiber: 5 g + Fat, saturated: 1 g

Cauliflower, Broccoli and Goat Cheese Bake

2½ cups	chopped cauliflower	625 mL
2½ cups	chopped broccoli	625 mL
1 tbsp	margarine	15 mL
1 tbsp	all-purpose flour	15 mL
½ cup	2% milk	125 mL
½ cup	chicken stock	125 mL
2 oz	goat cheese	50 g
2 tbsp	diced sweet red pepper	25 mL

Topping

⅓ cup	bran cereal*	75 mL
1 tsp	margarine, melted	5 mL
½ tsp	crushed garlic	2 mL

* Use a wheat bran breakfast cereal

The right roots: *As members of the cruciferous vegetable family, turnip and rutabaga are being studied for their ability to reduce the risk of breast, colon and kidney cancers. Cruciferous veggies contain more than 30 natural chemicals that can trigger the formation of enzymes that detoxify cancer-causing substances in the body. Want more crucifers on your dinner plate? Try bok choy, broccoli, Brussels sprouts, cabbage, cauliflower, kale, kohlrabi and mustard greens.*

When using margarine, choose a soft (non-hydrogenated) version to limit consumption of trans fats.

Serves 4
Preheat broiler
Baking dish sprayed with nonstick vegetable spray

1. Steam or microwave cauliflower and broccoli until just tender. Drain and place in baking dish.

2. In small saucepan, melt margarine; add flour and cook, stirring, for 1 minute. Add milk and stock; cook, stirring continuously, until thickened, approximately 5 minutes. Remove from stove. Stir in goat cheese until melted; pour over vegetables. Sprinkle red pepper over top.

3. *Topping:* In food processor, combine cereal, margarine and garlic; process using on/off motion until crumbly. Sprinkle over vegetables. Broil until browned, approximately 2 minutes.

Tips

✦ Cut the cauliflower and broccoli into florets and 2-inch (5 cm) stem pieces.

✦ The goat cheese can be replaced with mozzarella or cheddar.

✦ If in a hurry, omit the topping.

Make Ahead

✦ Sauce and topping can be prepared early in day. Warm sauce gently before pouring over vegetables. Add a little more milk to thin.

Nutritional Analysis (Per Serving)
✦ Calories: 148 ✦ Protein: 7 g ✦ Cholesterol: 15 mg
✦ Sodium: 405 mg ✦ Fat: 8 g ✦ Carbohydrates: 15 g
✦ Fiber: 5 g

Cauliflower, Leek and Sweet Potato Strudel

2 tsp	vegetable oil	10 mL
2 tsp	minced garlic	10 mL
2 1/2 cups	chopped leeks	625 mL
2 cups	finely chopped cauliflower	500 mL
2 cups	finely chopped peeled sweet potatoes	500 mL
1 cup	Basic Vegetable Stock (see recipe, page 52)	250 mL
3 tbsp	cornmeal	45 mL
2 tsp	dried basil	10 mL
1/4 tsp	freshly ground black pepper	1 mL
1	egg	1
1/2 cup	shredded sharp cheddar cheese (about 2 oz/50 g)	125 mL
2 tbsp	grated Parmesan cheese	25 mL
6	sheets phyllo pastry	6
2 tsp	melted margarine or butter	10 mL

When using margarine, choose a soft (non-hydrogenated) version to limit consumption of trans fats.

Serves 6 to 8
Preheat oven to 375°F (190°C)
Baking sheet sprayed with vegetable spray

1. In a large nonstick saucepan sprayed with vegetable spray, heat oil over medium heat. Cook garlic, leeks, cauliflower and sweet potatoes for 8 minutes, stirring often. Add stock, cornmeal, basil and pepper; reduce heat to low, cover and cook 15 minutes, stirring occasionally, or until vegetables are tender. Let cool.

2. Stir egg, cheddar and Parmesan into cooled vegetable mixture.

3. Layer 2 phyllo sheets on work surface and brush sparingly with melted margarine. Top with 2 more phyllo sheets and brush with margarine. Lay last 2 phyllo sheets on top. Spread vegetable mixture over surface leaving a 1-inch (2.5 cm) border on all sides. Starting at long end, roll up tightly. Tuck ends under.

4. Transfer to prepared baking sheet. Brush with remaining melted margarine. Bake 25 minutes or until golden brown.

Tips

✦ Cauliflower and sweet potatoes are a great combination. Substitute broccoli and white potato for a change.

✦ Phyllo pastry is a delicious low-fat alternative to other pastries and it's simple to use. Look for it in the freezer section of your grocery store. Work quickly and cover phyllo sheets with a towel until ready to use. Refreeze any remainders.

Make Ahead

✦ Prepare filling (to the end of Step 2) up to 1 day ahead. Fill a few hours before serving, cover and refrigerate. Bake just before serving.

Nutritional Analysis (Per Serving)
✦ Calories: 188   ✦ Protein: 6 g   ✦ Cholesterol: 37 mg
✦ Sodium: 166 mg   ✦ Fat, total: 6 g   ✦ Carbohydrates: 27 g
✦ Fiber: 3 g   ✦ Fat, saturated: 3 g

Tomatoes Stuffed with Spinach and Ricotta Cheese

4 cups	fresh spinach	1 L
4	medium tomatoes	4
2½ tsp	vegetable oil	12 mL
2 tsp	crushed garlic	10 mL
⅔ cup	chopped onion	150 mL
⅔ cup	ricotta cheese	150 mL
	Salt and pepper	

Topping

1 tbsp	dry bread crumbs	15 mL
1 tbsp	chopped fresh parsley	15 mL
1 tsp	margarine	5 mL
1 tsp	grated Parmesan cheese	5 mL

> *When using margarine, choose a soft (non-hydrogenated) version to limit consumption of trans fats.*

Serves 4
Preheat oven to 350°F (180°C)
Baking dish sprayed with nonstick vegetable spray

1. Rinse spinach and shake off excess water. With just the water clinging to leaves, cook until wilted. Squeeze out excess moisture; chop and set aside.

2. Slice off tops of tomatoes. Scoop out pulp, leaving shell of tomato intact. (Reserve pulp for another use.)

3. In nonstick skillet, heat oil; sauté garlic and onion until softened. Remove from heat. Add spinach, cheese, and salt and pepper to taste; mix well. Fill tomatoes with cheese mixture and place in baking dish.

4. *Topping:* Combine bread crumbs, parsley, margarine and cheese; sprinkle over tomatoes. Bake for 15 minutes or until heated through and topping is golden brown.

Tips

+ For a different texture, try crushed bran cereal for the topping instead of bread crumbs.

+ Use cottage cheese instead of ricotta to reduce the calories.

+ If frozen spinach is used, use ⅔ cup (150 mL) cooked and well drained.

Make Ahead

+ Make early in day and refrigerate. Bake just prior to serving.

Nutritional Analysis (Per Serving)
+ Calories: 132   + Protein: 7 g   + Cholesterol: 12 mg
+ Sodium: 108 mg   + Fat: 6 g   + Carbohydrates: 13 g
+ Fiber: 3 g

Spaghetti Squash with Vegetables and Tomato Sauce

1 to 2 lb	spaghetti squash	500 g to 1 kg
1 tbsp	margarine	15 mL
3/4 cup	chopped onions	175 mL
2 tsp	crushed garlic	10 mL
1 1/2 cups	sliced mushrooms	375 mL
3/4 cup	diced sweet green pepper	175 mL
1 cup	tomato sauce	250 mL
1 tsp	dried oregano	5 mL
1 tsp	dried basil	5 mL
1/4 cup	grated Parmesan cheese	50 mL

When using margarine, choose a soft (non-hydrogenated) version to limit consumption of trans fats.

Serves 4 to 6
Preheat broiler

1. Pierce squash in several places. In microwave, cook squash at high for 8 to 10 minutes or until soft. Cool and slice lengthwise in half. Discard seeds and with fork, scrape out spaghetti-like strands and set aside.

2. In large nonstick skillet, melt margarine; sauté onions, garlic, mushrooms and green pepper for about 5 minutes or until tender. Add spaghetti squash strands and cook for 2 more minutes.

3. Add tomato sauce, oregano and basil; combine well. Place in baking dish and sprinkle with Parmesan. Broil for 2 minutes or until browned.

Tips

✦ Instead of microwaving it, you can bake the squash in 350°F (180°C) oven for 40 to 50 minutes or until tender.

✦ For an attractive dish, serve in the spaghetti squash shells.

Make Ahead

✦ This can be prepared and baked ahead, then reheated in 325°F (160°C) oven until warm. It is best, however, if served immediately after baking.

Nutritional Analysis (Per Serving)
✦ Calories: 102   ✦ Protein: 3 g   ✦ Cholesterol: 3 mg
✦ Sodium: 337 mg   ✦ Fat: 4 g   ✦ Carbohydrates: 16 g
✦ Fiber: 4 g

Cheesy Ratatouille Bean Casserole

1 tbsp	vegetable oil	15 mL
2 tsp	crushed garlic	10 mL
1	medium onion, diced	1
1 cup	sliced mushrooms	250 mL
1 cup	thickly sliced zucchini	250 mL
2 cups	cubed eggplant	500 mL
1 cup	cubed peeled potatoes	250 mL
1	can (19 oz/540 mL) tomatoes, crushed	1
1 cup	drained cooked beans	250 mL
1 tsp	dried oregano	5 mL
1 tsp	dried basil	5 mL
1 cup	shredded mozzarella cheese	250 mL

For extra fiber, leave on the skins of the zucchini and eggplant.

Serves 4 or 5
Preheat oven to 400°F (200°C)

1. In large nonstick saucepan, heat oil over medium heat; cook garlic, onion, mushrooms, zucchini and eggplant, stirring constantly, for about 10 minutes or until softened.
2. Add potatoes, tomatoes, beans, oregano and basil; simmer for 30 minutes or until potatoes are tender.
3. Pour into large baking dish and sprinkle with mozzarella. Bake for 10 minutes or until cheese melts.

Make Ahead

✦ Prepare and refrigerate up to a day before and bake just before serving. This is delicious reheated.

Nutritional Analysis (Per Serving)
- ✦ Calories: 210
- ✦ Protein: 12 g
- ✦ Cholesterol: 12 mg
- ✦ Sodium: 395 mg
- ✦ Fat: 7 g
- ✦ Carbohydrates: 26 g
- ✦ Fiber: 6 g

Vegetarian Three-Bean Chili

1 tsp	vegetable oil	5 mL
2 tsp	minced garlic	10 mL
1 cup	chopped onions	250 mL
1 cup	chopped green peppers	250 mL
1 cup	chopped carrots	250 mL
1 cup	chopped zucchini	250 mL
1 tbsp	chili powder	15 mL
1 tsp	dried basil	5 mL
1 tsp	dried oregano	5 mL
2	cans (19 oz/540 mL) tomatoes, crushed	2
1 tbsp	tomato paste	15 mL
1 cup	canned red kidney beans, drained	250 mL
1 cup	canned black beans, drained	250 mL
1 cup	canned chickpeas, drained	250 mL

Serves 6

1. Over medium heat, heat oil in large nonstick saucepan sprayed with nonstick vegetable spray. Add garlic, onions, green peppers and carrots; cook for 5 minutes or until onions are softened. Add zucchini, chili powder, basil and oregano; cook for 2 minutes longer.
2. Add tomatoes and tomato paste; bring to a boil, reduce heat to medium-low, stir in beans and chickpeas, cover and cook for 35 minutes, or until thickened and carrots are tender.

Make Ahead

✦ Prepare up to 2 days ahead and gently reheat.

Nutritional Analysis (Per Serving)
- ✦ Calories: 236
- ✦ Protein: 12 g
- ✦ Cholesterol: 0 mg
- ✦ Sodium: 773 mg
- ✦ Fat: 3 g
- ✦ Carbohydrates: 47 g
- ✦ Fiber: 13 g

Corn, Leek and Red Pepper Casserole

1 tsp	vegetable oil	5 mL
1 tsp	minced garlic	5 mL
1 cup	sliced leeks	250 mL
1 cup	chopped red peppers	250 mL
2 cups	corn kernels	500 mL
2½ tbsp	all-purpose flour	35 mL
2	whole eggs	2
2	egg whites	2
1⅓ cups	2% evaporated milk	325 mL
¼ cup	chopped fresh dill (or 2 tsp/10 mL dried)	50 mL
¼ cup	bread crumbs	50 mL
½ tsp	margarine or butter	2 mL

Antioxidant all-stars: *An American study ranked the ability of fresh produce to act as antioxidants and neutralize harmful free radicals. The winners are:*

Vegetables	**Fruit**
kale	*blueberries*
beets	*strawberries*
red peppers	*plums*
broccoli	*oranges*
spinach	*red grapes*
potato	*kiwi*
sweet potato	*white grapes*
corn	*apples, tomatoes, bananas, pears and melons*

When using margarine, choose a soft (non-hydrogenated) version to limit consumption of trans fats.

Serves 6
Preheat oven to 350°F (180°C)
2-quart (2 L) casserole dish sprayed with vegetable spray

1. In nonstick skillet sprayed with vegetable spray, heat oil over medium heat. Add garlic, leeks and red peppers and cook for 7 minutes, or until tender, stirring occasionally; set aside.

2. Put 1 cup (250 mL) of corn in food processor with flour; purée. Add whole eggs, egg whites, evaporated milk and dill; process until smooth.

3. In large bowl, combine sautéed vegetables, corn purée and remaining 1 cup (250 mL) corn. Pour into prepared dish. Combine bread crumbs and margarine until crumbly. Sprinkle over top casserole and bake for 30 minutes or until set at center.

Tips

✦ Be sure to use evaporated milk — it's what gives this dish its creaminess.

✦ Leeks can have a lot of hidden dirt — to clean thoroughly, slice in half lengthwise and wash under cold running water, getting between the layers where dirt hides.

✦ Use fresh parsley, basil or coriander instead of dill.

✦ Reheat leftovers gently.

Make Ahead

✦ Cook vegetables early in day. Bake dish just before serving.

Nutritional Analysis (Per Serving)
✦ Calories: 194 ✦ Protein: 11 g ✦ Cholesterol: 76 mg
✦ Sodium: 340 mg ✦ Fat, total: 5 g ✦ Carbohydrates: 30 g
✦ Fiber: 2 g ✦ Fat, saturated: 1 g

Eggplant with Goat Cheese and Roasted Sweet Peppers

1	egg	1
1/4 cup	2% milk	50 mL
3/4 cup	seasoned bread crumbs	175 mL
2 tbsp	vegetable oil	25 mL
10	1/2-inch (1 cm) slices eggplant, skin on	10
3 oz	goat cheese	75 g
3 tbsp	2% milk	45 mL
3 tbsp	chopped roasted red peppers	45 mL
1/4 cup	chopped green onions (about 2 medium)	50 mL
1/2 tsp	minced garlic	2 mL

Serves 4 to 6
Preheat oven to 350°F (180°C)
Baking sheet sprayed with vegetable spray

1. Beat egg and milk together in small bowl. Put bread crumbs on plate. Dip the eggplant slices in egg wash then press into bread crumbs. In large nonstick skillet sprayed with vegetable spray, heat 1 tbsp (15 mL) of the oil over medium heat. Add half of the breaded eggplant slices and cook for 4 minutes or until golden brown on both sides. Add remaining 1 tbsp (15 mL) oil and respray skillet with vegetable spray. Repeat with remaining eggplant slices. Place on prepared baking sheet.

2. In small bowl, stir together goat cheese, milk, red peppers, green onions and garlic. Put a spoonful of topping on top of each eggplant slice. Bake for 10 minutes or until heated through.

Tip
✦ Feta cheese, grated cheddar or Swiss can replace goat cheese. A stronger tasting cheese suits this dish.

✦ Either use bottled-in-water roasted red peppers or, under a broiler, roast a small pepper for 15 to 20 minutes or until charred. Cool, then peel, deseed and chop. Use remainder for another purpose.

Make Ahead
✦ Prepare entire dish early in the day. Bake just before serving.

Nutritional Analysis (Per Serving)
✦ Calories: 150 ✦ Protein: 5 g ✦ Cholesterol: 37 mg
✦ Sodium: 399 mg ✦ Fat, total: 8 g ✦ Carbohydrates: 14 g
✦ Fiber: 1 g ✦ Fat, saturated: 1 g

Butternut Squash with Maple Syrup

1 lb	diced peeled butternut squash	500 g
1/3 cup	dried bread crumbs	75 mL
1/4 cup	light sour cream	50 mL
1/4 cup	maple syrup	50 mL
2 tsp	margarine or butter	10 mL
2 tsp	grated orange zest	10 mL
3/4 tsp	ground cinnamon	4 mL
1/4 tsp	ground ginger	1 mL
3	eggs, separated	3
1/2 cup	canned corn kernels, drained	125 mL
Pinch	salt	Pinch

When using margarine, choose a soft (non-hydrogenated) version to limit consumption of trans fats.

Serves 6 to 8
Preheat oven to 350°F (180°C)
8-inch (2 L) square baking dish sprayed with vegetable spray

1. In a pot of boiling water, cook squash 8 minutes or until tender; drain. Put in a food processor along with bread crumbs, sour cream, maple syrup, margarine, orange zest, cinnamon, ginger and 2 egg yolks. (Discard third egg yolk.) Process until smooth. Transfer to a large bowl; cool. Add corn.

2. In a bowl with an electric mixer, beat 3 egg whites with salt until stiff peaks form. Stir one-quarter of egg whites into squash mixture. Gently fold remaining egg whites into squash mixture. Pour into prepared pan. Bake 25 minutes or until set.

Tips

✦ Substitute sweet potato for squash.

✦ For a gingerbread taste, try adding 1 tbsp (15 mL) molasses and reducing maple syrup to 3 tbsp (45 mL).

✦ Egg whites can now be purchased in containers at grocery stores.

Make Ahead

✦ Prepare recipe to end of Step 1 up to 2 days in advance.

✦ Can be baked early in the day and reheated.

Nutritional Analysis (Per Serving)
✦ Calories: 99   ✦ Protein: 3 g   ✦ Cholesterol: 57 mg
✦ Sodium: 122 mg   ✦ Fat, total: 3 g ✦ Carbohydrates: 17 g
✦ Fiber: 0 g   ✦ Fat, saturated: 1 g

Acorn Squash with Rice, Pineapple and Molasses

1	acorn or pepper squash, slit several times with a knife	1
2 cups	vegetable or chicken stock	500 mL
½ cup	long-grain white rice	125 mL
½ cup	wild rice	125 mL
1 cup	diced carrots	250 mL
1 cup	canned crushed pineapple	250 mL
½ cup	raisins or dried cherries	75 mL
2 tbsp	orange juice concentrate	25 mL
1½ tbsp	molasses	20 mL
1 tbsp	packed brown sugar	15 mL
½ tsp	cinnamon	2 mL

Make room for molasses: *Not all sweeteners are empty calories. Take blackstrap molasses, for example. Just 1 tbsp (15 mL) gives you 179 mg calcium, 3.6 mg iron and 518 mg potassium. (It's a great source of calcium and iron for vegans.) Try swirling molasses into yogurt, adding it to baked beans or drizzling it over hot cereal.*

Serves 4

1. Microwave squash on high for 10 minutes or until tender; cool. Cut in half lengthwise. Scoop out cooked flesh; if desired, keep shell intact. Chop flesh.

2. Meanwhile, in a saucepan over medium-high heat, combine stock, white rice and wild rice; bring to a boil. Reduce heat to medium-low; cook, covered, for 20 minutes. Add carrots; cook, covered, for 10 minutes or until rice and carrots are tender and liquid is absorbed. (Wild rice will be crunchy.)

3. Add squash, pineapple, raisins, orange juice concentrate, molasses, brown sugar and cinnamon. Cook, uncovered and stirring often, for 5 minutes or until heated through. If desired, spoon squash mixture into reserved shell as a serving platter. Pour remaining squash into a serving dish.

Tip

✦ Acorn squash is named for its oblong shape (think of an acorn without its "hat"). That's about where the similarity ends, however; acorn squash is deeply ridged, usually green (although it can be yellow, brown, orange and/or black), with yellow-orange flesh. Like most squash, it is pretty bland on its own. But here, with addition of pineapple, raisins and molasses, the squash comes alive — providing a wonderful sweet-and-sour complement to the rice.

Nutritional Analysis (Per Serving)

✦ Calories: 330 ✦ Protein: 7 g ✦ Cholesterol: 0 mg
✦ Sodium: 99 mg ✦ Fat, total: 1 g ✦ Carbohydrates: 77 g
✦ Fiber: 5 g ✦ Fat, saturated: 0.3 g

Portobello Mushroom Sandwiches with Spinach Cheese Dressing

¼ cup	cooked spinach, well drained and finely chopped	50 mL
¼ cup	5% ricotta cheese	50 mL
¼ cup	shredded Swiss cheese (about 1 oz/25 g)	50 mL
2 tbsp	light mayonnaise	25 mL
1 tbsp	grated Parmesan cheese	15 mL
1½ tsp	freshly squeezed lemon juice	7 mL
1 tsp	Dijon mustard	5 mL
½ tsp	minced garlic	2 mL
4	portobello mushroom caps (about 2 oz/50 g each)	4
2 tsp	olive oil	10 mL
2	large pita breads, cut in half or 4 small pita breads, preferably whole wheat	2

Garnishes (optional)

Sliced tomatoes

Sliced onions

Lettuce leaves

Serves 4

1. In food processor or blender, purée spinach, ricotta, Swiss cheese, mayonnaise, Parmesan, lemon juice, mustard and garlic until smooth.
2. Wipe mushroom caps with a damp paper towel to clean. In a large nonstick frying pan sprayed with vegetable spray, heat oil over medium-high heat. Cook mushrooms 3 minutes per side or until tender when pierced with a fork and golden on both sides.
3. Put a hot mushroom cap into each pita and top with 2 tbsp (25 mL) spinach spread. If desired, garnish with tomatoes, onions and lettuce leaves. Serve hot.

Tips

✦ These mushroom sandwiches are almost beef-like in taste.

✦ If pitas are not available, try whole wheat hamburger buns.

✦ Portobello mushrooms can be refrigerated in a paper bag for several days in the refrigerator.

✦ If using whole portobello mushrooms, remove stems and save for soups or other dishes.

✦ Use 1½ cups (375 mL) fresh spinach to get ¼ cup (50 mL) finely chopped cooked spinach.

✦ Grill mushrooms if desired.

Make Ahead

✦ Prepare spinach dressing up to 2 days in advance.

✦ Sauté mushrooms early in day. Reheat before serving.

Nutritional Analysis (Per Serving)

✦ Calories: 263 ✦ Protein: 11 g ✦ Cholesterol: 10 mg
✦ Sodium: 328 mg ✦ Fat, total: 8 g ✦ Carbohydrates: 37 g
✦ Fiber: 1 g ✦ Fat, saturated: 2 g

Crustless Dill Spinach Quiche with Mushrooms and Cheese

10 oz	fresh spinach	300 g
2 tsp	vegetable oil	10 mL
1 tsp	minced garlic	5 mL
3/4 cup	chopped onions	175 mL
3/4 cup	chopped mushrooms	175 mL
2/3 cup	5% ricotta cheese	150 mL
2/3 cup	2% cottage cheese	150 mL
1/3 cup	grated cheddar cheese	75 mL
2 tbsp	grated Parmesan cheese	25 mL
1	whole egg	1
1	egg white	1
3 tbsp	chopped fresh dill (or 2 tsp/10 mL dried)	45 mL
1/4 tsp	ground black pepper	1 mL

Serves 6
Preheat oven to 350°F (180°C)
8-inch (2 L) springform pan sprayed with vegetable spray

1. Wash spinach and shake off excess water. In the water clinging to the leaves, cook the spinach over high heat just until it wilts. Squeeze out excess moisture, chop and set aside.

2. In large nonstick skillet, heat oil over medium heat; add garlic, onions and mushrooms and cook for 5 minutes or until softened. Remove from heat and add chopped spinach, ricotta, cottage, cheddar and Parmesan cheeses, whole egg, egg white, dill and pepper; mix well. Pour into prepared pan and bake for 35 to 40 minutes or until knife inserted in center comes out clean.

Tips

+ Use a 10-oz (300 g) package of frozen spinach instead of fresh spinach.

+ All ricotta or all cottage cheese can be used, but ricotta gives a creamy texture.

Make Ahead

+ Prepare mixture early in the day. Bake just before serving. Great reheated gently the next day.

Nutritional Analysis (Per Serving)
+ Calories: 134   + Protein: 13 g   + Cholesterol: 54 mg
+ Sodium: 259 mg   + Fat, total: 7 g   + Carbohydrates: 6 g
+ Fiber: 2 g   + Fat, saturated: 3 g

Zucchini and Roasted Pepper Quiche

2 tsp	vegetable oil	10 mL
1¹⁄₂ tsp	minced garlic	7 mL
1¹⁄₂ cups	chopped leeks	375 mL
4 cups	diced zucchini	1 L
1¹⁄₂ tsp	dried basil	7 mL
³⁄₄ cup	diced roasted red peppers	175 mL
¹⁄₄ cup	all-purpose flour	50 mL
¹⁄₄ cup	cornmeal	50 mL
1 tsp	baking powder	5 mL
¹⁄₄ tsp	salt	1 mL
¹⁄₄ tsp	freshly ground black pepper	1 mL
1	egg	1
1	egg white	1
¹⁄₂ cup	shredded cheddar cheese (about 2 oz/50 g)	125 mL
¹⁄₂ cup	2% milk	125 mL
¹⁄₂ cup	light sour cream	125 mL
3 tbsp	grated Parmesan cheese	45 mL

Serves 4 to 6
Preheat oven to 350°F (180°C)
8-inch (2 L) square baking dish spayed with vegetable spray

1. In a nonstick saucepan sprayed with vegetable spray, heat oil over medium heat. Add garlic and leeks; cook 4 minutes. Stir in zucchini and basil; cook 5 minutes longer or until vegetables are tender. Stir in roasted peppers; remove from heat and let cool.

2. In a large bowl, stir together flour, cornmeal, baking powder, salt and pepper. In a separate bowl, whisk together whole egg, egg white, cheddar, milk, sour cream and 2 tbsp (25 mL) of the Parmesan. Add wet ingredients and cooled vegetables to dry ingredients; stir to combine. Spoon into prepared baking dish. Sprinkle with remaining Parmesan.

3. Bake 30 to 35 minutes or until cake tester inserted at center comes out clean.

Tips

✦ This tastes like a rich quiche Lorraine — but without all the fat.

✦ Roast your own red bell peppers or buy water-packed roasted red peppers.

✦ If leeks are unavailable, substitute onions.

Make Ahead

✦ Prepare recipe to the end of Step 1 up to 2 days in advance.

✦ Bake quiche early in day and reheat gently.

Nutritional Analysis (Per Serving)
✦ Calories: 166 ✦ Protein: 9 g ✦ Cholesterol: 49 mg
✦ Sodium: 522 mg ✦ Fat, total: 7 g ✦ Carbohydrates: 18 g
✦ Fiber: 3 g ✦ Fat, saturated: 3 g

Zucchini Boats Stuffed with Cheese and Vegetables

3	medium zucchini	3
1 tbsp	vegetable oil	15 mL
2 tsp	crushed garlic	10 mL
½ cup	finely diced onions	125 mL
½ cup	finely diced mushrooms	125 mL
¼ cup	finely diced sweet red pepper	50 mL
2 tbsp	chopped fresh dill (or 1 tsp/5 mL dried dillweed)	25 mL
3 tbsp	dry bread crumbs	45 mL
4 tsp	grated Parmesan cheese	20 mL
	Salt and pepper	
¼ cup	shredded mozzarella cheese	50 mL

Serves 6
Preheat oven to 375°F (190°C)

1. Trim off ends of zucchini. Cook zucchini in boiling water for 3 minutes or until tender. Drain and rinse with cold water. Slice each lengthwise in half. With sharp knife, carefully remove pulp, leaving shell intact. Finely dice pulp and squeeze out excess moisture.

2. In nonstick skillet, heat oil; sauté garlic, onions, mushrooms, red pepper and zucchini until softened, approximately 10 minutes. Add dill, bread crumbs, Parmesan, and salt and pepper to taste; mix well.

3. Spoon filling evenly into zucchini shells and place in baking dish. Top each with mozzarella. Bake for 10 minutes or until hot and cheese melts.

Tip
✦ For a main course version, ¼ lb (125 g) ground beef, veal or chicken can be added when the vegetables are sautéed. Serve 2 boats per person.

Make Ahead
✦ Prepare early in the day and refrigerate. Bake just before serving.

Nutritional Analysis (Per Serving)
✦ Calories: 74 ✦ Protein: 4 g ✦ Cholesterol: 3 mg
✦ Sodium: 73 mg ✦ Fat: 4 g ✦ Carbohydrates: 7 g
✦ Fiber: 2 g

Mushrooms Stuffed with Goat Cheese and Leeks

16	medium mushrooms	16
1 tsp	vegetable oil	5 mL
1½ tsp	minced garlic	7 mL
⅓ cup	finely chopped leeks	75 mL
⅓ cup	finely chopped red peppers	75 mL
⅓ cup	crumbled goat cheese	75 mL
3 tbsp	light cream cheese	45 mL
2 tbsp	chopped fresh oregano (or ½ tsp/2 mL dried)	25 mL
2 tbsp	finely chopped green onions (about 1 medium)	25 mL

Serves 4 to 6
Preheat oven to 425°F (220°C)

1. Remove stems from mushrooms; set caps aside and dice stems.

2. In small nonstick saucepan sprayed with vegetable spray, heat oil over medium heat; add diced mushroom stems, garlic, leeks and peppers. Cook for 5 minutes, or until softened. Remove from heat.

3. Add goat and cream cheeses, oregano and green onions; mix well. Carefully stuff mixture into mushroom caps. Place in a baking dish and bake for 15 to 20 minutes or just until mushrooms release their liquid.

Nutritional Analysis (Per Serving)
- Calories: 72
- Protein: 4 g
- Cholesterol: 18 mg
- Sodium: 175 mg
- Fat: 5 g
- Carbohydrates: 4 g
- Fiber: 1 g

Basil and Roasted Red Pepper Stuffed Mushrooms

14 oz	large stuffing mushrooms (approximately 16)	400 g
¾ cup	packed basil leaves	175 mL
½ tsp	minced garlic	2 mL
1½ tbsp	olive oil	20 mL
2 tbsp	water	25 mL
1½ tbsp	toasted pine nuts	20 mL
1 tbsp	grated Parmesan cheese	15 mL
¼ cup	light cream cheese	50 mL
2 tbsp	finely diced roasted red peppers	25 mL

Toast pine nuts in a nonstick skillet for 2 minutes until browned, or in a 400°F (200°C) oven until browned, approximately 8 minutes.

Serves 6
Preheat oven to 425°F (220°C)
Baking sheet sprayed with vegetable spray

1. Wipe mushrooms clean and gently remove stems; reserve for another purpose. Put caps on baking sheet.

2. Put basil, garlic, olive oil, water, pine nuts, Parmesan and cream cheese into food processor; process until finely chopped, scraping down sides of bowl once. Process until smooth. Add red peppers and combine just until mixed.

3. Divide mixture evenly among mushroom caps. Bake for 15 minutes or until hot.

Nutritional Analysis (Per Serving)
- Calories: 95
- Protein: 4 g
- Cholesterol: 9 mg
- Sodium: 65 mg
- Fat: 7 g
- Carbohydrates: 4 g
- Fiber: 1 g

Cheddar Cheese Potato Skins

2	medium baking potatoes	2
4 tsp	margarine, melted	20 mL
1½ tsp	crushed garlic	7 mL
1 tbsp	finely chopped fresh parsley	15 mL
	Salt and pepper	
¼ cup	shredded cheddar cheese	50 mL

These taste great dipped in yogurt or low-fat sour cream. Sprinkle other herbs or diced vegetables over top.

When using margarine, choose a soft (non-hydrogenated) version to limit consumption of trans fats.

Serves 4
Preheat oven to 425°F (220°C)

1. Bake potatoes for 1 hour or until tender. (Or pierce skins and microwave at high for 8 to 10 minutes.) Cool and slice lengthwise in half; carefully remove pulp, leaving skin intact. (Reserve pulp for another use.) Place skins on baking sheet.

2. In small bowl, combine margarine, garlic, parsley, and salt and pepper to taste. Spread over potato shells. Top with cheese and bake for 20 minutes or until crisp.

Make Ahead

✦ Assemble and refrigerate potato shells early in day. Bake just prior to serving.

Nutritional Analysis (Per Serving)
- ✦ Calories: 114
- ✦ Protein: 3 g
- ✦ Cholesterol: 7 mg
- ✦ Sodium: 99 mg
- ✦ Fat: 6 g
- ✦ Carbohydrates: 12 g
- ✦ Fiber: 1 g

Baked French Wedge Potatoes

4	medium potatoes, unpeeled	4
2 tbsp	margarine, melted	25 mL
½ tsp	chili powder	2 mL
½ tsp	dried basil	2 mL
1 tsp	crushed garlic	5 mL
1½ tsp	chopped fresh parsley	7 mL
1 tbsp	grated Parmesan cheese	15 mL

These "French fries" beat those cooked in lots of oil. Children and adults can't stop eating them. Try different spices.

When using margarine, choose a soft (non-hydrogenated) version to limit consumption of trans fats.

Serves 6
Preheat oven to 375°F (190°C)
Baking sheet sprayed with nonstick vegetable spray

1. Scrub potatoes; cut each into 8 wedges. Place on baking sheet.

2. In small bowl, combine margarine, chili powder, basil, garlic and parsley; brush half over potatoes. Sprinkle with half of the Parmesan; bake for 30 minutes. Turn wedges over; brush with remaining mixture and sprinkle with remaining cheese. Bake for 30 minutes longer.

Tip

✦ Potatoes should be firm, heavy and smooth. Keep in a cool place for 2 to 3 weeks where there is ventilation to keep them dry.

Nutritional Analysis (Per Serving)
- ✦ Calories: 127
- ✦ Protein: 2 g
- ✦ Cholesterol: 1 mg
- ✦ Sodium: 73 mg
- ✦ Fat: 4 g
- ✦ Carbohydrates: 21 g
- ✦ Fiber: 2 g

Sweet Potato, Apple and Raisin Casserole

1 lb	sweet potatoes, peeled and cubed	500 g
¾ tsp	ground ginger	4 mL
¼ cup	honey or maple syrup	50 mL
¾ tsp	ground cinnamon	4 mL
2 tbsp	margarine, melted	25 mL
¼ cup	raisins	50 mL
2 tbsp	chopped walnuts	25 mL
¾ cup	cubed peeled sweet apples	175 mL

Sweet potatoes are sweet on their own. Lessen the honey or maple syrup if desired.

Chopped dates or apricots can replace the raisins.

When using margarine, choose a soft (non-hydrogenated) version to limit consumption of trans fats.

Serves 6
Preheat oven to 350°F (180°C)
Baking dish sprayed with nonstick vegetable spray

1. Steam or microwave sweet potatoes just until slightly underdone. Drain and place in baking dish.
2. In small bowl, combine ginger, honey, cinnamon, margarine, raisins, walnuts and apples; mix well. Pour over sweet potatoes and bake, uncovered, for 20 minutes or until tender.

Tip
✦ The darker the skin of the sweet potato, the moister it is.

Make Ahead
✦ Prepare casserole without apples up to the day before. Add apples, toss and bake just prior to serving.

Nutritional Analysis (Per Serving)
✦ Calories: 187   ✦ Protein: 2 g   ✦ Cholesterol: 0 mg
✦ Sodium: 62 mg   ✦ Fat: 5 g   ✦ Carbohydrates: 34 g
✦ Fiber: 3 g

Broccoli with Feta Cheese

4 cups	chopped broccoli florets and 2-inch (5 cm) stalk pieces	1 L
2 tsp	vegetable oil	10 mL
2 tsp	crushed garlic	10 mL
¾ cup	diced onion	175 mL
⅓ cup	sliced black olives	75 mL
1 cup	diced tomatoes	250 mL
2 tbsp	chicken stock	25 mL
1 tsp	dried oregano (or 2 tbsp/25 mL chopped fresh)	5 mL
1½ oz	feta cheese, crumbled	40 g

Serves 4

1. Steam or microwave broccoli just until barely tender. Drain and set aside.
2. In nonstick skillet, heat oil; sauté garlic and onion just until softened, approximately 3 minutes. Add broccoli, olives, tomatoes, chicken stock and oregano; cook for 3 minutes. Place in serving dish. Sprinkle with feta cheese.

Tip
✦ For a change, substitute asparagus for the broccoli, and goat cheese for the feta.

Nutritional Analysis (Per Serving)
✦ Calories: 111   ✦ Protein: 5 g   ✦ Cholesterol: 9 mg
✦ Sodium: 270 mg   ✦ Fat: 6 g   ✦ Carbohydrates: 11 g
✦ Fiber: 4 g

Fennel Gratin

1	medium fennel bulb, trimmed and sliced thinly	1
1½ tsp	vegetable oil	7 mL
2 tsp	crushed garlic	10 mL
½ cup	chopped onion	125 mL
2 cups	tomato sauce	500 mL
2 tbsp	chopped fresh dill (or 1 tsp/5 mL dried dillweed)	25 mL
½ cup	shredded mozzarella cheese	125 mL

The stalks and bulbs of fennel should be firm. If fennel is unavailable, replace with 1 large sliced zucchini or half a small sliced eggplant.

Serves 4
Preheat oven to 350°F (180°C)
8-inch (2 L) square baking dish

1. In saucepan of boiling water, cook fennel just until tender, 5 to 8 minutes. Drain and set aside.
2. In nonstick skillet, heat oil; sauté garlic and onion until softened. Add tomato sauce and dill.
3. Add half of the tomato sauce mixture to baking dish. Add fennel; pour remaining sauce over top. Top with cheese. Bake for 20 minutes or until hot and cheese melts.

Make Ahead
✦ Prepare and refrigerate early in day. Bake just before eating. This tastes great reheated.

Nutritional Analysis (Per Serving)
✦ Calories: 122   ✦ Protein: 7 g   ✦ Cholesterol: 7 mg
✦ Sodium: 928 mg   ✦ Fat: 4 g   ✦ Carbohydrates: 16 g
✦ Fiber: 4 g

Asparagus with Lemon and Garlic

½ lb	asparagus, trimmed	250 g
2 tsp	vegetable oil	10 mL
1 tsp	crushed garlic	5 mL
¼ cup	diced sweet red pepper	50 mL
1	green onion, sliced	1
2 tbsp	white wine	25 mL
4 tsp	lemon juice	20 mL
2 tbsp	chicken stock	25 mL
	Pepper	

If asparagus is not available, try broccoli or snow peas.

Serves 4

1. Steam or boil asparagus just until tender-crisp. Do not overcook. Drain and set aside.
2. In large nonstick skillet, heat oil; sauté garlic and red pepper until softened.
3. Reduce heat and add green onion, wine, lemon juice, chicken stock, pepper to taste and asparagus. Cook for 1 minute. Place asparagus mixture in serving dish.

Make Ahead
✦ Make this early in day if it is to be served cold, to allow the asparagus a chance to marinate.

Nutritional Analysis (Per Serving)
✦ Calories: 46   ✦ Protein: 2 g   ✦ Cholesterol: 0 mg
✦ Sodium: 29 mg   ✦ Fat: 2 g   ✦ Carbohydrates: 4 g
✦ Fiber: 1 g

Brussels Sprouts with Pecans and Sweet Potatoes

1 1/2 cups	cubed peeled sweet potatoes	375 mL
3/4 lb	brussels sprouts, cut in half	375 g
1 tbsp	margarine	15 mL
1/2 cup	chopped onion	125 mL
1 tsp	crushed garlic	5 mL
1/4 cup	chicken stock	50 mL
4 tsp	brown sugar or honey	20 mL
1/4 tsp	cinnamon	1 mL
2 tbsp	pecan pieces, toasted	25 mL

Brussels sprouts can have a slightly bitter taste, especially if overcooked. The addition of sweet potatoes and pecans balances the flavor.

Serves 4

1. In saucepan of boiling water, cook sweet potatoes until just tender; drain and reserve. Repeat with brussels sprouts. Set aside.
2. In nonstick skillet, melt margarine; sauté onion and garlic just until tender. Add sweet potatoes, brussels sprouts, stock, sugar, cinnamon and pecans; cook for 3 minutes or until vegetables are tender.

Tip

✦ Toast pecans in 400°F (200°C) oven or in skillet on top of stove for 2 minutes or until brown.

Nutritional Analysis (Per Serving)
✦ Calories: 182   ✦ Protein: 5 g   ✦ Cholesterol: 0 mg
✦ Sodium: 142 mg   ✦ Fat: 6 g   ✦ Carbohydrates: 30 g
✦ Fiber: 6 g

Carrots and Snow Peas with Maple Syrup and Pecans

1/2 lb	carrots, sliced thinly	250 g
1/2 lb	snow peas	250 g
1 1/2 tsp	margarine	7 mL
3 tbsp	maple syrup	45 mL
2 tbsp	chopped fresh parsley	25 mL
2 tbsp	chopped pecans, toasted	25 mL
1/2 tsp	cinnamon	2 mL

Green beans can be a good substitute for snow peas. Walnuts or pine nuts can replace pecans.

When using margarine, choose a soft (non-hydrogenated) version to limit consumption of trans fats.

Serves 4

1. Steam or microwave carrots at high just until barely tender, approximately 2 minutes. Drain and set aside.
2. Steam or microwave snow peas just until barely tender, approximately 2 minutes. Drain and set aside.
3. In nonstick skillet, heat margarine and maple syrup. Add carrots, snow peas and parsley; cook for 1 minute. Serve sprinkled with pecans and cinnamon.

Tips

✦ Toast pecans in small skillet on stove for 2 minutes or in 400°F (200°C) oven until golden.

✦ Smaller carrots are more tender and sweeter than larger ones.

Nutritional Analysis (Per Serving)
✦ Calories: 125   ✦ Protein: 3 g   ✦ Cholesterol: 0 mg
✦ Sodium: 72 mg   ✦ Fat: 4 g   ✦ Carbohydrates: 20 g
✦ Fiber: 3 g

Chocolate Cheesecake with Sour Cream Topping (page 345) ➤

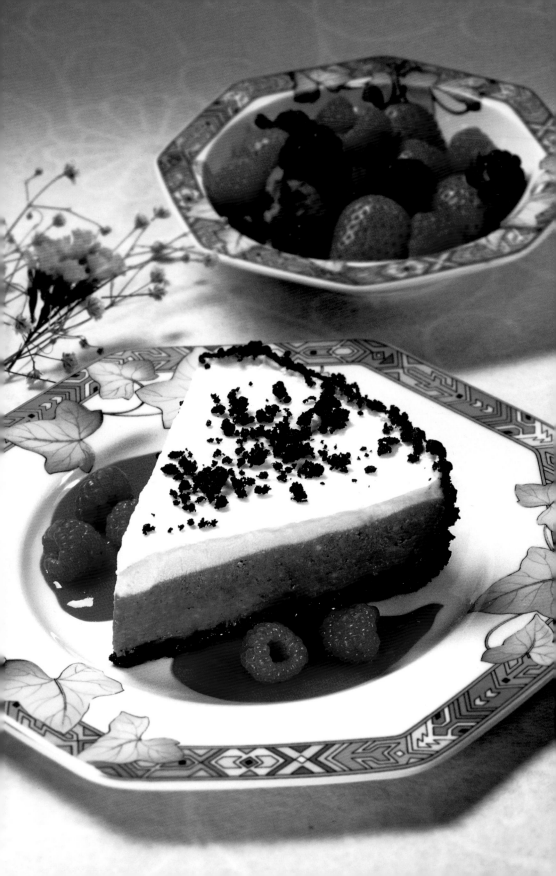

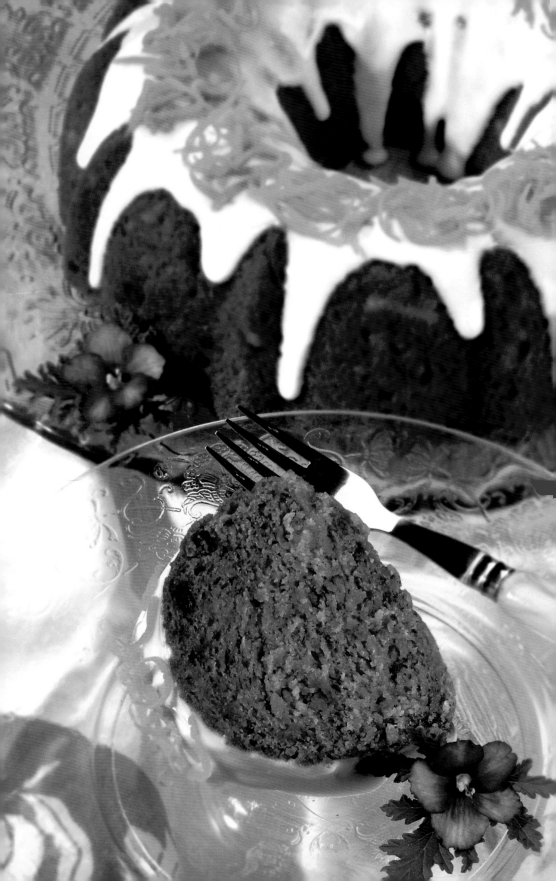

Snow Peas with Sesame Seeds

1 tbsp	vegetable oil	15 mL
1½ tsp	crushed garlic	7 mL
1 lb	snow peas, trimmed	500 g
½ cup	diced sweet red peppers	125 mL
2 tsp	sesame oil	10 mL
1½ tsp	sesame seeds, toasted	7 mL
4	medium green onions, sliced	4

Nuts such as toasted pine nuts can be substituted for the sesame seeds.

Serves 4

1. In nonstick skillet, heat vegetable oil; sauté garlic, snow peas and red peppers until tender-crisp.
2. Add sesame oil and seeds and green onions; cook for 1 minute. Serve immediately.

Tips

✦ This dish is also great with asparagus instead of snow peas.

✦ Toast sesame seeds in small skillet on high heat for 2 minutes until brown, stirring continuously.

Make Ahead

✦ If serving cold as a salad, prepare early in the day and stir just before serving.

Nutritional Analysis (Per Serving)
✦ Calories: 112 ✦ Protein: 4 g ✦ Cholesterol: 0 mg
✦ Sodium: 8 mg ✦ Fat: 6 g ✦ Carbohydrates: 10 g
✦ Fiber: 3 g

Green Beans and Diced Tomatoes

8 oz	green beans, trimmed	250 g
1½ tsp	vegetable oil	7 mL
1 tsp	crushed garlic	5 mL
¾ cup	chopped onion	175 mL
⅓ cup	chopped sweet red or yellow pepper	75 mL
1½ cups	diced tomatoes	375 mL
½ tsp	dried basil (or 1 tbsp/15 mL fresh)	2 mL
½ tsp	dried oregano	2 mL
2 tbsp	chicken stock	25 mL
2 tsp	lemon juice	10 mL
2 tsp	grated Parmesan cheese (optional)	10 mL

Serves 4

1. Steam or microwave green beans just until tender. Set aside.
2. In nonstick skillet, heat oil; sauté garlic, onion and red pepper just until tender.
3. Add green beans, tomatoes, basil, oregano, stock and lemon juice; cook for 2 minutes, stirring constantly. Serve sprinkled with Parmesan (if using).

Tip

✦ Snow peas or asparagus can replace the green beans.

Make Ahead

✦ If serving cold, prepare early in day and allow flavors to blend.

Nutritional Analysis (Per Serving)
✦ Calories: 65 ✦ Protein: 2 g ✦ Cholesterol: 1 mg
✦ Sodium: 55 mg ✦ Fat: 2 g ✦ Carbohydrates: 10 g
✦ Fiber: 3 g

◄ Carrot Cake with Cream Cheese Frosting (page 348)

Teriyaki Sesame Vegetable

1½ tsp	vegetable oil	7 mL
1 tsp	crushed garlic	5 mL
Half	large sweet red or yellow pepper, sliced thinly	Half
Half	large sweet green pepper, sliced thinly	Half
1½ cups	snow peas	375 mL
1	large carrot, sliced thinly	1
½ tsp	sesame seeds	2 mL
Sauce		
1 tsp	crushed garlic	5 mL
1 tbsp	soya sauce	15 mL
1 tbsp	rice wine vinegar or white wine vinegar	15 mL
½ tsp	minced gingerroot	2 mL
½ tsp	sesame oil	2 mL
1 tbsp	water	15 mL
1 tbsp	brown sugar	15 mL
1½ tsp	vegetable oil	7 mL

Serves 4

1. *Sauce:* In small saucepan, combine garlic, soya sauce, vinegar, ginger, sesame oil, water, sugar and vegetable oil; cook for 3 to 5 minutes or until thickened and syrupy.
2. In large nonstick skillet, heat oil; sauté garlic, red and green peppers, snow peas and carrot, stirring constantly, for 2 minutes.
3. Add sauce; sauté for 2 minutes or just until vegetables are tender-crisp. Place in serving dish and sprinkle with sesame seeds.

Tip

✦ Remember to cook over high heat and not to overcook.

Nutritional Analysis (Per Serving)
✦ Calories: 96 ✦ Protein: 2 g ✦ Cholesterol: 0 mg
✦ Sodium: 271 mg ✦ Fat: 4 g ✦ Carbohydrates: 12 g
✦ Fiber: 2 g

Tomatoes Stuffed with Corn, Black Beans and Pine Nuts

4	medium tomatoes	4
½ cup	canned corn kernels, drained	125 mL
½ cup	canned black beans, rinsed and drained	125 mL
¼ cup	chopped fresh coriander	50 mL
¼ cup	chopped green onions	50 mL
¼ cup	chopped red bell peppers	50 mL
2 tbsp	light mayonnaise	25 mL
2 tbsp	toasted pine nuts	25 mL
1 tbsp	grated Parmesan cheese	15 mL
2 tsp	freshly squeezed lemon juice	10 mL
1 tsp	Dijon mustard	5 mL

Serves 4

1. Slice tops off tomatoes and reserve. Scoop out and discard seeds and core.
2. In a small bowl, mix together corn, black beans, coriander, green onions, red peppers, mayonnaise, pine nuts, Parmesan, lemon juice and Dijon.
3. Divide mixture evenly between tomato shells, about ⅓ cup (75 mL) per tomato. Cover with reserved tomato tops and serve.

Make Ahead

✦ Prepare filling up to 1 day in advance. Stuff tomatoes a few hours before serving.

Nutritional Analysis (Per Serving)
✦ Calories: 136 ✦ Protein: 6 g ✦ Cholesterol: 1 mg
✦ Sodium: 238 mg ✦ Fat, total: 6 g ✦ Carbohydrates: 19 g
✦ Fiber: 5 g ✦ Fat, saturated: 1 g

Caramelized Balsamic Onions with Chopped Dates

2 tsp	margarine or butter	10 mL
2 tsp	minced garlic	10 mL
1½ lbs	onions, thinly sliced	750 g
½ cup	chopped dates	125 mL
3 tbsp	balsamic vinegar	45 mL
1 tbsp	brown sugar	15 mL

On non-vegetarian days these onions make a great topping for chicken, fish or beef.

When using margarine, choose a soft (non-hydrogenated) version to limit consumption of trans fats.

Serves 4

1. In a large nonstick saucepan, melt margarine over medium heat. Add garlic and onions; cook, stirring occasionally, until soft and brown, about 20 minutes.
2. Stir in dates, vinegar and brown sugar; cook 10 minutes, stirring occasionally.

Tip

✦ Use this wonderful onion dish as a vegetable side dish or as a topping over cooked pasta or other grains.

Make Ahead

✦ Prepare early in day and reheat before serving.

Nutritional Analysis (Per Serving)

✦ Calories: 153 ✦ Protein: 3 g ✦ Cholesterol: 0 mg
✦ Sodium: 32 mg ✦ Fat, total: 2 g ✦ Carbohydrates: 34 g
✦ Fiber: 5 g ✦ Fat, saturated: 0.3 g

Sugar Snap Peas with Sesame Sauce

1 tbsp	honey	15 mL
1 tbsp	rice wine vinegar	15 mL
1 tbsp	sesame oil	15 mL
1 tbsp	soya sauce	15 mL
½ tsp	minced garlic	2 mL
1 lb	sugar snap peas, trimmed	500 g
1 tsp	vegetable oil	5 mL
1 tbsp	toasted sesame seeds	15 mL

Serves 4

1. In a small bowl, combine honey, vinegar, sesame oil, soya sauce and garlic; set aside.
2. Steam or boil sugar peas 2 minutes. In a large nonstick skillet sprayed with vegetable spray, heat oil over medium-high heat; cook peas for 3 minutes or until tender-crisp. Pour sauce over peas; cook until heated through. Serve immediately, sprinkled with sesame seeds.

Tip

✦ Use snow peas or green beans instead of the sugar snap peas.

Make Ahead

✦ Prepare sauce up to 2 days in advance.
✦ Best cooked right before serving.

Nutritional Analysis (Per Serving)

✦ Calories: 116 ✦ Protein: 3 g ✦ Cholesterol: 0 mg
✦ Sodium: 269 mg ✦ Fat, total: 6 g ✦ Carbohydrates: 15 g
✦ Fiber: 2 g ✦ Fat, saturated: 1 g

Roasted Garlic Sweet Pepper Strips

4	large sweet peppers (combination of green, red and yellow)	4
2 tbsp	olive oil	25 mL
1½ tsp	crushed garlic	7 mL
1 tbsp	grated Parmesan cheese	15 mL

Serves 4
Preheat oven to 400°F (200°C)

1. On baking sheet, bake whole peppers for 15 to 20 minutes, turning occasionally, or until blistered and blackened. Place in paper bag; seal and let stand for 10 minutes.
2. Peel off charred skin from peppers; cut off tops and bottoms. Remove seeds and ribs; cut into 1-inch (2.5 cm) wide strips and place on serving platter.
3. Mix oil with garlic; brush over peppers. Sprinkle with cheese.

Tip
+ Add a sprinkle of fresh herbs such as parsley or basil to oil mixture.

Make Ahead
+ These peppers can be prepared ahead of time and served cold.

Nutritional Analysis (Per Serving)
+ Calories: 95
+ Protein: 1 g
+ Cholesterol: 1 mg
+ Sodium: 26 mg
+ Fat: 7 g
+ Carbohydrates: 7 g
+ Fiber: 2 g

Desserts

continued on next page

Chocolate Marble Vanilla Cheesecake

Crust

2 cups	chocolate wafer crumbs	500 mL
3 tbsp	water	45 mL
1½ tbsp	margarine or butter, melted	20 mL

Filling

2 cups	ricotta cheese	500 mL
2 cups	2% cottage cheese	500 mL
1¾ cups	granulated sugar	425 mL
2	large eggs	2
⅓ cup	all-purpose flour	75 mL
⅔ cup	light sour cream	150 mL
2 tsp	vanilla	10 mL
2 oz	semi-sweet chocolate	50 g
2 tbsp	water	25 mL

When using margarine, choose a soft (non-hydrogenated) version to limit consumption of trans fats.

Serves 20
Preheat oven to 350°F (180°C)
9-inch (2.5 L) springform pan sprayed with vegetable spray

1. *Crust:* In bowl, combine crumbs, water and margarine; mix well. Press onto sides and bottom of springform pan; refrigerate.

2. In food processor, combine ricotta and cottage cheeses, sugar and eggs; process until completely smooth. Add flour, sour cream and vanilla; process until well combined. Pour into pan. Melt chocolate with water and stir until smooth. Spoon onto cake in several places and swirl through lightly with a knife. Bake for 65 minutes or until set around edge but still slightly loose in center. Let cool; refrigerate until well chilled.

Tips

✦ This recipe can be cut in half, but use only 2 tbsp (25 mL) flour. Bake for 35 minutes, or until slightly loose at the center.

✦ For a mocha flavor, dissolve 2 tsp (10 mL) instant coffee in same amount of water and add to batter.

Make Ahead

✦ Prepare up to 2 days ahead. Freeze for up to 6 weeks.

Nutritional Analysis (Per Serving)
✦ Calories: 215 ✦ Protein: 7 g ✦ Cholesterol: 31 mg
✦ Sodium: 230 mg ✦ Fat: 5 g ✦ Carbohydrates: 31 g
✦ Fiber: 1 g

Marble Mocha Cheesecake

Crust

1½ cups	chocolate wafer crumbs	375 mL
2 tbsp	granulated sugar	25 mL
2 tbsp	water	25 mL
1 tbsp	margarine or butter	15 mL

Filling

1⅔ cups	5% ricotta cheese	400 mL
⅓ cup	softened light cream cheese	75 mL
¾ cup	granulated sugar	175 mL
1	egg	1
⅓ cup	light sour cream or 2% yogurt	75 mL
1 tbsp	all-purpose flour	15 mL
1 tsp	vanilla	5 mL
1½ tsp	instant coffee granules	7 mL
1½ tsp	hot water	7 mL
3 tbsp	semi-soft chocolate chips, melted	45 mL

> *When using margarine, choose a soft (non-hydrogenated) version to limit consumption of trans fats.*

Serves 12
Preheat oven to 350°F (180°C)
8-inch (2 L) springform pan sprayed with vegetable spray

1. Combine chocolate crumbs, sugar, water and margarine; mix thoroughly. Press into bottom and up sides of springform pan.

2. In large bowl or food processor, beat together ricotta cheese, cream cheese, sugar, egg, sour cream, flour and vanilla until well blended. Dissolve coffee granules in hot water; add to batter and mix until incorporated.

3. Pour batter into springform pan and smooth top. Drizzle melted chocolate on top. Draw knife or spatula through the chocolate and batter several times to create marbling. Bake for 35 to 40 minutes; center will be slightly loose. Let cool, and refrigerate several hours before serving.

Tips

+ Serve with chocolate-dipped strawberries. Melt 2 oz (50 g) chocolate with 1 tsp (5 mL) vegetable oil. Dip the bottom half of the berry in chocolate.

+ Graham crackers or other cookie crumbs can be used for the crust.

+ Melt chocolate in microwave on defrost or in a double boiler.

+ If instant coffee is unavailable, use 2 tsp (10 mL) prepared strong coffee.

Make Ahead

+ Bake up to 2 days ahead and keep refrigerated.

+ Freeze for up to 6 weeks.

Nutritional Analysis (Per Serving)

+ Calories: 210   + Protein: 8 g   + Cholesterol: 34 mg
+ Sodium: 178 mg + Fat, total: 7 g + Carbohydrates: 29 g
+ Fiber: 1 g   + Fat, saturated: 4 g

Chocolate Cheesecake with Sour Cream Topping

8 oz	ricotta cheese	250 g
8 oz	2% cottage cheese	250 g
1 cup	granulated sugar	250 mL
1	large egg	1
1 tsp	vanilla	5 mL
1/4 cup	sifted unsweetened cocoa powder	50 mL
1 tbsp	all-purpose flour	15 mL

Crust

1 1/2 cups	graham or chocolate wafer crumbs	375 mL
2 tbsp	water	25 mL
1 tbsp	margarine, melted	15 mL

Topping

1 cup	light sour cream	250 mL
2 tbsp	granulated sugar	25 mL
1 tsp	vanilla	5 mL

When using margarine, choose a soft (non-hydrogenated) version to limit consumption of trans fats.

Makes 12 servings
Preheat oven to 350°F (180°C)
8-inch (2 L) springform pan sprayed with nonstick vegetable spray

1. *Crust:* In bowl, combine crumbs, water and margarine; mix well. Pat onto bottom and sides of springform pan. Refrigerate.

2. In food processor, combine ricotta and cottage cheeses, sugar, egg and vanilla; process until smooth. Add cocoa and flour; process just until combined. Pour into pan and bake for 30 minutes or until set around edge but still slightly loose in center.

3. *Topping:* Meanwhile, stir together sour cream, sugar and vanilla; pour over cheesecake. Bake for 10 more minutes. (Topping will be loose.) Let cool and refrigerate for at least 3 hours or until set.

Tips
+ Garnish with fresh berries or sifted cocoa.
+ Cooking with cocoa rather than chocolate has a major advantage. One ounce of semisweet chocolate has 140 calories and 9 g of fat. One ounce of cocoa has 90 calories and 3 g of fat.

Make Ahead
+ Prepare a day before or freeze for up to 3 weeks.

Nutritional Analysis (Per Serving)
+ Calories: 209 + Protein: 8 g + Cholesterol: 32 mg
+ Sodium: 206 mg + Fat: 5 g + Carbohydrates: 32 g
+ Fiber: 1 g

Tangy Banana Cheesecake

1 cup	low-fat cottage cheese	250 mL
1 cup	low-fat yogurt	250 mL
2	egg whites	2
2 tbsp	lemon juice	25 mL
1 tsp	vanilla extract	5 mL
1/3 cup	whole wheat flour	75 mL
1/4 cup	honey	50 mL
2	ripe bananas	2
	Berries or sliced bananas	

Serves 6 to 8
Preheat oven to 375°F (190°C)
9-inch (23 cm) pie plate sprayed with baking spray

1. In a blender or food processor, combine cottage cheese, yogurt, egg whites, lemon juice and vanilla; purée until smooth. Add flour; blend until well mixed. With motor running, add honey through feed tube; process until smooth. Add bananas; blend until smooth. Pour into prepared pie plate.

2. Bake 30 to 40 minutes or until firm to the touch. Cool on wire rack. Chill at least 1 hour. Serve garnished with berries or sliced bananas.

Tip

✦ For an extra-nutritious dessert with a nutty flavor, coat pie plate with wheat germ after spraying with baking spray.

Nutritional Analysis (Per Serving)
✦ Calories: 100   ✦ Protein: 6 g   ✦ Cholesterol: 3 mg
✦ Sodium: 120 mg   ✦ Fat: 1 g   ✦ Carbohydrates: 18 g

Raspberry Cheesecake

1 cup	5% ricotta cheese	250 mL
1 cup	low-fat cottage cheese	250 mL
1/3 cup	granulated sugar or 1/4 cup (50 mL) fructose	75 mL
1/3 cup	low-fat yogurt	75 mL
2	eggs	2
1 tsp	grated lemon zest	5 mL
1/2 tsp	vanilla extract	2 mL
1 tbsp	all-purpose flour	15 mL
1 1/2 tsp	cornstarch	7 mL
1 cup	raspberries	250 mL
	Raspberry purée (optional)	

Serves 12
Preheat oven to 350°F (180°C)
8-inch (2 L) springform pan sprayed with baking spray

1. In a food processor, beat together ricotta cheese, cottage cheese, sugar, yogurt, eggs, lemon zest and vanilla until smooth. Beat in flour and cornstarch. Transfer to a bowl; gently fold in raspberries. Pour into prepared pan.

2. Bake 35 minutes or until a tester inserted in center comes out clean. Cool on a wire rack. Chill. Serve plain or, if desired, with raspberry purée.

Nutritional Analysis (Per Serving)
✦ Calories: 91   ✦ Protein: 6 g   ✦ Cholesterol: 57 mg
✦ Sodium: 109 mg   ✦ Fat: 3 g   ✦ Carbohydrates: 9 g

You can substitute whole frozen raspberries for fresh. Thaw and drain before using.

La Costa Cheesecake with Strawberry Sauce

Cheesecake

2 cups	low-fat cottage cheese	500 mL
3 tbsp	fructose	45 mL
2 tbsp	lemon juice	25 mL
2 tsp	vanilla extract	10 mL
2	eggs	2
2 tbsp	low-fat milk powder	25 mL

Strawberry Sauce

2 cups	strawberries	500 mL
1	ripe banana	1
	Fresh strawberries (optional)	

Thaw unsweetened frozen strawberries for sauce or use fresh ripe berries; if using frozen, drain excess liquid before puréeing.

The milk powder gives an extra calcium boost to this cheesecake.

Serves 12
Preheat oven to 325° F (160° C)
9-inch (23 cm) pie plate

1. *Make the cheesecake:* In a blender or food processor, combine cottage cheese, fructose, lemon juice, vanilla and eggs; purée until smooth. Add milk powder; blend just until mixed. Pour into pie plate. Set pie plate in larger pan; pour in enough hot water to come half way up sides. Bake 30 to 35 minutes. Remove from water bath; cool on wire rack. Chill.

2. *Make the strawberry sauce:* In a blender or food processor, purée strawberries with banana until smooth.

3. To serve, drizzle 2 tbsp (25 mL) strawberry sauce over each slice of cheesecake. Garnish with strawberries, if desired.

Nutritional Analysis (Per Serving)
- Calories: 84
- Protein: 6 g
- Cholesterol: 53 mg
- Sodium: 168 mg
- Fat: 2 g
- Carbohydrates: 9 g

Blueberry Peach Cake

1 cup	granulated sugar	250 mL
3/4 cup	applesauce	175 mL
1/4 cup	vegetable oil	50 mL
2	eggs	2
1 tsp	vanilla	5 mL
1 1/2 cups	all-purpose flour	375 mL
1/2 cup	whole wheat flour	125 mL
2 tsp	cinnamon	10 mL
1 1/2 tsp	baking powder	7 mL
1 tsp	baking soda	5 mL
1/2 cup	2% yogurt	125 mL
1 cup	sliced peeled peaches	250 mL
1 cup	blueberries	250 mL
	Icing sugar	

If using frozen blueberries, thaw first, then drain off the excess liquid.

Makes 16 slices
Preheat oven to 350°F (180°C)
9-inch (3 L) Bundt pan sprayed with nonstick vegetable spray

1. In large bowl, beat together sugar, applesauce, oil, eggs and vanilla, mixing well.

2. Combine all-purpose and whole wheat flours, cinnamon, baking powder and baking soda; stir into bowl just until blended. Stir in yogurt; fold in peaches and blueberries. Pour into pan.

3. Bake for 40 to 45 minutes or until cake tester inserted into center comes out clean. Let cool; dust with icing sugar.

Make Ahead
- Bake a day before or freeze for up to 6 weeks.

Nutritional Analysis (Per Serving)
- Calories: 171
- Protein: 3 g
- Cholesterol: 27 mg
- Sodium: 102 mg
- Fat: 4 g
- Carbohydrates: 31 g
- Fiber: 1 g

Carrot Cake with Cream Cheese Frosting

⅓ cup	margarine or butter	75 mL
1 cup	granulated sugar	250 mL
2	eggs	2
1 tsp	vanilla	5 mL
1	large ripe banana, mashed	1
2 cups	grated carrots	500 mL
⅔ cup	raisins	150 mL
½ cup	canned pineapple, drained and crushed	125 mL
½ cup	2% yogurt	125 mL
2 cups	all-purpose flour	500 mL
1½ tsp	baking powder	7 mL
1½ tsp	baking soda	7 mL
1½ tsp	cinnamon	7 mL
¼ tsp	nutmeg	1 mL

Icing

⅓ cup	light cream cheese, softened	75 mL
⅔ cup	icing sugar	150 mL
1 tbsp	2% milk	15 mL

> *When using margarine, choose a soft (non-hydrogenated) version to limit consumption of trans fats.*

Serves 16

Preheat oven to 350°F (180°C)

9-inch (3 L) Bundt pan sprayed with vegetable spray

1. In large bowl, cream together margarine and sugar until smooth; add eggs and vanilla and beat well (mixture may look curdled). Add mashed banana, carrots, raisins, pineapple and yogurt; stir until well combined.

2. In bowl, stir together flour, baking powder, baking soda, cinnamon and nutmeg. Add to the carrot mixture; stir just until combined. Pour into prepared pan and bake for 40 to 45 minutes or until cake tester inserted in the center comes out clean. Let cool for 10 minutes before inverting onto serving plate.

3. In bowl or food processor, beat together cream cheese, icing sugar and milk until smooth; drizzle over top of cake. Decorate with grated carrots if desired.

Tips

♦ Very ripe bananas can be kept frozen for up to 3 months.

♦ Raisins can be replaced with chopped, pitted dates, apricots or prunes.

♦ Food processor can be used to mix cake. Do not over-process.

Make Ahead

♦ Bake up to 2 days ahead.

♦ Freeze for up to 6 weeks.

Nutritional Analysis (Per Serving)

♦ Calories: 223   ♦ Protein: 4 g   ♦ Cholesterol: 30 mg
♦ Sodium: 218 mg   ♦ Fat, total: 5 g   ♦ Carbohydrates: 41 g
♦ Fiber: 1 g   ♦ Fat, saturated: 1 g

Date Cake with Coconut Topping

Cake

12 oz	chopped, pitted dried dates	300 g
1¾ cups	water	425 mL
¼ cup	margarine or butter	50 mL
1 cup	granulated sugar	250 mL
2	eggs	2
1½ cups	all-purpose flour	375 mL
1½ tsp	baking powder	7 mL
1 tsp	baking soda	5 mL

Topping

⅓ cup	unsweetened coconut	75 mL
¼ cup	brown sugar	50 mL
3 tbsp	2% milk	45 mL
2 tbsp	margarine or butter	25 mL

When using margarine, choose a soft (non-hydrogenated) version to limit consumption of trans fats.

Serves 16
Preheat oven to 350°F (180°C)
9-inch square (2.5 L) cake pan sprayed with vegetable spray

1. Put dates and water in saucepan; bring to a boil, cover and reduce heat to low. Cook for 10 minutes, stirring often, or until dates are soft and most of the liquid has been absorbed. Set aside to cool for 10 minutes.

2. In large bowl or food processor, beat together margarine and sugar. Add eggs and mix well. Add cooled date mixture and mix well.

3. In bowl, combine flour, baking powder and baking soda. Stir into date mixture just until blended. Pour into cake pan and bake for 35 to 40 minutes or until cake tester inserted in center comes out dry.

4. In small saucepan, combine coconut, brown sugar, milk and margarine; cook over medium heat, stirring, for 2 minutes, or until sugar dissolves. Pour over cake.

Tips

✦ To chop dates easily, use kitchen shears. Whole pitted dates can be used, but then use food processor to finely chop dates after they are cooked.

✦ Chopped pitted prunes can replace dates.

Make Ahead

✦ Prepare up to 2 days ahead, or freeze for up to 6 weeks. The dates keep this cake moist.

Nutritional Analysis (Per Serving)

✦ Calories: 217   ✦ Protein: 3 g   ✦ Cholesterol: 27 mg
✦ Sodium: 136 mg   ✦ Fat, total: 5 g   ✦ Carbohydrates: 41 g
✦ Fiber: 2 g   ✦ Fat, saturated: 2 g

Prune Orange Spice Cake

8 oz	chopped pitted prunes	250 g
1 cup	orange juice	250 mL
1/3 cup	margarine or butter	75 mL
3/4 cup	granulated sugar	175 mL
2	eggs	2
2 tsp	grated orange zest	10 mL
1 tsp	vanilla	5 mL
1 cup	all-purpose flour	250 mL
1/2 cup	whole wheat flour	125 mL
1 tsp	baking powder	5 mL
3/4 tsp	cinnamon	4 mL
1/2 tsp	baking soda	2 mL
1/8 tsp	nutmeg	0.5 mL
1/3 cup	2% yogurt	75 mL

Icing

4 tsp	orange juice	20 mL
1/2 cup	icing sugar	125 mL

When using margarine, choose a soft (non-hydrogenated) version to limit consumption of trans fats.

Serves 16
Preheat oven to 350°F (180°C)
9-inch square (2.5 L) baking dish sprayed with vegetable spray

1. Put prunes and orange juice in saucepan; bring to a boil, cover and reduce heat to low. Cook for 10 to 12 minutes, stirring often, or until prunes are soft and most of the liquid has been absorbed. Set aside.

2. In large bowl, cream together margarine and sugar; add eggs, orange zest and vanilla and mix well. Stir in prune mixture and mix well.

3. In bowl, combine flour, whole wheat flour, baking powder, cinnamon, baking soda and nutmeg. Add to wet ingredients alternately with yogurt. Pour into cake pan and bake for 30 to 35 minutes or until cake tester inserted in center comes out clean.

4. In small bowl, combine orange juice and icing sugar until well mixed. Pour over cake.

Tips

✦ To cut prunes easily, use kitchen shears, or you can use whole pitted prunes, but you'll need to finely chop prunes in food processor after they are cooked.

✦ Chopped dried dates can replace prunes.

Make Ahead

✦ Bake up to 2 days ahead or freeze for up to 6 weeks. The dried fruit keeps this cake very moist.

Nutritional Analysis (Per Serving)
✦ Calories: 179
✦ Protein: 3 g
✦ Cholesterol: 27 mg
✦ Sodium: 90 mg
✦ Fat, total: 4 g
✦ Carbohydrates: 33 g
✦ Fiber: 2 g
✦ Fat, saturated: 1 g

Chocolate Espresso Cake

½ cup	semi-sweet chocolate chips	125 mL
¼ cup	espresso or strong brewed coffee	50 mL
2	eggs, separated	2
¾ cup	granulated sugar	175 mL
¾ cup	2% evaporated milk	175 mL
½ cup	cocoa	125 mL
3 tbsp	all-purpose flour	45 mL
1 tsp	vanilla extract	5 mL
3 tbsp	granulated sugar	45 mL

Serves 10 to 12
Preheat oven to 350°F (180°C)
8-inch (2 L) springform pan sprayed with vegetable spray

1. Melt chocolate chips with coffee; stir until smooth. Allow to cool.

2. In a large bowl, beat together egg yolks, ¾ cup (175 mL) sugar, evaporated milk, cocoa, flour and vanilla until smooth. Beat in chocolate-coffee mixture.

3. With an electric mixer in a separate bowl, beat egg whites until soft peaks form. Gradually add 3 tbsp (45 mL) sugar and continue beating until stiff peaks form.

4. Stir one-quarter of egg whites into chocolate batter. Gently fold in remaining egg whites. Spoon into prepared pan. Bake 30 to 35 minutes or until cake is set at the center. Chill before serving.

Tips

✦ To make cutting easier, dip knife in hot water before slicing.

✦ For a chocolate liqueur flavor, try using half coffee and half chocolate liqueur.

✦ This cake seems so dense and rich you'll never believe it is light. A small piece goes a long way.

✦ Decorate with fresh berries and serve with a puréed berry sauce.

Make Ahead

✦ Prepare up to 2 days in advance or freeze up to 6 weeks.

Nutritional Analysis (Per Serving)
✦ Calories: 136   ✦ Protein: 3 g   ✦ Cholesterol: 37 mg
✦ Sodium: 29 mg   ✦ Fat, total: 4 g   ✦ Carbohydrates: 24 g
✦ Fiber: 2 g   ✦ Fat, saturated: 2 g

Chocolate Angel Food Cake

1 cup	cake and pastry flour	250 mL
¼ cup	cocoa	50 mL
1⅓ cups	granulated sugar	325 mL
12	egg whites, at room temperature	12
½ tsp	cream of tartar	2 mL
1 tsp	vanilla extract	5 mL
½ tsp	almond extract	2 mL
	Strawberry purée or sliced strawberries	

Serves 12
Preheat oven to 375°F (190°C)
10-inch (4 L) tube pan sprayed with baking spray

1. Into a bowl, sift together flour, cocoa and ⅓ cup (75 mL) of the sugar; set aside.

2. In a large bowl, beat egg whites until foamy. Add cream of tartar; beat until soft peaks form. Gradually add remaining sugar, beating until stiff peaks form. In two additions, gently fold cocoa mixture into egg whites until well blended. Fold in vanilla and almond extracts. Pour batter into prepared pan.

3. Bake 35 to 40 minutes or until cake springs back when lightly touched. Turn pan upside down and place over a bottle or an inverted funnel. Cool cake completely before removing from pan. Serve with strawberry purée or sliced strawberries.

Tip

✦ Eggs separate more easily when cold. Use 3 bowls — one to separate eggs over, one for the yolks and one to which perfectly clean whites are transferred. Make sure there's not a speck of yolk in the whites or they won't beat properly. Egg whites beat to a greater volume when at room temperature.

Nutritional Analysis (Per Serving)
✦ Calories: 170   ✦ Protein: 4 g   ✦ Cholesterol: 0 mg
✦ Sodium: 58 mg   ✦ Fat: 1 g   ✦ Carbohydrates: 38 g

Strawberry Shortcake

Shortcakes

2	eggs	2
³/₄ cup	granulated sugar or ½ cup (125 mL) fructose	175 mL
¼ tsp	vanilla extract	1 mL
⅛ tsp	ground cardamom (optional)	0.5 mL
Pinch	nutmeg	Pinch
⅓ cup	all-purpose flour	75 mL

Toppings

6 oz	dessert topping mix	175 g
1 cup	ice water	250 mL
2 cups	halved fresh strawberries	500 mL
	Mint leaves	

Serves 6
Preheat oven to 350°F (180°C)
6-cup muffin tin sprayed with baking spray

1. *Make shortcakes:* In a bowl, beat eggs with sugar for 5 minutes or until thickened and creamy. Beat in vanilla, cardamom (if desired) and nutmeg. Fold in flour until well mixed. Divide batter among muffin cups. Bake for 10 to 12 minutes or until golden and tester inserted in center comes out clean. Remove from muffin tins; cool on wire rack.

2. Split cooled shortcakes in half horizontally; place bottom halves on six individual dessert dishes. Beat dessert topping mix with ice water until soft peaks form. Spoon some dessert topping onto each shortcake bottom, top each with a few strawberries and replace shortcake tops. Divide remaining dessert topping and strawberries among shortcakes. Serve garnished with mint leaves.

Tip

✦ Instead of making shortcakes, use 2 large lady fingers per serving. Or, use 12 oz (375 g) store-bought sponge cake; divide into 6 pieces, then cut each piece in half to form a sandwich.

Nutritional Analysis (Per Serving)
✦ Calories: 149   ✦ Protein: 4 g   ✦ Cholesterol: 80 mg
✦ Sodium: 39 mg   ✦ Fat: 2 g   ✦ Carbohydrates: 26 g

Chiffon Cake

1 cup	cake and pastry flour	250 mL
1/2 cup	granulated sugar	125 mL
1 1/2 tsp	baking powder	7 mL
3	medium eggs	3
2	medium egg whites	2
1/3 cup	water	75 mL
1 tsp	grated lemon zest	5 mL
1 tsp	grated orange zest	5 mL
1/2 tsp	vanilla extract	2 mL
1/2 cup	egg whites (about 4 medium egg whites)	125 mL
1/4 tsp	cream of tartar	1 mL
	Sliced fresh fruit	

Eggs separate more easily when cold. Use 3 bowls — one to separate eggs over, one for the yolks and one to hold the perfectly clean whites. Make sure there's not a speck of yolk in the whites or they won't beat properly.

Serves 10

Preheat oven to 350°F (180°C)

9-inch (2.5 L) springform pan sprayed with baking spray

1. Sift flour, sugar and baking powder into a bowl. In another bowl, beat together whole eggs, 2 egg whites, water, lemon zest, orange zest and vanilla until well mixed. Slowly add wet ingredients to dry ingredients, mixing until combined. Set aside.

2. In a separate bowl, beat egg whites until foamy. Add cream of tartar; beat until stiff peaks form. Gently fold egg whites into batter. Pour into prepared pan. Bake 25 to 30 minutes or until tester inserted in center comes out clean. Cool on wire rack.

3. Serve garnished with sliced fresh fruit.

Nutritional Analysis (Per Serving)
- Calories: 143
- Protein: 5 g
- Cholesterol: 90 mg
- Sodium: 56 mg
- Fat: 2 g
- Carbohydrates: 26 g

Applesauce Carrot Cake

2 1/3 cups	whole wheat flour	575 mL
4 tsp	cinnamon	20 mL
2 tsp	baking powder	10 mL
1 tsp	baking soda	5 mL
1/2 tsp	nutmeg	2 mL
1/4 tsp	allspice	1 mL
1/4 tsp	salt	1 mL
1 cup	unsweetened applesauce	250 mL
3/4 cup	honey	175 mL
1/3 cup	corn oil	75 mL
3	eggs	3
2 cups	grated carrots	500 mL
	Lemon Cream Frosting (optional) (see recipe, page 355)	
	Lemon, orange and/or lime zest cut into thin strips (optional)	

Serves 32

Preheat oven to 350°F (180°C)

8-cup (2 L) bundt pan sprayed with baking spray

1. In a large bowl, stir together flour, cinnamon, baking powder, baking soda, nutmeg, allspice and salt. In another bowl, beat together applesauce, honey, oil and eggs; gradually stir into flour mixture until well mixed. Stir in grated carrots. Pour into prepared pan.

2. Bake 35 minutes or until tester inserted in center comes out clean. Cool in pan for 5 minutes; invert and cool completely on wire rack. Ice with lemon cream frosting and garnish with zest, if desired. Store in refrigerator.

Nutritional Analysis (Per Serving)
- Calories: 75
- Protein: 2 g
- Cholesterol: 11 mg
- Sodium: 90 mg
- Fat: 2 g
- Carbohydrates: 28 g

Banana Cake with Lemon Cream Frosting

Cake

1¾ cups	whole wheat flour	425 mL
2 tsp	baking powder	10 mL
¾ tsp	baking soda	4 mL
½ cup	buttermilk	125 mL
½ cup	honey	125 mL
¼ cup	walnut oil or vegetable oil	50 mL
3	ripe bananas	3
4	egg whites	4

Lemon Cream Frosting

1 cup	5% ricotta cheese	250 mL
1½ tbsp	honey	22 mL
1 tbsp	grated lemon zest	15 mL
1 tbsp	lemon juice	15 mL
1½ tsp	cornstarch or arrowroot	7 mL
¼ cup	chopped walnuts	50 mL
	Lemon zest cut into thin strips	

Serves 25
Preheat oven to 350°F (180°C)
13- by 9-inch (3.5 L) cake pan sprayed with baking spray

1. *Make the cake:* In a bowl stir together flour, baking powder and baking soda; set aside. In a food processor or blender, purée buttermilk, honey, oil and bananas until smooth; stir into flour mixture just until mixed. In another bowl, beat egg whites until stiff peaks form; fold into batter. Pour into prepared pan. Bake 20 to 30 minutes or until tester inserted in center comes out clean. Cool in pan on wire rack.

2. *Make the frosting:* In a food processor, purée ricotta, honey, lemon zest, lemon juice and cornstarch until smooth. Transfer to a saucepan. Cook over medium heat, stirring constantly, until steaming hot. Remove from heat. Chill.

3. Spread cold frosting over cooled cake. Sprinkle with walnuts and strips of lemon zest.

Tips

✦ For the smoothest frosting, use extra-smooth ricotta cheese.

✦ For the most intense walnut flavor, use walnut oil in the cake and toast the walnuts for garnishing the cake.

Nutritional Analysis (Per Serving)
✦ Calories: 85   ✦ Protein: 2 g   ✦ Cholesterol: 2 mg
✦ Sodium: 64 mg   ✦ Fat: 2 g   ✦ Carbohydrates: 14 g

Blueberry Honey Cake

1 cup	fresh or frozen blueberries	250 mL
1/3 cup	honey	75 mL
1/3 cup	water	75 mL
1 tbsp	cornstarch or arrowroot	15 mL
1 tbsp	water	15 mL
1 1/2 cups	whole wheat flour	375 mL
1 tsp	baking powder	5 mL
1 cup	2% milk	250 mL
1/3 cup	honey	75 mL
1 tbsp	vegetable oil	15 mL

Serves 6 to 8
Preheat oven to 350°F (180°C)
9-inch (1.5 L) round cake pan sprayed with baking spray

1. In a saucepan combine blueberries, honey and 1/3 cup (75 mL) water; bring to a boil over medium heat. Stir together cornstarch and 1 tbsp (15 mL) water; add to simmering blueberry mixture. Cook, stirring constantly, until thickened. Remove from heat; set aside.

2. In a large bowl, stir together flour and baking powder. In another bowl, whisk together milk, honey and oil until smooth; add to flour mixture, stirring to combine. Pour into prepared pan. Pour blueberry mixture on top of batter. Bake 25 to 35 minutes or until tester inserted in center comes out clean.

Nutritional Analysis (Per Serving)
- Calories: 176
- Protein: 5 g
- Cholesterol: 2 mg
- Sodium: 24 mg
- Fat: 3 g
- Carbohydrates: 36 g

Banana Date Cake

1 tsp	baking soda	5 mL
1 cup	boiling water	250 mL
2 cups	chopped dates (about 10 oz/280 g)	500 mL
1/2 cup	brown sugar	125 mL
3 tbsp	margarine	45 mL
1	egg	1
1	ripe banana, mashed	1
1 1/2 cups	all-purpose flour	375 mL
1 cup	bran cereal*	250 mL
1/3 cup	chopped pecans or walnuts	75 mL
2 tsp	cinnamon	10 mL

* Use a wheat bran breakfast cereal.

For easier preparation, use scissors to cut dates. Be sure to buy pitted dates.

When using margarine, choose a soft (non-hydrogenated) version.

Makes 25 squares
Preheat oven to 350°F (180°C)
9-inch (2.5 L) square cake pan sprayed with nonstick vegetable spray

1. In bowl, stir baking soda into water; add dates and let stand for 10 minutes.

2. In large bowl or food processor, beat together sugar, margarine, egg and banana until well blended.

3. Combine flour, cereal, pecans and cinnamon; add to banana mixture alternately with soaked dates, mixing well. Pour into cake pan; bake for 25 to 30 minutes or until cake tester comes out dry.

Make Ahead
- Prepare up to 2 days in advance or freeze for up to 6 weeks.

Nutritional Analysis (Per Serving)
- Calories: 121
- Protein: 2 g
- Cholesterol: 8 mg
- Sodium: 87 mg
- Fat: 3 g
- Carbohydrates: 24 g
- Fiber: 2 g

Banana Spice Cake with Cream Cheese Frosting

Cake

1/3 cup	margarine or butter	75 mL
3/4 cup	granulated sugar	175 mL
1/2 cup	packed brown sugar	125 mL
2	eggs	2
3/4 cup	light sour cream	175 mL
2 tsp	vanilla extract	10 mL
1	medium ripe banana, mashed	1
1 1/2 cups	all-purpose flour	375 mL
2 tsp	baking powder	10 mL
1 1/2 tsp	ground cinnamon	7 mL
1 tsp	baking soda	5 mL
1/8 tsp	ground allspice	0.5 mL
1/8 tsp	ground ginger	0.5 mL
1/8 tsp	ground nutmeg	0.5 mL

Icing

1/3 cup	light cream cheese, softened	75 mL
2/3 cup	icing sugar	150 mL
1 tbsp	2% milk	15 mL

When using margarine, choose a soft (non-hydrogenated) version to limit consumption of trans fats.

Serves 12
Preheat oven to 350°F (180°C)
12-cup (3 L) Bundt pan sprayed with vegetable spray

1. *Make the cake:* In a food processor or in a bowl with an electric mixer, cream together margarine, sugar and brown sugar. Add eggs one at a time, beating well after each; beat in sour cream, vanilla and banana. In a separate bowl, stir together flour, baking powder, cinnamon, baking soda, allspice, ginger and nutmeg. Add liquid ingredients to dry ingredients, blending just until mixed. Pour into prepared pan.

2. Bake 35 minutes or until cake tester inserted in center comes out clean. Cool in pan on wire rack.

3. *Make icing:* In a bowl or food processor, beat together cream cheese, icing sugar and milk until smooth.

4. Invert cake and drizzle icing over top.

Tips

+ Increase amount of spices to your taste — or omit any not on hand.

+ Freeze overripe bananas in their skins up to 3 months. Defrost and use mashed in baking.

+ Use as a muffin batter. Bake 15 to 20 minutes or until tester comes out clean.

Make Ahead

+ Bake up to 2 days in advance. Freeze for up to 6 weeks.

Nutritional Analysis (Per Serving)

+ Calories: 250
+ Protein: 4 g
+ Cholesterol: 41 mg
+ Sodium: 269 mg
+ Fat, total: 6 g
+ Carbohydrates: 43 g
+ Fiber: 1 g
+ Fat, saturated: 2 g

Apricot Date Streusel Cake

3 tbsp	margarine	45 mL
3/4 cup	granulated sugar	175 mL
1	egg	1
2	egg whites	2
3 tbsp	lemon juice	45 mL
1 tsp	vanilla	5 mL
1 3/4 cups	all-purpose flour	425 mL
1/2 cup	wheat bran breakfast cereal	125 mL
1 tsp	cinnamon	5 mL
1 tsp	baking powder	5 mL
1 tsp	baking soda	5 mL
1 1/3 cups	2% yogurt	325 mL
1/3 cup	finely chopped dates	75 mL
1/3 cup	finely chopped dried apricots	75 mL

Topping

1/4 cup	brown sugar	50 mL
2 tbsp	all-purpose flour	25 mL
2 tbsp	wheat bran cereal, crushed	25 mL
1 tsp	cinnamon	5 mL
1 tbsp	margarine	15 mL

Dried fruits offer a concentrated sweetness that is completely different from that of their fresh counterparts. Just compare grapes and raisins, or plums and prunes, and you can imagine the sweet intensity of dried cranberries, cherries, blueberries, pineapple and mangoes. Try them all!

When using margarine, choose a soft (non-hydrogenated) version to limit consumption of trans fats.

Makes 16 slices
Preheat oven to 350°F (180°C)
9-inch (3 L) Bundt pan sprayed with nonstick vegetable spray

1. *Topping:* In small bowl, combine sugar, flour, cereal and cinnamon; cut in margarine until crumbly. Set aside.

2. In large bowl or food processor, cream together margarine and sugar; beat in egg, egg whites, lemon juice and vanilla until well mixed.

3. Combine flour, cereal, cinnamon, baking powder and baking soda; stir into bowl just until incorporated. Stir in yogurt; fold in dates and apricots.

4. Pour half of batter into pan. Sprinkle with half of topping. Pour remaining batter over top; sprinkle with remaining topping. Bake for 35 to 45 minutes or until tester inserted into center comes out clean.

Tips

✦ It's easy to chop dried fruit when you use scissors.

✦ Feel free to use all dates or all apricots. Dried prunes are delicious.

Make Ahead

✦ Bake up to a day before or freeze up to 6 weeks.

Nutritional Analysis (Per Serving)
✦ Calories: 173   ✦ Protein: 4 g   ✦ Cholesterol: 14 mg
✦ Sodium: 171 mg   ✦ Fat: 4 g   ✦ Carbohydrates: 32 g
✦ Fiber: 2 g

Apple Pecan Streusel Cake

1/4 cup	soft margarine	50 mL
1 cup	brown sugar	250 mL
2	eggs	2
2 tsp	vanilla	10 mL
1 1/4 cups	all-purpose flour	300 mL
3/4 cup	whole wheat flour	175 mL
2 1/2 tsp	cinnamon	12 mL
1 1/2 tsp	baking powder	7 mL
1 tsp	baking soda	5 mL
1 cup	2% yogurt or light sour cream	250 mL
2 3/4 cups	diced peeled apples	675 mL
1/4 cup	raisins	50 mL

Topping

1/4 cup	chopped pecans	50 mL
1/4 cup	all-purpose flour	50 mL
3 tbsp	brown sugar	45 mL
1 tbsp	margarine, melted	15 mL
1 1/2 tsp	cinnamon	7 mL

When using margarine, choose a soft (non-hydrogenated) version to limit consumption of trans fats.

1. *Topping:* In small bowl, combine pecans, flour, sugar, margarine and cinnamon until crumbly. Set aside.

2. In large bowl or food processor, cream together margarine and sugar. Beat in eggs and vanilla until well blended.

3. Combine all-purpose and whole wheat flours, cinnamon, baking powder and baking soda; add to bowl alternately with yogurt, mixing just until blended. Fold in apples and raisins. Pour into pan.

4. Sprinkle with topping; bake for 40 to 45 minutes or until cake tester inserted into center comes out clean.

Tips

✦ Try substituting pears for the apples and chopped dates for the raisins.

✦ When measuring flour, fill a dry measure to overflowing, then level off with a knife.

Make Ahead

✦ Bake a day before or freeze for up to 6 weeks.

Nutritional Analysis (Per Serving)
✦ Calories: 207 ✦ Protein: 4 g ✦ Cholesterol: 27 mg
✦ Sodium: 161 mg ✦ Fat: 6 g ✦ Carbohydrates: 36 g
✦ Fiber: 2 g

Chocolate Marble Coffee Cake

¼ cup	margarine	50 mL
¾ cup	granulated sugar	175 mL
1	egg	1
1	egg white	1
1½ tsp	vanilla	7 mL
1¼ cups	all-purpose flour	300 mL
1½ tsp	baking powder	7 mL
1 tsp	cinnamon	5 mL
½ tsp	baking soda	2 mL
1 cup	2% yogurt	250 mL

Chocolate Marble

¼ cup	granulated sugar	50 mL
3 tbsp	sifted unsweetened cocoa powder	45 mL
3 tbsp	2% milk	45 mL

When using margarine, choose a soft (non-hydrogenated) version to limit consumption of trans fats.

Makes 16 slices
Preheat oven to 350°F (180°C)
8-inch (2 L) square cake pan sprayed with nonstick vegetable spray

1. In large bowl or food processor, cream together margarine and sugar. Beat in egg, egg white and vanilla.

2. Combine flour, baking powder, cinnamon and baking soda; add to bowl alternately with yogurt, mixing just until blended. Do not overmix. Pour all but 1 cup (250 mL) into cake pan.

3. *Chocolate Marble:* In small bowl, stir together sugar, cocoa and milk until blended. Add to reserved batter, mixing well. Pour over batter in pan; draw knife through mixture to create marbled effect. Bake for 35 to 40 minutes or until cake tester inserted into center comes out clean.

Tips

✦ One ounce of unsweetened cocoa has 3 g of fat, compared to 1 oz of semi-sweet chocolate, which has 9 g of fat.

✦ Sift icing sugar over top of cooled cake to decorate.

Make Ahead

✦ Bake a day before or freeze for up to 6 weeks.

Nutritional Analysis (Per Serving)
✦ Calories: 130　✦ Protein: 3 g　✦ Cholesterol: 14 mg
✦ Sodium: 119 mg　✦ Fat: 3 g　✦ Carbohydrates: 22 g
✦ Fiber: 1 g

Orange Coffee Cake

2 cups	orange juice	500 mL
2 tsp	grated orange zest	10 mL
1 cup	granulated sugar	250 mL
1/4 cup	butter	50 mL
3	medium eggs	3
1 cup	all-purpose flour	250 mL
1 cup	whole wheat flour	250 mL
2 tsp	baking soda	10 mL
	Icing sugar	
	Sliced fresh strawberries	

Serves 10 to 12
Preheat oven to 350°F (180°C)
8-cup (2 L) bundt pan sprayed with baking spray

1. In a saucepan combine orange juice and orange zest; bring to a boil. Remove from heat, transfer to a bowl and refrigerate until cool.

2. In a bowl, cream sugar with butter; add eggs, one at a time, beating well after each. In another bowl, stir together flour, whole-wheat flour and baking soda. Add to creamed mixture alternately with orange juice, making three additions of flour and two of orange juice. Pour into prepared pan. Bake 35 to 40 minutes or until tester inserted in center comes out clean. Cool in pan for 5 minutes; invert and cool completely on wire rack.

3. Serve dusted with sifted icing sugar and garnished with sliced strawberries.

Nutritional Analysis (Per Serving)
✦ Calories: 136   ✦ Protein: 3 g   ✦ Cholesterol: 51 mg
✦ Sodium: 225 mg ✦ Fat: 3 g   ✦ Carbohydrates: 24 g

Orange-Glazed Coffee Cake

1/4 cup	soft margarine	50 mL
1 cup	granulated sugar	250 mL
2	eggs	2
1	egg white	1
1 1/2 cups	orange juice	375 mL
1 1/2 tsp	grated orange rind	7 mL
1 cup	whole wheat flour	250 mL
1 cup	all-purpose flour	250 mL
1 tsp	cinnamon	5 mL
1 tsp	baking powder	5 mL
1 tsp	baking soda	5 mL
Glaze		
1/2 cup	icing sugar	125 mL
4 tsp	frozen orange juice concentrate, thawed	20 mL

Makes 16 slices
Preheat oven to 350°F (180°C)
9-inch (3 L) Bundt pan sprayed with nonstick vegetable spray

1. In large bowl or food processor, cream together margarine and sugar. Beat in eggs, egg white, orange juice and rind until well blended.

2. Combine whole wheat and all-purpose flours, cinnamon, baking powder and baking soda; add to creamed mixture and mix until well blended. Pour into pan. Bake for 35 to 40 minutes or until cake tester inserted into center comes out clean. Let cool.

3. *Glaze:* Mix icing sugar with orange juice concentrate; pour over cake, allowing to drip down sides.

If you pierce the cake with a fork when warm and pour glaze over top, the icing will filter through the cake.

Nutritional Analysis (Per Serving)
✦ Calories: 166   ✦ Protein: 3 g   ✦ Cholesterol: 26 mg
✦ Sodium: 125 mg ✦ Fat: 4 g   ✦ Carbohydrates: 31 g
✦ Fiber: 1 g

Cinnamon Date Coffee Cake

³/₄ cup	granulated sugar	175 mL
3 tbsp	softened butter	45 mL
2	egg whites	2
1	egg	1
1¹/₃ cups	low-fat yogurt	325 mL
3 tbsp	lemon juice	45 mL
1 tsp	vanilla extract	5 mL
2 cups	all-purpose flour	500 mL
1 tsp	baking powder	5 mL
1 tsp	baking soda	5 mL
1 tsp	cinnamon	5 mL
¹/₈ tsp	nutmeg	0.5 mL
²/₃ cup	chopped dates	150 mL
¹/₄ cup	packed brown sugar	50 mL
	Icing sugar	
	Extra sliced dates (optional)	

Serves 16
Preheat oven to 350° F (180° C)
8-cup (2 L) bundt pan sprayed with baking spray

1. In a bowl, beat together sugar, butter, egg whites and egg until smooth. Beat in yogurt, lemon juice and vanilla. In another bowl, sift together flour, baking powder, baking soda, cinnamon and nutmeg; stir into yogurt mixture just until combined.

2. In a small bowl, stir together brown sugar and dates. Pour half of cake batter into prepared pan and sprinkle with half of date mixture. Repeat. Bake 40 minutes or until tester inserted in center comes out clean. Cool in pan for 5 minutes; invert and cool completely on wire rack. Serve dusted with sifted icing sugar and garnished with sliced dates, if desired.

Nutritional Analysis (Per Serving)
+ Calories: 163   + Protein: 4 g   + Cholesterol: 34 mg
+ Sodium: 69 mg   + Fat: 2 g   + Carbohydrates: 24 g

Sour Cream Brownies

²/₃ cup	granulated sugar	150 mL
¹/₃ cup	soft margarine	75 mL
1	egg	1
1 tsp	vanilla	5 mL
¹/₃ cup	unsweetened cocoa powder	75 mL
¹/₃ cup	all-purpose flour	75 mL
1 tsp	baking powder	5 mL
¹/₄ cup	light sour cream	50 mL

If desired, sprinkle 2 tbsp (25 mL) chopped nuts over the batter before baking.

Garnish with a sprinkling of icing sugar after baking.

When using margarine, choose a soft (non-hydrogenated) version to limit consumption of trans fats.

Makes 16 squares
Preheat oven to 350°F (180°C)
8-inch (2 L) square cake pan sprayed with nonstick vegetable spray

1. In bowl, beat together sugar and margarine until smooth. Beat in egg and vanilla, mixing well.

2. Combine cocoa, flour and baking powder; stir into bowl just until blended. Stir in sour cream. Pour into pan.

3. Bake for 20 to 25 minutes or until edges start to pull away from pan and center is still slightly soft.

Make Ahead
+ Bake a day before or freeze for up to 6 weeks.

Nutritional Analysis (Per Serving)
+ Calories: 90   + Protein: 1 g   + Cholesterol: 14 mg
+ Sodium: 83 mg   + Fat: 4 g   + Carbohydrates: 12 g
+ Fiber: 1 g

Triple Chocolate Brownies

½ cup	granulated sugar	125 mL
⅓ cup	margarine or butter	75 mL
1	egg	1
1 tsp	vanilla	5 mL
½ cup	all-purpose flour	125 mL
⅓ cup	cocoa	75 mL
1 tsp	baking powder	5 mL
¼ cup	2% milk	50 mL
¼ cup	chocolate chips	50 mL
Icing		
¼ cup	icing sugar	50 mL
1½ tbsp	cocoa	20 mL
1 tbsp	milk	15 mL

When using margarine, choose a soft (non-hydrogenated) version to limit consumption of trans fats.

Makes 16 brownies
Preheat oven to 350°F (180°C)
8-inch square (2 L) cake pan sprayed with vegetable spray

1. In bowl, beat together sugar and margarine. Beat in egg and vanilla, mixing well.
2. In another bowl, combine flour, cocoa and baking powder; stir into sugar and butter mixture just until blended. Stir in milk and chocolate chips. Pour into prepared pan and bake approximately 18 minutes or until edges start to pull away from pan and center is still a little wet. Let cool slightly before glazing.
3. In small bowl, whisk together icing sugar, cocoa and milk; pour over brownies in pan.

Nutritional Analysis (Per Serving)
- Calories: 102
- Protein: 2 g
- Cholesterol: 14 mg
- Sodium: 69 mg
- Fat, total: 5 g
- Carbohydrates: 14 g
- Fiber: 1 g
- Fat, saturated: 1 g

Cream Cheese–Filled Brownies

Filling		
4 oz	light cream cheese, softened	125 g
2 tbsp	granulated sugar	25 mL
2 tbsp	2% milk	25 mL
1 tsp	vanilla extract	5 mL
Cake		
1 cup	packed brown sugar	250 mL
⅓ cup	light sour cream	75 mL
¼ cup	vegetable oil	50 mL
1	egg	1
1	egg white	1
¾ cup	all-purpose flour	175 mL
½ cup	cocoa	125 mL
1 tsp	baking powder	5 mL

This tastes like a low-fat Twinkie cupcake. Children and adults devour this dessert. When pouring batter, don't worry if there's a swirling pattern — the result will be attractive.

Makes 12 to 16 squares
Preheat oven to 350°F (180°C)
8-inch (2 L) square baking dish sprayed with vegetable spray

1. *Make the filling:* In a food processor or in a bowl with an electric mixer, beat together cream cheese, sugar, milk and vanilla until smooth. Set aside.
2. *Make the cake:* In a large bowl whisk together brown sugar, sour cream, oil, whole egg and egg white. In a separate bowl, stir together flour, cocoa and baking powder. Add liquid ingredients to dry, blending just until mixed.
3. Pour half the cake batter into prepared pan. Spoon filling on top; spread with a wet knife. Pour remaining batter into pan. Bake 20 to 25 minutes or until just barely loose at center.

Make Ahead
- Prepare up to 2 days in advance. Freeze up to 4 weeks

Nutritional Analysis (Per Serving)
- Calories: 133
- Protein: 3 g
- Cholesterol: 19 mg
- Sodium: 84 mg
- Fat, total: 5 g
- Carbohydrates: 20 g
- Fiber: 1 g
- Fat, saturated: 2 g

Cocoa Roll with Creamy Cheese and Berries

5	egg whites	5
1/8 tsp	cream of tartar	0.5 mL
2/3 cup	granulated sugar	150 mL
1/2 cup	cake-and-pastry flour	125 mL
4 tsp	unsweetened cocoa powder	20 mL
1 1/2 tsp	vanilla	7 mL
	Icing sugar	

Filling

1 1/4 cups	ricotta cheese	300 mL
1/4 cup	light sour cream	50 mL
3 tbsp	icing sugar	45 mL
1 1/4 cups	sliced strawberries and/or blueberries	300 mL

To cut back on calories and fat, avoid eating too many high-fat snacks. Cookies, snack crackers and chips are okay once in a while, but in small amounts. Try measuring out a cup of chips and see if that satisfies your craving. If not, go for the fruit bowl.

Makes 10 slices
Preheat oven to 325°F (160°C)
Jelly roll pan lined with parchment paper and sprayed with nonstick vegetable spray

1. In medium bowl, beat egg whites and cream of tartar until soft peaks form. Gradually beat in 1/3 cup (75 mL) of sugar until stiff peaks form.
2. Sift together remaining sugar, flour and cocoa; sift over egg whites and fold in gently along with vanilla. Do not overmix. Pour onto baking sheet and spread evenly. Bake for 15 to 20 minutes or until top springs back when lightly touched.
3. *Filling:* In bowl or food processor, mix together cheese, sour cream and sugar until smooth. Fold in berries. Set aside.
4. Sprinkle cake lightly with icing sugar. Carefully invert onto surface sprinkled with icing sugar. Carefully remove parchment paper. Spread filling over cake and roll up. Place on serving dish. Sprinkle with icing sugar.

Tips
✦ Decorate roll with fresh berries.
✦ Substitute other fresh berries of your choice.

Make Ahead
✦ Prepare cake early in day and keep covered until ready to roll with filling.

Nutritional Analysis (Per Serving)
✦ Calories: 152 ✦ Protein: 6 g ✦ Cholesterol: 11 mg
✦ Sodium: 72 mg ✦ Fat: 3 g ✦ Carbohydrates: 25 g
✦ Fiber: 1 g

Date Oatmeal Squares

1/2 lb	pitted dates, chopped	250 g
1 cup	water or orange juice	250 mL
1 cup	all-purpose flour	250 mL
1 cup	rolled oats	250 mL
2/3 cup	brown sugar	150 mL
1/2 cup	bran cereal*	125 mL
1/2 tsp	baking powder	2 mL
1/2 tsp	baking soda	2 mL
1/2 cup	soft margarine	125 mL

* Use a wheat bran breakfast cereal.

Use scissors to cut the dates for easier preparation. Try half dates and half pitted, chopped prunes for a change.

When using margarine, choose a soft (non-hydrogenated) version.

Makes 16 squares
Preheat oven to 350°F (180°C)
8-inch (2 L) square cake pan sprayed with nonstick vegetable spray

1. In saucepan, cover and cook dates and water over low heat, stirring often, for approximately 15 minutes or until dates are soft and liquid absorbed. Set aside.
2. In bowl, combine flour, rolled oats, sugar, cereal, baking powder and baking soda; cut in margarine until crumbly.
3. Pat half onto bottom of cake pan; spoon date mixture over top. Pat remaining crumb mixture over date mixture. Bake for 20 to 25 minutes or until golden.

Nutritional Analysis (Per Serving)
- ✦ Calories: 187
- ✦ Protein: 2 g
- ✦ Cholesterol: 0 mg
- ✦ Sodium: 142 mg
- ✦ Fat: 6 g
- ✦ Carbohydrates: 32 g
- ✦ Fiber: 2 g

Lemon Poppy Seed Squares

Cake

1/2 cup	granulated sugar	125 mL
1 tbsp	margarine or butter	15 mL
2 tsp	poppy seeds	10 mL
1 1/2 tsp	grated lemon zest	7 mL
1	egg	1
3/4 cup	cake and pastry flour	175 mL

Topping

2/3 cup	granulated sugar	150 mL
2 tsp	grated lemon zest	10 mL
1/3 cup	freshly squeezed lemon juice	75 mL
1 tbsp	cornstarch	15 mL
1	egg	1
1	egg white	1

Try substituting lime juice and zest for the lemon.

When using margarine, choose a soft (non-hydrogenated) version.

Makes 16 squares
Preheat oven to 350°F (180°C)
8-inch square (2 L) baking pan sprayed with vegetable spray

1. *Make the cake:* In a bowl whisk together sugar, margarine, poppy seeds, lemon zest and egg until smooth. Add wet ingredients to flour and stir just until mixed. Pat into prepared pan; set aside.
2. *Make the topping:* In a bowl stir together sugar, lemon zest, lemon juice, cornstarch, whole egg and egg white. Pour over cake batter in pan.
3. Bake 20 to 25 minutes or until set with center still slightly soft. Cool to room temperature on a wire rack.

Make Ahead
- ✦ Prepare up to 2 days in advance.

Nutritional Analysis (Per Serving)
- ✦ Calories: 96
- ✦ Protein: 2 g
- ✦ Cholesterol: 27 mg
- ✦ Sodium: 21 mg
- ✦ Fat, total: 2 g
- ✦ Carbohydrates: 19 g
- ✦ Fiber: 0 g
- ✦ Fat, saturated: 0.3 g

Peanut Butter-Coconut-Raisin Granola Bars

1⅓ cups	rolled oats	325 mL
⅔ cup	raisins	150 mL
½ cup	bran flakes	125 mL
⅓ cup	unsweetened coconut	75 mL
3 tbsp	chocolate chips	45 mL
2 tbsp	chopped pecans	25 mL
1 tsp	baking soda	5 mL
¼ cup	peanut butter	50 mL
¼ cup	brown sugar	50 mL
3 tbsp	margarine or butter	45 mL
3 tbsp	honey	45 mL
1 tsp	vanilla	5 mL

Corn flakes can replace bran flakes. Don't worry if you only have raisin bran on hand. Chopped dates can replace raisins.

When using margarine, choose a soft (non-hydrogenated) version to limit consumption of trans fats.

Makes 25 bars
Preheat oven to 350°F(180°C)
9-inch square (2.5 L) pan sprayed with vegetable spray

1. Put oats, raisins, bran flakes, coconut, chocolate chips, pecans and baking soda in bowl. Combine until well mixed.

2. In small saucepan, whisk together peanut butter, brown sugar, margarine, honey and vanilla over medium heat for approximately 30 seconds or just until sugar dissolves and mixture is smooth. Pour over dry ingredients and stir to combine. Press into prepared pan and bake for 15 to 20 minutes or until browned. Let cool completely before cutting into bars.

Make Ahead
✦ Prepare these up to 2 days ahead and keep tightly closed in a cookie tin. These freeze for up to 2 weeks.

Nutritional Analysis (Per Serving)
✦ Calories: 88   ✦ Protein: 2 g   ✦ Cholesterol: 0 mg
✦ Sodium: 77 mg   ✦ Fat, total: 4 g   ✦ Carbohydrates: 12 g
✦ Fiber: 1 g   ✦ Fat, saturated: 1 g

Date Nut Bar

1⅓ cups	chopped dates	325 mL
¼ cup	walnut pieces	50 mL
¼ cup	whole almonds	50 mL
½ cup	granola	125 mL

Eat a balanced breakfast every day. Skipping breakfast is linked to weight gain and greater food intake later in the day. If you don't have a lot of time, at least have a small healthy snack.

Serves 16
8-inch square (2 L) baking dish

1. In a food processor, combine dates, walnuts and almonds; process until mixture begins to come together.

2. Sprinkle half of granola over bottom of baking dish. Press date mixture firmly and evenly over granola. Top with remaining granola, pressing down slightly to embed in date mixture. Chill.

3. Cut into squares.

Tip
✦ For an extra calcium boost, try using part or all dried figs instead of dates.

Nutritional Analysis (Per Serving)
✦ Calories: 83   ✦ Protein: 1 g   ✦ Cholesterol: 0 mg
✦ Sodium: 1 mg   ✦ Fat: 3 g   ✦ Carbohydrates: 13 g

Carrot Pineapple Zucchini Loaf

1/4 cup	margarine	50 mL
1 cup	granulated sugar	250 mL
1	egg	1
1	egg white	1
2 tsp	cinnamon	10 mL
1 1/2 tsp	vanilla	7 mL
1/4 tsp	nutmeg	1 mL
3/4 cup	grated carrot	175 mL
3/4 cup	grated zucchini	175 mL
1/2 cup	drained crushed pineapple	125 mL
1/3 cup	raisins	75 mL
1 1/4 cups	all-purpose flour	300 mL
1/2 cup	whole wheat flour	125 mL
1 tsp	baking powder	5 mL
1 tsp	baking soda	5 mL

If you like muffins, fill 12 muffin cups and bake for 20 minutes or until tops are firm to the touch.

Makes 20 slices
Preheat oven to 350°F (180°C)
9- x 5-inch (2 L) loaf pan sprayed with nonstick vegetable spray

1. In large bowl or food processor, cream margarine with sugar. Add egg, egg white, cinnamon, vanilla and nutmeg; beat well. Stir in carrot, zucchini, pineapple and raisins, blending until well combined.

2. Combine all-purpose and whole wheat flours, baking powder and soda; add to bowl and mix just until combined. Pour into loaf pan and bake for 35 to 45 minutes or until tester inserted into center comes out dry.

Make Ahead
✦ Make up to 2 days in advance or freeze for up to 2 months.

Nutritional Analysis (Per Serving)
✦ Calories: 117   ✦ Protein: 2 g   ✦ Cholesterol: 11 mg
✦ Sodium: 99 mg   ✦ Fat: 3 g   ✦ Carbohydrates: 22 g
✦ Fiber: 1 g

Pumpkin Molasses Raisin Loaf

1 1/4 cups	brown sugar	300 mL
1/3 cup	margarine or butter	75 mL
2	eggs	2
2 tbsp	molasses	25 mL
1 tsp	vanilla	5 mL
1 cup	canned pumpkin purée	250 mL
1 cup	raisins	250 mL
1 1/3 cups	all-purpose flour	325 mL
2/3 cup	whole wheat flour	150 mL
2 1/4 tsp	cinnamon	11 mL
1 1/2 tsp	baking powder	7 mL
1/2 tsp	baking soda	2 mL
1/4 tsp	ginger	1 mL
1/2 cup	2% yogurt	125 mL

When using margarine, choose a soft (non-hydrogenated) version to limit consumption of trans fats.

Makes 20 half-slices
Preheat oven to 350°F (180°C)
9- by 5-inch (2 L) loaf pan sprayed with vegetable spray

1. In large bowl, beat sugar and margarine together until crumbly. Add eggs and mix until smooth. Beat in molasses, vanilla and pumpkin. (Mixture may appear curdled.) Stir in raisins.

2. In bowl, combine flour, whole wheat flour, cinnamon, baking powder, baking soda and ginger. Add to wet ingredients alternately with the yogurt; stir just until combined. Pour into pan and bake for 55 to 60 minutes or until cake tester inserted in center comes out clean.

Make Ahead
✦ Can be prepared up to 2 days ahead.

Nutritional Analysis (Per Serving)
✦ Calories: 160   ✦ Protein: 3 g   ✦ Cholesterol: 22 mg
✦ Sodium: 79 mg   ✦ Fat, total: 4 g   ✦ Carbohydrates: 31 g
✦ Fiber: 1 g   ✦ Fat, saturated: 1 g

Lemon Poppy Seed Loaf

3/4 cup	granulated sugar	175 mL
1/3 cup	soft margarine	75 mL
1	egg	1
2 tsp	grated lemon rind	10 mL
3 tbsp	lemon juice	45 mL
1/3 cup	2% milk	75 mL
1 1/4 cups	all-purpose flour	300 mL
1 tbsp	poppy seeds	15 mL
1 tsp	baking powder	5 mL
1/2 tsp	baking soda	2 mL
1/3 cup	2% yogurt or light sour cream	75 mL

Glaze

1/4 cup	icing sugar	50 mL
2 tbsp	lemon juice	25 mL

When using margarine, choose a soft (non-hydrogenated) version to limit consumption of trans fats.

Makes 20 half-slices
Preheat oven to 350°F (180°C)
9- x 5- inch (2 L) loaf pan sprayed with nonstick vegetable spray

1. In large bowl or food processor, beat together sugar, margarine, egg, lemon rind and juice, mixing well. Add milk, mixing well.

2. Combine flour, poppy seeds, baking powder and baking soda; add to bowl alternately with yogurt, mixing just until incorporated. Do not overmix. Pour into pan and bake for 35 to 40 minutes or until tester inserted into center comes out dry.

3. *Glaze:* Prick holes in top of loaf with fork. Combine icing sugar with lemon juice; pour over loaf.

Make Ahead

✦ Bake a day before or freeze for up to 6 weeks.

Nutritional Analysis (Per Serving)
✦ Calories: 101   ✦ Protein: 1 g   ✦ Cholesterol: 11 mg
✦ Sodium: 89 mg   ✦ Fat: 3 g   ✦ Carbohydrates: 15 g
✦ Fiber: 0.5 g

Banana Walnut Bread

2	ripe bananas, mashed	2
1/2 cup	butter, softened	125 mL
1/2 cup	granulated sugar	125 mL
1	egg	1
1	egg white	1
1 1/3 cups	whole wheat flour	325 mL
1/3 cup	chopped walnuts	75 mL
1 tsp	baking soda	5 mL
1/4 tsp	salt	1 mL
1/4 cup	hot water	50 mL
	Sesame seeds or extra chopped walnuts (optional)	

Serves 20
Preheat oven to 375°F (190°C)
9- by 5-inch (2 L) loaf pan sprayed with baking spray

1. In a bowl, beat bananas with butter until well mixed. Beat in sugar, whole egg and egg white until fluffy.

2. In another bowl, stir together flour, walnuts, baking soda and salt. Stir into banana mixture along with hot water just until blended. Pour into prepared loaf pan. If desired, sprinkle with sesame seeds or extra chopped walnuts.

3. Bake for 35 to 45 minutes or until cake tester inserted in center comes out clean. Cool in pan for 5 minutes. Remove from pan and cool on wire rack.

Nutritional Analysis (Per Serving)
✦ Calories: 124   ✦ Protein: 2 g   ✦ Cholesterol: 28 mg
✦ Sodium: 147 mg   ✦ Fat: 6 g   ✦ Carbohydrates: 15 g

Banana Nut Raisin Loaf

2	large ripe bananas	2
1/3 cup	soft margarine	75 mL
1/2 cup	granulated sugar	125 mL
1	egg	1
1	egg white	1
1/4 cup	hot water	50 mL
1 1/3 cups	whole wheat flour	325 mL
3/4 tsp	baking soda	4 mL
1/4 cup	raisins	50 mL
1/3 cup	chopped pecans or walnuts	75 mL

When using margarine, choose a soft (non-hydrogenated) version to limit consumption of trans fats.

Buy firm, plump bananas that are green at the stem. Ripen them in a bowl at room temperature, then refrigerate. The skin will turn brown, but the fruit will be unaffected.

Makes 20 half-slices
Preheat oven to 375°F (190°C)
9- x 5-inch (2 L) loaf pan sprayed with nonstick vegetable spray

1. In bowl or food processor, beat bananas and margarine; beat in sugar, egg, egg white and water until smooth.
2. Combine flour and baking soda; stir into batter along with raisins and all but a few of the pecans, mixing just until blended. Do not overmix. Pour into pan; arrange reserved nuts down middle of mixture. Bake for 35 to 45 minutes or until tester inserted into center comes out dry.

Make Ahead
✦ Bake up to 2 days in advance or freeze for up to 6 weeks.

Nutritional Analysis (Per Serving)
✦ Calories: 108 ✦ Protein: 2 g ✦ Cholesterol: 10 mg
✦ Sodium: 78 mg ✦ Fat: 5 g ✦ Carbohydrates: 15 g
✦ Fiber: 1 g

Pineapple Carrot Date Muffins

3/4 cup	granulated sugar	175 mL
1/3 cup	vegetable oil	75 mL
1	egg	1
1 tsp	vanilla	5 mL
1/2 cup	grated carrots	75 mL
1/2 cup	canned pineapple, drained and crushed	75 mL
1/3 cup	finely chopped dates	75 mL
1/3 cup	light sour cream or 2% yogurt	75 mL
1 cup	all-purpose flour	250 mL
2/3 cup	rolled oats	150 mL
1 tsp	baking powder	5 mL
1 tsp	baking soda	5 mL
1 tsp	cinnamon	5 mL
1/4 tsp	nutmeg	1 mL

Makes 12 muffins
Preheat oven to 375°F (190°C)
12 muffin cups sprayed with vegetable spray

1. In large bowl, combine sugar, oil, egg and vanilla; mix well.
2. Stir in carrots, pineapple, dates and sour cream.
3. In bowl, combine flour, oats, baking powder, baking soda, cinnamon and nutmeg. Add to wet ingredients and mix just until combined. Spoon into prepared muffin cups and bake for 15 to 18 minutes or until tops are firm to the touch and tester inserted in center comes out clean.

Make Ahead
✦ Prepare up to a day ahead. Freeze for up to 6 weeks.

Nutritional Analysis (Per Serving)
✦ Calories: 189 ✦ Protein: 3 g ✦ Cholesterol: 20 mg
✦ Sodium: 118 mg ✦ Fat, total: 7 g ✦ Carbohydrates: 30 g
✦ Fiber: 1 g ✦ Fat, saturated: 1 g

Blueberry Lemon Cornmeal Muffins

¾ cup	granulated sugar	175 mL
¼ cup	margarine or butter	50 mL
1	egg	1
3 tbsp	freshly squeezed lemon juice	45 mL
3 tbsp	2% milk	45 mL
1½ tsp	grated lemon zest	7 mL
1 cup	all-purpose flour	250 mL
¼ cup	cornmeal	50 mL
1½ tsp	baking powder	7 mL
1 tsp	baking soda	5 mL
½ cup	2% plain yogurt	125 mL
1¼ cups	fresh or frozen blueberries	300 mL
2 tsp	all-purpose flour	10 mL

Fresh blueberries are always best tasting, especially the small ones available in the summer. If using frozen berries, do not thaw. The flour will help to absorb the excess liquid.

When using margarine, choose a soft (non-hydrogenated) version.

Makes 12
Preheat oven to 350°F (180°C)
12 muffin cups sprayed with vegetable spray

1. In a large bowl with an electric mixer, beat sugar, margarine, egg, lemon juice, milk and lemon zest until well blended. (Mixture may appear curdled.)
2. In another bowl, stir together flour, cornmeal, baking powder and baking soda. Add flour mixture and yogurt alternately to creamed mixture. In a small bowl, toss blueberries with flour; fold into batter. Divide batter among muffin cups.
3. Bake 20 to 25 minutes or until tops are firm to the touch and tester inserted in center comes out clean.

Make Ahead
✦ Bake up to 2 days in advance; store in an airtight container.
✦ Freeze for up to 6 weeks.

Nutritional Analysis (Per Serving)
✦ Calories: 149 ✦ Protein: 3 g ✦ Cholesterol: 19 mg
✦ Sodium: 189 mg ✦ Fat, total: 4 g ✦ Carbohydrates: 26 g
✦ Fiber: 1 g ✦ Fat, saturated: 1 g

Yogurt Bran Muffins

½ cup	brown sugar	125 mL
¼ cup	margarine	50 mL
1 tbsp	molasses	15 mL
1	egg	1
1 tsp	vanilla	5 mL
¾ cup	bran cereal*	175 mL
½ cup	all-purpose flour	125 mL
⅓ cup	whole wheat flour	75 mL
¾ tsp	baking powder	4 mL
½ tsp	baking soda	2 mL
½ cup	2% yogurt	125 mL
⅓ cup	raisins	75 mL

* Use a wheat bran breakfast cereal

Makes 12 muffins
Preheat oven to 375°F (190°C)
12 muffin cups sprayed with nonstick vegetable spray

1. In large bowl, combine sugar, margarine, molasses, egg and vanilla until well blended.
2. Combine cereal, all-purpose and whole wheat flours, baking powder and baking soda; add to bowl alternately with yogurt. Stir in raisins. Pour into muffin cups; bake for 15 to 18 minutes or until tops are firm to the touch.

Nutritional Analysis (Per Serving)
✦ Calories: 157 ✦ Protein: 3 g ✦ Cholesterol: 18 mg
✦ Sodium: 177 mg ✦ Fat: 4 g ✦ Carbohydrates: 28 g
✦ Fiber: 2 g

Banana Date Muffins

¼ cup	margarine or butter	50 mL
1	medium banana, mashed	1
¾ cup	granulated sugar	175 mL
1	egg	1
1 tsp	vanilla	5 mL
¾ cup	all-purpose flour	175 mL
½ cup	bran or corn flakes cereal	125 mL
1 tsp	baking powder	5 mL
1 tsp	baking soda	5 mL
¾ cup	pitted, dried and chopped dates	175 mL
½ cup	2% yogurt	125 mL

These muffins will be fairly flat due to the weight of the dates.

When using margarine, choose a soft (non-hydrogenated) version.

Makes 12 muffins
Preheat oven to 375°F (190°C)
12 muffin cups sprayed with vegetable spray

1. In large bowl, combine margarine, banana, sugar, egg and vanilla; mix well.
2. In bowl, combine flour, bran flakes cereal, baking powder and baking soda. Add to wet ingredients and stir just until mixed. Stir in dates and yogurt, just until smooth.
3. Spoon batter into prepared muffin cups and bake for 15 to 20 minutes, or until tops are firm and tester inserted in center comes out clean.

Make Ahead
✦ Prepare up to a day ahead, or freeze up to 3 weeks.

Nutritional Analysis (Per Serving)
✦ Calories: 158   ✦ Protein: 2 g   ✦ Cholesterol: 19 mg
✦ Sodium: 176 mg   ✦ Fat, total: 4 g   ✦ Carbohydrates: 30 g
✦ Fiber: 1 g   ✦ Fat, saturated: 1 g

Streusel Apple Muffins

½ cup	brown sugar	125 mL
½ cup	applesauce	125 mL
¼ cup	vegetable oil	50 mL
1	egg	1
1 tsp	vanilla	5 mL
1 cup	all-purpose flour	250 mL
1 tsp	baking soda	5 mL
1 tsp	baking powder	5 mL
½ tsp	cinnamon	2 mL
¾ cup	diced peeled apple	175 mL

Topping

2 tbsp	brown sugar	25 mL
2 tsp	all-purpose flour	10 mL
½ tsp	cinnamon	2 mL
1 tsp	margarine	5 mL

When using margarine, choose a soft (non-hydrogenated) version to limit consumption of trans fats.

Makes 12 muffins
Preheat oven to 375°F (190°C)
12 muffin cups sprayed with nonstick vegetable spray

1. In large bowl, combine sugar, applesauce, oil, egg and vanilla until well mixed. Combine flour, baking soda, baking powder and cinnamon; stir into bowl just until incorporated. Stir in apple. Pour into muffin cups, filling two-thirds full.
2. *Topping:* In small bowl, combine sugar, flour and cinnamon; cut in margarine until crumbly. Sprinkle evenly over muffins. Bake for 20 minutes or until tops are firm to the touch.

Make Ahead
✦ Prepare up to a day before. Freeze for up to 6 weeks.

Nutritional Analysis (Per Serving)
✦ Calories: 141   ✦ Protein: 1 g   ✦ Cholesterol: 17 mg
✦ Sodium: 114 mg   ✦ Fat: 5 g   ✦ Carbohydrates: 22 g
✦ Fiber: 1 g

Rugelach (Cinnamon Chocolate Twist Cookies)

Dough

2¼ cups	all-purpose flour	550 mL
⅔ cup	granulated sugar	150 mL
½ cup	cold margarine or butter	125 mL
⅓ cup	2% yogurt	75 mL
3 to 4 tbsp	water	45 to 50 mL
½ cup	brown sugar	125 mL
⅓ cup	raisins	75 mL
2 tbsp	semi-sweet chocolate chips	25 mL
1 tbsp	cocoa	15 mL
½ tsp	cinnamon	2 mL

When using margarine, choose a soft (non-hydrogenated) version to limit consumption of trans fats.

Makes 26 cookies
Preheat oven to 350°F (180°C)
Baking sheets sprayed with vegetable spray

1. In bowl, combine flour and sugar. Cut in margarine until crumbly. Add yogurt and water, and mix until combined. Roll into a smooth ball, wrap and place in refrigerator for 30 minutes.

2. Put brown sugar, raisins, chocolate chips, cocoa and cinnamon in food processor; process until crumbly, approximately 20 seconds.

3. Divide dough in half. Roll one portion into a rectangle of ¼-inch (5 mm) thickness on a well-floured surface. Sprinkle half of the filling on top of the dough rectangle. Roll up tightly, long end to long end, jelly-roll fashion; pinch ends together. Cut into 1-inch (2.5 cm) thick pieces; some filling will fall out. Place on baking sheets cut side up. Repeat with remaining dough and filling.

4. With the back of a spoon or your fingers, gently flatten each cookie. Bake for 25 minutes, turning the cookies over at the halfway mark (12½ minutes).

Tips

✦ These traditionally high-fat cookies are lower in fat and calories because we've used yogurt instead of cream cheese, and cocoa instead of chocolate.

✦ These are best eaten the day they are made; any leftover cookies are best eaten biscotti fashion, dipped in coffee.

Make Ahead

✦ Prepare dough and freeze for up to 2 weeks. Bake cookies up to a day ahead, keeping tightly covered.

Nutritional Analysis (Per Serving)

✦ Calories: 117 ✦ Protein: 2 g ✦ Cholesterol: 0 mg
✦ Sodium: 53 mg ✦ Fat, total: 4 g ✦ Carbohydrates: 19 g
✦ Fiber: 1 g ✦ Fat, saturated: 1 g

Oatmeal Orange Coconut Cookies

¼ cup	margarine or butter	50 mL
¼ cup	brown sugar	50 mL
½ cup	granulated sugar	125 mL
1	egg	1
1 tsp	vanilla	5 mL
2 tbsp	orange juice concentrate, thawed	25 mL
½ tsp	grated orange zest	2 mL
⅔ cup	all-purpose flour	150 mL
½ tsp	baking powder	2 mL
½ tsp	baking soda	2 mL
½ tsp	cinnamon	2 mL
1 cup	corn flakes or bran flakes cereal	250 mL
⅔ cup	raisins	150 mL
½ cup	rolled oats	125 mL
¼ cup	coconut	50 mL

If using bran flakes cereal, do not use All-Bran or raw bran.

When using margarine, choose a soft (non-hydrogenated) version to limit consumption of trans fats.

Makes 40 cookies
Preheat oven to 350°F (180°C)
Baking sheets sprayed with vegetable spray

1. In large bowl, cream together margarine, brown sugar and granulated sugar. Add egg, vanilla, orange juice concentrate and orange zest and mix well.
2. In another bowl, combine flour, baking powder, baking soda, cinnamon, corn flakes, raisins, rolled oats and coconut just until combined. Add to sugar mixture and mix until just combined
3. Drop by heaping teaspoons (5 mL) onto prepared baking sheets 2 inches (5 cm) apart and press down with back of fork; bake approximately 10 minutes or until browned.

Make Ahead
✦ Bake cookies up to a day ahead, keeping tightly covered in a cookie tin. Freeze cookie dough for up to 2 weeks.

Nutritional Analysis (Per Serving)
✦ Calories: 51   ✦ Protein: 1 g   ✦ Cholesterol: 5 mg
✦ Sodium: 34 mg   ✦ Fat, total: 1 g   ✦ Carbohydrates: 9 g
✦ Fiber: 0 g   ✦ Fat, saturated: 1 g

Oatmeal Date Cookies

⅓ cup	margarine or butter	75 mL
⅓ cup	granulated sugar	75 mL
1	egg	1
1 tsp	vanilla	5 mL
⅔ cup	all-purpose flour	150 mL
1 tsp	baking powder	5 mL
¾ tsp	cinnamon	4 mL
¾ cup	rolled oats	175 mL
¾ cup	bran flakes cereal or corn flakes	175 mL
⅔ cup	chopped, pitted and dried dates	150 mL

You can use Raisin Bran cereal. Do not use All-Bran or raw bran.

Makes 32 cookies
Preheat oven to 350°F (180°C)
Baking sheets sprayed with vegetable spray

1. In large bowl, cream together margarine and sugar. Add egg and vanilla and mix well.
2. In another bowl, combine flour, baking powder, cinnamon, rolled oats, cereal and dates. Add to sugar mixture and mix until just combined.
3. Drop by heaping teaspoonfuls (5 mL) onto prepared baking sheets 2 inches (5 cm) apart and press down with back of fork; bake for approximately 10 minutes or until browned.

Nutritional Analysis (Per Serving)
✦ Calories: 54   ✦ Protein: 1 g   ✦ Cholesterol: 7 mg
✦ Sodium: 36 mg   ✦ Fat, total: 2 g   ✦ Carbohydrates: 8 g
✦ Fiber: 1 g   ✦ Fat, saturated: 0.4 g

Peanut Butter Fudge Cookies

¼ cup	softened margarine or butter	50 mL
⅓ cup	peanut butter	75 mL
¾ cup	granulated sugar	175 mL
¼ cup	brown sugar	50 mL
1	egg	1
1 tsp	vanilla	5 mL
1 cup	all-purpose flour	250 mL
¼ cup	cocoa	50 mL
1 tsp	baking powder	5 mL
¼ cup	2% yogurt	50 mL
¾ cup	raisins	175 mL
3 tbsp	chocolate chips	45 mL

If you are not hungry for breakfast, chances are you had too much to eat before you went to bed. Your total calorie intake over the course of the day is what matters to your weight, so try not to overdo it.

When using margarine, choose a soft (non-hydrogenated) version to limit consumption of trans fats.

Makes 40 cookies
Preheat oven to 350°F (180°C)
Baking sheets sprayed with vegetable spray

1. In large bowl, cream together margarine, peanut butter, sugar and brown sugar. Add egg and vanilla and beat well.
2. In another bowl, combine flour, cocoa and baking powder; add to peanut butter mixture and stir just until combined. Stir in yogurt, raisins and chocolate chips. Drop by heaping teaspoonfuls (5 mL) onto prepared sheets 2 inches (5 cm) apart, and press down slightly with back of fork. Bake approximately 12 minutes, or until firm to the touch and slightly browned.

Tips
+ Chopped dates can replace raisins.
+ Use a natural peanut butter, smooth or chunky.

Make Ahead
+ Cookies never last long, but these can be made up to a day ahead, kept tightly covered in a cookie jar or tin.
+ Prepare cookie dough and freeze up to 2 weeks, then bake.

Nutritional Analysis (Per Serving)
+ Calories: 67
+ Protein: 1 g
+ Cholesterol: 5 mg
+ Sodium: 20 mg
+ Fat, total: 2 g
+ Carbohydrates: 11 g
+ Fiber: 1 g
+ Fat, saturated: 0.6 g

Date Roll-Up Cookies

Filling

8 oz	pitted dried dates	250 g
1 cup	orange juice	250 mL
1/4 tsp	ground cinnamon	1 mL

Dough

2 1/4 cups	all-purpose flour	· 550 mL
2/3 cup	granulated sugar	150 mL
1/4 cup	margarine or butter	50 mL
1/4 cup	vegetable oil	50 mL
1/4 cup	2% plain yogurt	50 mL
3 tbsp	water	45 mL
1 tsp	vanilla extract	5 mL
1 tsp	grated orange zest	5 mL

For quick and easy snacks, try bagels with low-fat cream cheese, bran or oatmeal muffins with a serving of yogurt, pita bread stuffed with salad, cereal with milk, fresh fruit and yogurt, hard-cooked eggs, raw vegetables, rice cakes, fig bars or pretzels.

When using margarine, choose a soft (non-hydrogenated) version to limit consumption of trans fats.

Makes about 32 cookies
Preheat oven to 350°F (180°C)
Large baking sheet sprayed with vegetable spray

1. *Make the filling:* In a saucepan bring dates, orange juice and cinnamon to a boil; reduce heat to medium-low and cook 10 minutes or until soft. Mash with a fork until liquid is absorbed. Refrigerate.

2. *Make the dough:* In a food processor, combine flour, sugar, margarine, oil, yogurt, water, vanilla and orange zest; process until dough forms. Add up to 1 tbsp (15 mL) more water, if necessary. Divide dough in half; form each half into a ball, wrap and refrigerate for 15 minutes or until chilled.

3. Between 2 sheets of waxed paper sprinkled with flour, roll one of the dough balls into a rectangle, approximately 12 by 10 inches (30 by 25 cm) and 1/8 inch (5 mm) thick. Remove top sheet of waxed paper. Spread half of date mixture over rolled dough. Starting at short end and using the waxed paper as an aid, roll up tightly. Cut into 1/2-inch (1 cm) slices and place on prepared baking sheet. Repeat with remaining dough and filling.

4. Bake 25 minutes or until lightly browned.

Tips

✦ For maximum freshness, store cookies in airtight containers in the freezer; remove as needed.

✦ Try this recipe with dried figs or apricots.

Make Ahead

✦ Prepare date mixture and freeze until needed.

Nutritional Analysis (Per Serving)
✦ Calories: 93   ✦ Protein: 1 g   ✦ Cholesterol: 0 mg
✦ Sodium: 16 mg   ✦ Fat, total: 2 g ✦ Carbohydrates: 18 g
✦ Fiber: 1 g   ✦ Fat, saturated: 0.3 g

Double Chocolate Raisin Cookies

¼ cup	soft margarine	50 mL
¾ cup	granulated sugar	175 mL
1	egg	1
1 tsp	vanilla	5 mL
3 tbsp	unsweetened cocoa powder	45 mL
½ tsp	baking soda	2 mL
½ tsp	baking powder	2 mL
½ cup	whole wheat flour	125 mL
¾ cup	all-purpose flour	175 mL
¼ cup	chocolate chips	50 mL
¼ cup	raisins	50 mL

Try white chocolate or peanut butter chips for a change.

When using margarine, choose a soft (non-hydrogenated) version to limit consumption of trans fats.

Makes 40 cookies
Preheat oven to 350°F (180°C)
Baking sheets sprayed with nonstick vegetable spray

1. In large bowl or food processor, beat together margarine, sugar, egg and vanilla until well blended.
2. Combine cocoa, baking soda, baking powder, whole wheat and all-purpose flours; add to bowl and mix until just combined. Stir in chocolate chips and raisins.
3. Drop by heaping teaspoonfuls (5 mL) 2 inches (5 cm) apart onto baking sheets. Bake for 12 to 15 minutes or until browned.

Make Ahead
✦ Dough can be frozen for up to 2 weeks.

Nutritional Analysis (Per Serving)
✦ Calories: 49   ✦ Protein: 1 g   ✦ Cholesterol: 5 mg
✦ Sodium: 32 mg   ✦ Fat: 1 g   ✦ Carbohydrates: 8 g
✦ Fiber: 0.5 g

Oatmeal Raisin Pecan Cookies

½ cup	brown sugar	125 mL
¼ cup	soft margarine	50 mL
1	egg	1
1 tsp	vanilla	5 mL
½ cup	rolled oats	125 mL
¼ cup	whole wheat flour	50 mL
¼ cup	wheat germ	50 mL
¼ cup	pecan pieces	50 mL
¼ cup	raisins	50 mL
½ tsp	baking powder	2 mL

These cookies are soft and chewy if baked for a shorter time; crisp if baked longer.

If wheat germ is not available, substitute another ¼ cup (50 mL) rolled oats.

When using margarine, choose a soft (non-hydrogenated) version.

Makes 30 cookies
Preheat oven to 350°F (180°C)
Baking sheets sprayed with nonstick vegetable spray

1. In large bowl or food processor, beat together sugar, margarine, egg and vanilla until well blended.
2. Add rolled oats, flour, wheat germ, pecans, raisins and baking powder; mix just until incorporated.
3. Drop by heaping teaspoonfuls (5 mL) 2 inches (5 cm) apart onto baking sheets. Bake for 12 to 15 minutes or until browned.

Make Ahead
✦ Dough can be frozen for up to 2 weeks.

Nutritional Analysis (Per Serving)
✦ Calories: 55   ✦ Protein: 1 g   ✦ Cholesterol: 7 mg
✦ Sodium: 31 mg   ✦ Fat: 3 g   ✦ Carbohydrates: 7 g
✦ Fiber: 0.5 g

Vanilla Almond Snaps

³/₄ cup	whole blanched almonds	175 mL
¹/₄ cup	granulated sugar	50 mL
¹/₄ tsp	salt	1 mL
2	egg whites	2
2 tbsp	granulated sugar	25 mL
¹/₂ tsp	vanilla extract	2 mL
	Sliced almonds (optional)	

Use a pastry bag with a star tip and pipe the mixture onto baking sheet for an elegant cookie.

Makes about 30
Preheat oven to 275°F (140°C)
Baking sheet lined with parchment paper and sprayed with baking spray

1. In a food processor, grind almonds with ¹/₄ cup (50 mL) sugar and salt until as fine as possible. Transfer to a bowl and set aside.
2. In another bowl, beat egg whites until soft peaks form. Gradually add 2 tbsp (25 mL) sugar, beating until stiff peaks form. Fold in vanilla. Fold into ground nut mixture until blended. Drop by teaspoonfuls (5 mL) onto prepared baking sheet. If desired, sprinkle with a few sliced almonds.
3. Bake for 25 minutes or until golden.

Nutritional Analysis (Per Serving)
- Calories: 34
- Protein: 0.9 g
- Cholesterol: 0 mg
- Sodium: 19 mg
- Fat: 2 g
- Carbohydrates: 3 g

Crisp Nut Cookies

2	eggs	2
³/₄ cup	granulated sugar	175 mL
6 tbsp	melted butter	90 mL
¹/₄ cup	water	50 mL
2 tsp	vanilla extract	10 mL
1 tsp	almond extract	5 mL
2¹/₂ cups	all-purpose flour	625 mL
¹/₂ cup	chopped nuts	125 mL
2¹/₄ tsp	baking powder	11 mL

These resemble the classic Jewish cookie mandelbrot.

Makes about 45
Preheat oven to 350°F (180°C)
Baking sheet sprayed with baking spray

1. In a bowl, beat eggs with sugar until well mixed. Beat in butter, water, vanilla and almond extract.
2. In another bowl, stir together flour, nuts and baking powder. Stir into egg-sugar mixture until dough forms a ball. Divide dough in half. Form each half into a log 12 inches (30 cm) long. Put on prepared baking sheet.
3. Bake for 20 minutes. Cool for 5 minutes. Cut on the diagonal into ¹/₂-inch (1 cm) thick slices. Bake for 20 minutes or until golden.

Tip
- Use almonds, pecans, pine nuts or a combination.

Nutritional Analysis (Per Serving)
- Calories: 63
- Protein: 1 g
- Cholesterol: 17 mg
- Sodium: 20 mg
- Fat: 2 g
- Carbohydrates: 10 g

Oatmeal Raisin Cookies

6 tbsp	packed brown sugar	90 mL
1/4 cup	butter, softened	50 mL
1	egg	1
1 tsp	vanilla extract	5 mL
1/2 cup	rolled oats	125 mL
1/2 cup	raisins	125 mL
1/4 cup	whole wheat flour	50 mL
1/4 cup	wheat germ	50 mL
1/2 tsp	baking powder	2 mL

Makes about 18
Preheat oven to 375°F (190°C)
Baking sheet sprayed with baking spray

1. In a bowl cream brown sugar with butter. Beat in egg and vanilla. In another bowl, stir together oats, raisins, whole wheat flour, wheat germ and baking powder. Stir into creamed mixture just until blended.

2. Drop batter by teaspoonfuls (5 mL) onto prepared baking sheet, leaving 2 inches (5 cm) between cookies. Bake for 10 to 12 minutes or until golden. Cool on wire racks.

Nutritional Analysis (Per Serving)
- Calories: 49
- Protein: 0.9 g
- Cholesterol: 10 mg
- Sodium: 56 mg
- Fat: 2 g
- Carbohydrates: 6 g

Peanut Butter Cookies

1/2 cup	peanut butter	125 mL
1/2 cup	packed brown sugar	125 mL
1/3 cup	margarine	75 mL
1	egg	1
1 tsp	vanilla extract	5 mL
1/2 cup	all-purpose flour	125 mL
2 tbsp	sesame seeds	25 mL
3/4 tsp	baking soda	4 mL
1/2 tsp	nutmeg	2 mL
Coating (optional)		
1	egg white, beaten	1
1/2 cup	wheat germ	125 mL

When using margarine, choose a soft (non-hydrogenated) version to limit consumption of trans fats.

Makes about 40
Preheat oven to 350°F (180°C)
Baking sheet sprayed with baking spray

1. In a bowl, beat peanut butter, brown sugar, margarine, egg and vanilla until light and fluffy. In another bowl, stir together flour, sesame seeds, baking soda and nutmeg. Stir flour mixture into peanut butter mixture just until combined. Form into 1-inch (2.5 cm) balls. If desired, dip balls in egg white, then roll in wheat germ. Put on prepared baking sheet.

2. Bake for 10 to 12 minutes or until golden.

Tip
- Use a natural, all-peanut type of peanut butter.

Nutritional Analysis (Per Serving)
- Calories: 103
- Protein: 2 g
- Cholesterol: 18 mg
- Sodium: 9 mg
- Fat: 3 g
- Carbohydrates: 16 g

Gingerbread Biscotti

³/₄ cup	packed brown sugar	175 mL
¹/₄ cup	margarine or butter	50 mL
¹/₄ cup	molasses	50 mL
2	eggs	2
1 tsp	vanilla extract	5 mL
2¹/₃ cups	all-purpose flour	575 mL
2¹/₄ tsp	baking powder	11 mL
1 tsp	ground cinnamon	5 mL
1 tsp	ground ginger	5 mL
¹/₂ tsp	ground allspice	2 mL
¹/₄ tsp	ground nutmeg	1 mL

To add fiber, use ²/₃ cup (150 mL) whole wheat flour and 1²/₃ cups (400 mL) all-purpose flour.

For a decadent treat, melt 2 oz (50 g) semi-sweet chocolate and dip ends of cookies. Let harden.

Makes 40 to 48
Preheat oven to 350°F (180°C)
Baking sheet sprayed with vegetable spray

1. In a food processor or in a bowl with an electric mixer, beat together brown sugar, margarine, molasses, eggs and vanilla until smooth. In a separate bowl, stir together flour, baking powder, cinnamon, ginger, allspice and nutmeg. Add wet ingredients to dry ingredients, mixing just until combined.
2. Divide dough in half. Form each half into a log 12 inches (30 cm) long and 2 inches (5 cm) around; transfer to prepared baking sheet. Bake 20 minutes. Cool 10 minutes.
3. Cut logs on an angle into ¹/₂-inch (1 cm) slices. Bake 20 minutes or until lightly browned.

Nutritional Analysis (Per Serving)
- ✦ Calories: 207
- ✦ Protein: 1 g
- ✦ Cholesterol: 9 mg
- ✦ Sodium: 27 mg
- ✦ Fat, total: 1 g
- ✦ Carbohydrates: 9 g
- ✦ Fiber: 0 g
- ✦ Fat, saturated: 0.2 g

Pecan Biscotti

2	eggs	2
³/₄ cup	granulated sugar	175 mL
¹/₃ cup	margarine	75 mL
¹/₄ cup	water	50 mL
2 tsp	vanilla	10 mL
1 tsp	almond extract	5 mL
2³/₄ cups	all-purpose flour	675 mL
¹/₂ cup	chopped pecans	125 mL
2¹/₄ tsp	baking powder	11 mL

Instead of pecans, you can use almonds, hazelnuts, pine nuts or a combination.

When using margarine, choose a soft (non-hydrogenated) version to limit consumption of trans fats.

Makes 45 cookies
Preheat oven to 350°F (180°C)
Baking sheet sprayed with nonstick vegetable spray

1. In large bowl, blend eggs with sugar; beat in margarine, water, vanilla and almond extract until smooth.
2. Add flour, pecans and baking powder; mix until dough forms ball. Divide dough in half; shape each portion into 12-inch (30 cm) long log and place on baking sheet. Bake for 20 minutes. Let cool for 5 minutes.
3. Cut logs on angle into ¹/₂-inch (1 cm) thick slices. Place slices on sides on baking sheet; bake for 20 minutes or until lightly browned.

Nutritional Analysis (Per Serving)
- ✦ Calories: 60
- ✦ Protein: 1 g
- ✦ Cholesterol: 9 mg
- ✦ Sodium: 40 mg
- ✦ Fat: 2 g
- ✦ Carbohydrates: 8 g
- ✦ Fiber: 0.5 g

Lemon and Lime Poppy Seed Biscotti

1 cup	granulated sugar	250 mL
1/4 cup	margarine or butter	50 mL
2	eggs	2
1 1/2 tsp	grated lime zest	7 mL
1 1/2 tsp	grated lemon zest	7 mL
2 tbsp	freshly squeezed lime juice	25 mL
2 tbsp	freshly squeezed lemon juice	25 mL
1 tsp	vanilla extract	5 mL
2 1/2 cups	all-purpose flour	625 mL
2 1/4 tsp	baking powder	11 mL
2 tsp	poppy seeds	10 mL

When using margarine, choose a soft (non-hydrogenated) version to limit consumption of trans fats.

Makes about 40 cookies
Preheat oven to 350°F (180°C)
Baking sheet sprayed with vegetable spray

1. In a food processor or in a bowl with an electric mixer, beat sugar, margarine and eggs until smooth. Beat in lime zest, lemon zest, lime juice, lemon juice and vanilla.

2. In a separate bowl, stir together flour, baking powder and poppy seeds. Add wet ingredients to dry ingredients, mixing just until combined. Dough will be stiff.

3. Divide dough in half. Form each half into a log 12 inches (30 cm) long and 1 1/2 inches (4 cm) around; transfer to prepared baking sheet. Bake 20 minutes. Cool 10 minutes.

4. Cut logs on an angle into 1/2-inch (1 cm) slices. Bake 20 minutes.

Tips

✦ If desired, omit lime and use double the quantity of lemon juice and zest.

✦ If dough is sticky when forming into logs, try wetting your fingers.

Make Ahead

✦ Store cookies in air-tight containers for up to 1 week.

✦ Freeze in air-tight containers up to 6 weeks.

Nutritional Analysis (Per Serving)
✦ Calories: 61   ✦ Protein: 1 g   ✦ Cholesterol: 0 mg
✦ Sodium: 28 mg   ✦ Fat, total: 1 g   ✦ Carbohydrates: 12 g
✦ Fiber: 0 g   ✦ Fat, saturated: 0.2 g

Two-Tone Chocolate Orange Biscotti

1¼ cups	granulated sugar	300 mL
⅓ cup	margarine or butter	75 mL
2	eggs	2
2 tbsp	orange juice concentrate	25 mL
1 tbsp	grated orange zest	15 mL
2⅔ cups	all-purpose flour	650 mL
2½ tsp	baking powder	12 mL
3 tbsp	cocoa	45 mL

When using margarine, choose a soft (non-hydrogenated) version to limit consumption of trans fats.

Makes 40 to 48
Preheat oven to 350°F (180°C)
Baking sheet sprayed with vegetable spray

1. In a food processor or in a bowl with an electric mixer, beat together sugar, margarine, eggs, orange juice concentrate and orange zest until smooth. Add flour and baking powder; mix just until combined.

2. Divide dough in half; to one half, add cocoa and mix well. Divide chocolate and plain doughs in half to produce 4 doughs. Roll each piece into a long thin rope approximately 12 inches (30 cm) long and 1 inch (2.5 cm) wide. Use extra flour if too sticky. Place 1 cocoa dough on top of (or beside) each plain dough. (Ensure the plain and cocoa doughs touch one another.)

3. Bake 20 minutes. Cool 10 minutes. Cut logs on an angle into ½-inch (1 cm) slices. Bake another 20 minutes.

Tips

✦ If dough is sticky when forming into logs, try wetting your fingers.

✦ Two colors of dough make these cookies very attractive.

Make Ahead

✦ Freeze in containers for up to 6 weeks.

Nutritional Analysis (Per Serving)

✦ Calories: 72   ✦ Protein: 1 g   ✦ Cholesterol: 11 mg
✦ Sodium: 42 mg   ✦ Fat, total: 2 g ✦ Carbohydrates: 13 g
✦ Fiber: 0 g   ✦ Fat, saturated: 0.4 g

Apricot Date Biscotti

1/3 cup	margarine or butter	75 mL
3/4 cup	granulated sugar	175 mL
2	eggs	2
2 tbsp	orange juice concentrate, thawed	25 mL
2 tbsp	water	25 mL
2 tsp	grated orange zest	10 mL
1 tsp	vanilla	5 mL
2 2/3 cups	all-purpose flour	650 mL
2 1/4 tsp	baking powder	11 mL
1 tsp	cinnamon	5 mL
2/3 cup	pitted, dried and chopped dates	150 mL
2/3 cup	chopped dried apricots	150 mL

When using margarine, choose a soft (non-hydrogenated) version to limit consumption of trans fats.

Makes 48 cookies
Preheat oven to 350°F (180°C)
Baking sheet sprayed with vegetable spray

1. In large bowl, cream together margarine and sugar; add eggs, orange juice concentrate, water, orange zest and vanilla and mix well.

2. In bowl, combine flour, baking powder, cinnamon, dates and apricots; add to wet ingredients and stir just until mixed. Divide dough into 3 portions; shape each portion into a 12-inch (30-cm) long log, 2 inches wide (5 cm), and put on prepared baking sheet. Bake for 20 minutes. Let cool for 10 minutes.

3. Cut logs on an angle into 1/2-inch (1-cm) thick slices. Put slices flat on baking sheet and bake for another 20 minutes or until lightly browned.

Tips

+ Use a serrated knife to cut the logs into slices.

+ Dried prunes or raisins can replace, or be used in combination with, the apricots and dates.

+ Orange juice concentrate gives a more intense flavor than just orange juice. Use frozen concentrate, then refreeze the remainder.

Make Ahead

+ Bake cookies up to 2 days ahead for best flavor, keeping tightly covered in cookie tin.

+ Freeze cookie dough for up to 2 weeks.

Nutritional Analysis (Per Serving)
+ Calories: 62   + Protein: 1 g   + Cholesterol: 9 mg
+ Sodium: 19 mg   + Fat, total: 1 g   + Carbohydrates: 11 g
+ Fiber: 1 g   + Fat, saturated: 0.3 g

Chocolate Seashells

2 tbsp	apple juice concentrate	25 mL
2 tbsp	honey	25 mL
1 tsp	vanilla extract	5 mL
1/4 cup	cocoa	50 mL
9 tbsp	granulated sugar or 7 tbsp (110 mL) fructose	140 mL
1 tbsp	butter	15 mL
1	egg	1
6 tbsp	apple juice	90 mL
2 tsp	instant coffee granules	10 mL
1/2 cup	all-purpose flour	125 mL
1/4 cup	whole wheat flour	50 mL
1/4 cup	cocoa	50 mL
1/2 tsp	baking soda	2 mL
1/2 cup	sorbet, ice milk or frozen yogurt (optional)	125 mL
	Icing sugar	

Makes about 18
Preheat oven to 350°F (180°C)
Madeleine cookie forms sprayed with baking spray

1. In a small saucepan, heat apple juice concentrate, honey and vanilla over medium-low heat, stirring until blended. Whisk in cocoa until smooth and thickened. Set aside to cool.

2. In a bowl cream sugar with butter; beat in egg until well mixed. Stir in cooled cocoa sauce. In a separate bowl, stir together coffee granules and apple juice until dissolved; stir into cocoa mixture. Sift together flour, whole wheat flour, cocoa and baking soda directly onto cocoa mixture; gently fold in until well mixed. Fill cookie forms two-thirds full.

3. Bake 12 minutes or until cookies spring back when lightly touched. Cool. Dust with sifted icing sugar. If desired, slit cookie lengthwise without cutting all the way through and prop open with a small ball of sorbet.

Nutritional Analysis (Per Serving)
- Calories: 45
- Protein: 1 g
- Cholesterol: 18 mg
- Sodium: 64 mg
- Fat: 1 g
- Carbohydrates: 7 g

Cocoa Kisses

3	egg whites, at room temperature	3
1 cup	granulated sugar	250 mL
1/8 tsp	salt	0.5 mL
1 tsp	vanilla extract	5 mL
3 tbsp	cocoa	45 mL
1/2 cup	chopped pecans	125 mL

It's easier to separate eggs when they're cold, but egg whites beat to a greater volume when at room temperature.

Makes about 40
Preheat oven to 250°F (120°C)
Baking sheet sprayed with baking spray

1. In a large bowl, beat egg whites until soft peaks form; gradually add sugar and salt, beating until mixture is glossy and stiff peaks form. Beat in vanilla. Sift cocoa into bowl; fold into meringue along with pecans.

2. Put mixture in a pastry bag fitted with star tip; pipe small kisses onto prepared baking sheet (alternatively, drop mixture by teaspoonfuls [5 mL] onto baking sheet). Bake 1 hour or until firm and dry.

Nutritional Analysis (Per Serving)
- Calories: 35
- Protein: 1 g
- Cholesterol: 0 mg
- Sodium: 8 mg
- Fat: 1 g
- Carbohydrates: 6 g

Sour Cream Orange Apple Cake

Topping

1/3 cup	packed brown sugar	75 mL
3 tbsp	chopped pecans	45 mL
1 1/2 tbsp	all-purpose flour	20 mL
2 tsp	margarine or butter	10 mL
1/2 tsp	ground cinnamon	2 mL

Filling

2 cups	chopped peeled apples	500 mL
1/2 cup	raisins	125 mL
1 tbsp	granulated sugar	15 mL
1 tsp	ground cinnamon	5 mL

Cake

2/3 cup	packed brown sugar	150 mL
1/2 cup	granulated sugar	125 mL
1/3 cup	vegetable oil	75 mL
2	eggs	2
1 tbsp	grated orange zest	15 mL
2 tsp	vanilla extract	10 mL
1 2/3 cups	all-purpose flour	400 mL
2 tsp	baking powder	10 mL
1 tsp	baking soda	5 mL
1/2 cup	orange juice	125 mL
1/2 cup	light sour cream	125 mL

If you don't want to layer the cake, just mix apples with batter, then add topping.

When using margarine, choose a soft (non-hydrogenated) version to limit consumption of trans fats.

Serves 14
Preheat oven to 350°F (180°C)
10-inch (3 L) springform pan sprayed with vegetable spray

1. *Make the topping:* In a small bowl, combine brown sugar, pecans, flour, margarine and cinnamon. Set aside.

2. *Make the filling:* In a bowl mix together apples, raisins, sugar and cinnamon. Set aside.

3. *Make the cake:* In a food processor or in a large bowl with an electric mixer, beat together brown sugar, granulated sugar and oil. Add eggs, one at a time, beating well after each. Mix in orange zest and vanilla.

4. In a separate bowl, stir together flour, baking powder and baking soda. In another bowl, stir together orange juice and sour cream. Add flour mixture and sour cream mixture alternately to beaten sugar mixture, mixing just until blended. Spoon half of batter into prepared pan. Top with half of apple mixture. Spoon remaining batter into pan. Top with remaining apple mixture; sprinkle with topping.

5. Bake 45 to 50 minutes, or until cake tester inserted in center comes out clean. Cool on a wire rack.

Tips

✦ Try chopped pears or peaches instead of apples.

✦ To increase fiber, use 2/3 cup (150 mL) whole wheat and 1 cup (250 mL) all-purpose flour.

✦ Makes two 9- by 5-inch (2 L) loaves. Bake approximately 35 minutes or until tester comes out clean.

Make Ahead

✦ Prepare up to 2 days in advance.

✦ Freeze up to 6 weeks.

Nutritional Analysis (Per Serving)
- ✦ Calories: 284
- ✦ Protein: 4 g
- ✦ Cholesterol: 36 mg
- ✦ Sodium: 187 mg
- ✦ Fat, total: 9 g
- ✦ Carbohydrates: 49 g
- ✦ Fiber: 2 g
- ✦ Fat, saturated: 1 g

Cream Cheese–Filled Brownies (page 363) ➤

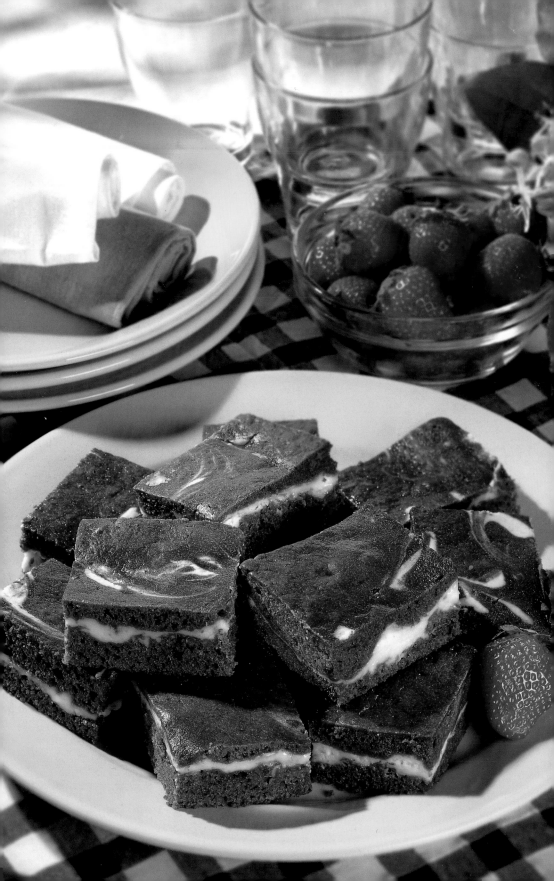

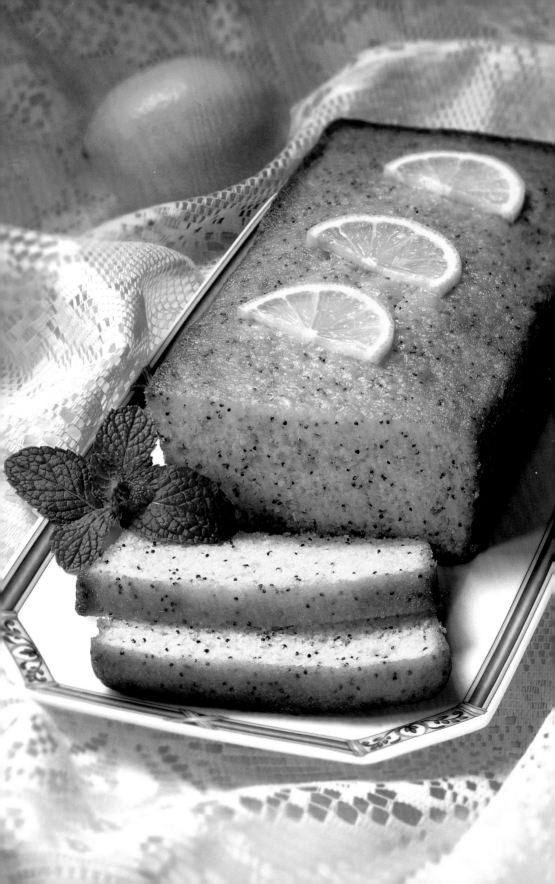

Sour Cream Apple Pie

5½ cups	sliced peeled apples (5 to 6 apples)	1.375 L
½ cup	granulated sugar	125 mL
½ cup	2% yogurt	125 mL
½ cup	light sour cream	125 mL
¼ cup	raisins	50 mL
2 tbsp	all-purpose flour	25 mL
1 tsp	cinnamon	5 mL
1	egg, lightly beaten	1
1 tsp	vanilla	5 mL

Crust

1½ cups	graham wafer crumbs	375 mL
2 tbsp	margarine, melted	25 mL
1 tbsp	brown sugar	15 mL
1 tbsp	water	15 mL

Topping

¼ cup	brown sugar	50 mL
3 tbsp	all-purpose flour	45 mL
2 tbsp	rolled oats	25 mL
½ tsp	cinnamon	2 mL
1 tbsp	margarine	15 mL

When using margarine, choose a soft (non-hydrogenated) version to limit consumption of trans fats.

Makes 16 slices
Preheat oven to 350°F (180°C)
8-inch (2 L) springform pan

1. *Crust:* In bowl, combine graham crumbs, margarine, sugar and water; pat onto bottom and sides of pan. Refrigerate.

2. In large bowl, combine apples, sugar, yogurt, sour cream, raisins, flour, cinnamon, egg and vanilla; toss together until well mixed. Pour over crust.

3. *Topping:* In small bowl, combine sugar, flour, rolled oats and cinnamon; cut in margarine until crumbly. Sprinkle over pie; bake for 30 to 40 minutes or until topping is browned and apples are tender.

Tips

✦ For an attractive presentation, sprinkle a little icing sugar over top.

✦ Substitute vanilla wafer crumbs for the graham crumbs for a change.

Make Ahead

✦ Prepare early in the day and warm slightly before serving. Or freeze for up to 2 weeks.

Nutritional Analysis (Per Serving)
✦ Calories: 153   ✦ Protein: 2 g   ✦ Cholesterol: 17 mg
✦ Sodium: 98 mg   ✦ Fat: 4 g   ✦ Carbohydrates: 28 g
✦ Fiber: 1 g

Tropical Fruit Tart

1³/₄ cups	2% yogurt	425 mL
²/₃ cup	granulated sugar	150 mL
¹/₂ cup	light sour cream	125 mL
3 tbsp	frozen orange juice concentrate, thawed	45 mL
2 tbsp	all-purpose flour	25 mL
1¹/₂ tsp	orange rind	7 mL
Crust		
1¹/₄ cups	all-purpose flour	300 mL
¹/₄ cup	icing sugar	50 mL
¹/₃ cup	margarine	75 mL
3 tbsp	(approx) cold water	45 mL
Topping		
3 cups	sliced fruit (kiwi, mangos, papayas, star fruit)	750 mL

When using margarine, choose a soft (non-hydrogenated) version to limit consumption of trans fats.

Makes 12 servings
Preheat oven to 400°F (200°C)
9-inch (2 L) tart or springform pan sprayed with nonstick vegetable spray

1. *Crust:* In bowl, combine flour with sugar; cut in margarine until crumbly. With fork, gradually stir in water, adding 1 tbsp (15 mL) more if necessary to make dough hold together. Pat into pan and bake for 15 minutes or until browned. Reduce heat to 375°F (190°C).

2. Meanwhile, in bowl, combine yogurt, sugar, sour cream, orange juice concentrate, flour and orange rind; mix well and pour over crust. Bake for 35 to 45 minutes or until filling is set. Let cool and refrigerate until chilled.

3. *Topping:* Decoratively arrange sliced fruit over filling.

Nutritional Analysis (Per Serving)
- Calories: 221
- Protein: 4 g
- Cholesterol: 5 mg
- Sodium: 103 mg
- Fat: 6 g
- Carbohydrates: 37 g
- Fiber: 2 g

Pear, Apple and Raisin Strudel

2²/₃ cups	chopped peeled apples	650 mL
2²/₃ cups	chopped peeled pears	650 mL
¹/₃ cup	raisins	75 mL
2 tbsp	chopped pecans or walnuts	25 mL
2 tbsp	brown sugar	25 mL
1 tbsp	lemon juice	15 mL
1 tbsp	honey	15 mL
1 tsp	cinnamon	5 mL
6	phyllo sheets (see sidebar, page 387)	6
4 tsp	margarine, melted	20 mL

Sprinkle with icing sugar for a finishing touch.

Ripen pears at room temperature in a bowl or paper bag.

Makes 12 slices
Preheat oven to 350°F (180°C)
Baking sheet sprayed with nonstick vegetable spray

1. In bowl, combine apples, pears, raisins, pecans, sugar, lemon juice, honey and cinnamon; mix well.

2. Lay out 2 sheets of phyllo; brush with some margarine. Place 2 more sheets over top; brush with margarine again. Top with remaining 2 sheets phyllo.

3. Spread filling over phyllo, leaving 1-inch (2.5 cm) border uncovered. Roll up like jelly roll and place seam down on baking sheet. Brush with remaining margarine. Bake for 40 to 50 minutes or until golden and fruit is tender.

Nutritional Analysis (Per Serving)
- Calories: 114
- Protein: 1 g
- Cholesterol: 0 mg
- Sodium: 65 mg
- Fat: 2 g
- Carbohydrates: 23 g
- Fiber: 2 g

Mango Blueberry Strudel

2 cups	fresh blueberries (or frozen, thawed and drained)	500 mL
1 tbsp	all-purpose flour	15 mL
2½ cups	peeled chopped ripe mango	625 mL
¼ cup	granulated sugar	50 mL
1 tbsp	lemon juice	15 mL
½ tsp	cinnamon	2 mL
6	sheets phyllo pastry	6
2 tsp	melted margarine or butter	10 mL

Phyllo pastry is located in the freezer section of store. Handle quickly so the sheets do not dry out. Cover those not being used with a slightly damp cloth.

Serves 8
Preheat oven to 375°F (190°C)
Baking sheet sprayed with vegetable spray

1. Toss blueberries with flour. In large bowl, combine mango, blueberries, sugar, lemon juice and cinnamon.

2. Lay 2 phyllo sheets one on top of the other; brush with melted margarine. Layer another 2 phyllo sheets on top and brush with melted margarine. Layer last 2 sheets on top. Put fruit filling along long end of phyllo; gently roll over until all of filling is enclosed, fold sides in, and continue to roll. Put on prepared baking sheet, brush with remaining margarine and bake for 20 to 25 minutes or until golden. Sprinkle with icing sugar.

Nutritional Analysis (Per Serving)
- Calories: 146
- Protein: 2 g
- Cholesterol: 0 mg
- Sodium: 65 mg
- Fat, total: 2 g
- Carbohydrates: 31 g
- Fiber: 3 g
- Fat, saturated: 0.4 g

Peach and Blueberry Crisp

½ cup	granulated sugar	125 mL
2 tbsp	all-purpose flour	25 mL
2 tsp	lemon juice	10 mL
1 tsp	grated lemon rind	5 mL
1 tsp	cinnamon	5 mL
3 cups	sliced peeled ripe peaches	750 mL
2 cups	blueberries	500 mL
Topping		
½ cup	rolled oats	125 mL
⅓ cup	all-purpose flour	75 mL
3 tbsp	brown sugar	45 mL
½ tsp	cinnamon	2 mL
3 tbsp	soft margarine	45 mL

Blueberries should be removed from their carton and placed in a moisture-proof container in the refrigerator. Do not wash until just before using.

Serves 6 to 8
Preheat oven to 350°F (180°C)
9-inch (2.5 L) square cake pan

1. In large bowl, combine sugar, flour, lemon juice, rind and cinnamon; stir in peaches and blueberries until well mixed. Spread in cake pan.

2. *Topping:* In small bowl, combine rolled oats, flour, sugar and cinnamon; cut in margarine until crumbly. Sprinkle over fruit. Bake for 30 to 35 minutes or until topping is browned and fruit is tender. Serve warm.

Make Ahead
- Although best straight from the oven, crisp can be prepared early in day and reheated slightly before serving.

Nutritional Analysis (Per Serving)
- Calories: 199
- Protein: 2 g
- Cholesterol: 0 mg
- Sodium: 60 mg
- Fat: 5 g
- Carbohydrates: 38 g
- Fiber: 2 g

Blueberry Apple Crisp

3	medium apples, peeled, cored and sliced	3
1 cup	fresh blueberries	250 mL
1/4 cup	apple juice	50 mL
2 tbsp	granulated sugar	25 mL
1 tbsp	lemon juice	15 mL
1 tsp	cinnamon	5 mL
Topping		
1 cup	rolled oats	250 mL
1/3 cup	whole wheat flour	75 mL
1/4 cup	packed brown sugar	50 mL
2 tbsp	apple juice	25 mL
2 tbsp	softened butter	25 mL
1/2 tsp	cinnamon	2 mL

Serves 10
Preheat oven to 350°F (180°C)
9-inch (2.5 L) square baking dish

1. In a bowl, mix together apples, blueberries, apple juice, sugar, lemon juice and cinnamon. Transfer to baking dish.
2. *Make topping:* In a bowl, stir together rolled oats, flour, brown sugar, apple juice, butter and cinnamon until crumbly. Sprinkle over blueberry mixture.
3. Bake 30 minutes or until golden. Serve warm or cold.

Tip

✦ In season, substitute pears for the apples and use ground ginger instead of cinnamon.

Nutritional Analysis (Per Serving)
✦ Calories: 115   ✦ Protein: 1 g   ✦ Cholesterol: 5 mg
✦ Sodium: 20 mg   ✦ Fat: 2 g   ✦ Carbohydrates: 23 g

Blueberry Strawberry Pear Crisp

1 1/2 cups	fresh blueberries (or frozen, thawed and drained)	375 mL
1 1/2 cups	sliced strawberries	375 mL
1 1/2 cups	chopped peeled pears	375 mL
1/2 cup	granulated sugar	125 mL
2 tbsp	all-purpose flour	25 mL
2 tsp	orange juice	10 mL
1 tsp	grated orange zest	5 mL
1/2 tsp	cinnamon	2 mL
Topping		
3/4 cup	brown sugar	175 mL
3/4 cup	all-purpose flour	175 mL
1/2 cup	rolled oats	125 mL
1/2 tsp	cinnamon	2 mL
1/4 cup	cold butter	50 mL

Other fruits can be substituted, such as peaches, apples or mangoes.

Serves 8
Preheat oven to 350°F (180°C)
9-inch square (2.5 L) cake pan sprayed with vegetable spray

1. In large bowl, combine blueberries, strawberries, pears, sugar, flour, orange juice, orange zest and cinnamon; toss gently to mix. Spread in cake pan.
2. In small bowl, combine brown sugar, flour, oats and cinnamon; cut butter in until crumbly. Sprinkle over fruit mixture. Bake for 30 to 35 minutes or until topping is browned and fruit is tender.

Tip

✦ Serve with frozen yogurt.

Make Ahead

✦ Can be baked earlier in the day, but best if baked just ahead serving.

Nutritional Analysis (Per Serving)
✦ Calories: 267   ✦ Protein: 3 g   ✦ Cholesterol: 0 mg
✦ Sodium: 69 mg   ✦ Fat, total: 5 g   ✦ Carbohydrates: 54 g
✦ Fiber: 3 g   ✦ Fat, saturated: 1 g

Creamy Pumpkin Cheese Pie

1½ cups	graham cracker crumbs	375 mL
2 tbsp	granulated sugar	25 mL
2 tbsp	water	25 mL
1 tbsp	vegetable oil	15 mL
4 oz	light cream cheese	125 g
½ cup	5% ricotta cheese	125 mL
⅓ cup	granulated sugar	75 mL
1	egg	1
1 tsp	vanilla extract	5 mL
1 cup	canned pumpkin or mashed cooked butternut squash	250 mL
⅔ cup	2% evaporated milk	150 mL
¾ cup	packed brown sugar	175 mL
1 tsp	ground cinnamon	5 mL
¼ tsp	ground ginger	1 mL
¼ tsp	ground nutmeg	1 mL
3 tbsp	light sour cream	45 mL
2½ tsp	granulated sugar	12 mL

Serves 12
Preheat oven to 350° F (180° C)
9-inch (2.5 L) springform pan or 9-inch (23 cm)
  deep dish pie plate

1. In a bowl combine graham crumbs, sugar, water and oil; press into bottom and sides of pan; set aside.

2. In a food processor, combine cream cheese, ricotta, sugar, egg and vanilla; process until smooth. Pour into prepared crust.

3. In a food processor, combine pumpkin, evaporated milk, sugar, cinnamon, ginger and nutmeg until well blended. Spoon carefully over cheese filling.

4. In a small bowl, stir together sour cream and sugar. Put in a squeeze bottle or in a small plastic sandwich bag with the very tip of corner cut off. Draw 4 concentric circles on top of pumpkin filling. Run a toothpick through the circles at regular intervals.

5. Bake 50 minutes or until just slightly loose at the center. Cool on wire rack. Chill before serving.

Tips

✦ In the fall use fresh pumpkin. Bake pumpkin or squash in a 400°F (200°C) oven until tender, approximately 1 hour.

✦ The topping is simple but highly decorative.

Make Ahead

✦ Bake up to 2 days in advance. Freeze up to 6 weeks.

Nutritional Analysis (Per Serving)

✦ Calories: 203   ✦ Protein: 6 g   ✦ Cholesterol: 29 mg
✦ Sodium: 209 mg   ✦ Fat, total: 5 g   ✦ Carbohydrates: 34 g
✦ Fiber: 1 g   ✦ Fat, saturated: 2 g

Orange Cappuccino Pudding Cake

1 cup	all-purpose flour	250 mL
1 cup	packed brown sugar	250 mL
2 tsp	baking powder	10 mL
2 tsp	grated orange zest	10 mL
½ cup	orange juice	125 mL
2 tbsp	vegetable oil	25 mL
1	egg	1
2 tsp	vanilla extract	10 mL
¼ cup	semi-sweet chocolate chips	50 mL
⅓ cup	granulated sugar	75 mL
¼ cup	instant coffee mix powder or hot chocolate mix	50 mL
¼ cup	cocoa	50 mL

Use a flavored coffee mix powder, like Irish cream or vanilla, or a cappuccino mix.

Pudding cakes are fantastic because they give you the added bonus of a low-fat sauce.

Serves 8 to 10
Preheat oven to 350°F (180°C)
8-inch square (2 L) baking dish sprayed with vegetable spray

1. In a bowl stir together flour, brown sugar and baking powder. In a separate bowl, whisk together orange zest, orange juice, oil, egg and vanilla. Add the wet ingredients to the dry, blending just until mixed. Batter will be thick. Pour into prepared pan. Sprinkle chocolate chips over top.

2. In a bowl whisk together 1¼ cups (300 mL) hot water, sugar, coffee mix and cocoa. Pour carefully over cake batter. Bake 35 minutes or until cake springs back when touched lightly in center. Serve warm; spoon cake and underlying sauce into individual dessert dishes.

Make Ahead

✦ Best served right out of the oven. But can be reheated in microwave for similar texture.

Nutritional Analysis (Per Serving)
✦ Calories: 210   ✦ Protein: 3 g   ✦ Cholesterol: 22 mg
✦ Sodium: 82 mg   ✦ Fat, total: 5 g   ✦ Carbohydrates: 40 g
✦ Fiber: 2 g   ✦ Fat, saturated: 1 g

Banana-Strawberry Mousse

3	small ripe bananas	3
1 cup	orange juice	250 mL
1 cup	strawberries	250 mL
6 tbsp	lemon juice	90 mL
1/2 cup	cold water	125 mL
1	package (1 tbsp/7 g) gelatin	1
	Orange segments or sliced strawberries	

For attractive orange segments, peel a whole orange with a sharp knife, removing zest, pith and membrane; cut on both sides of dividing membranes to release segments.

Serves 6

1. In a blender, combine bananas, orange juice, strawberries and lemon juice; purée until smooth. Put water in a small saucepan; sprinkle with gelatin. Let stand 1 minute. Heat gently, stirring until gelatin dissolves. With motor running, pour hot gelatin through blender feed tube; purée until smooth. Divide among 6 individual dessert dishes or champagne coupes.

2. Chill 2 hours. Serve garnished with orange segments or sliced strawberries.

Nutritional Analysis (Per Serving)
- Calories: 82
- Protein: 2 g
- Cholesterol: 0 mg
- Sodium: 5 mg
- Fat: 0.4 g
- Carbohydrates: 19 g

Key Lime Dessert

Filling

3/4 cup	fructose	175 mL
1/4 cup	cornstarch	50 mL
1 1/2 cups	water	375 mL
2	egg whites, at room temperature	2
1	egg, at room temperature	1
2 tsp	grated lime zest	10 mL
1/4 cup	freshly squeezed lime juice	50 mL

Meringue

2	egg whites	2
1/4 tsp	cream of tartar	1 mL
4 tsp	fructose	20 mL

To get the most juice from limes or other citrus fruit, bring fruit to room temperature before juicing.

Make sure the egg whites for the meringue are perfectly pure, without a speck of yolk, or they will not beat properly.

Serves 8
Preheat oven to 400°F (200°C)
4-cup (1 L) soufflé dish or eight 1/2-cup (125 mL) ramekins

1. *Make the filling:* In a saucepan, stir together fructose and cornstarch. Gradually whisk in water until smooth. Bring to a boil over medium heat, stirring constantly. Continue to boil for 1 minute, stirring constantly, or until thickened. Remove from heat.

2. In a bowl beat egg whites with egg. Gradually whisk half of hot cornstarch mixture into egg mixture. Pour back into remaining cornstarch mixture. Return saucepan to medium heat; cook, stirring, 1 minute. Remove from heat. Stir in lime zest and juice. Pour into soufflé dish.

3. *Make the meringue:* In a bowl, beat egg whites until foamy. Add cream of tartar and beat until soft peaks form. Gradually add fructose, beating until stiff peaks form. Spoon over hot filling. Bake 8 to 10 minutes or until golden brown.

Nutritional Analysis (Per Serving)
- Calories: 120
- Protein: 3 g
- Cholesterol: 37 mg
- Sodium: 43 mg
- Fat: 1 g
- Carbohydrates: 25 g

Fluffy Apricot Soufflé with Raspberry Sauce

Soufflé

8 oz	dried apricots	250 g
1/4 cup	water	50 mL
1/4 cup	granulated sugar	50 mL
1/4 tsp	almond extract	1 mL
5	egg whites	5

Sauce

1 cup	raspberries	250 mL
Half	ripe banana	Half
1 tbsp	fruit jam (any flavor)	15 mL
1 tsp	lemon juice	5 mL

Serves 6
Preheat oven to 300°F (150°C)
8-cup (2 L) soufflé dish sprayed with baking spray

1. In a saucepan combine apricots and water; cook over medium heat 5 minutes or until all the water is absorbed. Transfer hot apricots to a food processor or blender; purée just until finely chopped. Add sugar and almond extract; purée until well mixed. Transfer to a bowl; cool mixture to room temperature.

2. In another bowl, beat egg whites until stiff peaks form. Stir one-third of egg whites into cooled apricot mixture until well mixed. Gently fold in remaining egg whites. Apricot pieces will still be evident. Pour into prepared dish.

3. Set soufflé dish in larger pan; pour in enough hot water to come half way up sides. Bake 20 minutes. Reduce oven temperature to 250°F (120°C); bake 12 minutes longer or until light brown and no longer loose. Meanwhile, make the raspberry sauce: In a blender or food processor, combine raspberries, banana, jam and lemon juice; purée until smooth. Strain to remove seeds.

4. Serve soufflé hot, drizzled with raspberry sauce.

Tips

✦ For a strawberry sauce, substitute strawberries for the raspberries.

✦ Thaw unsweetened frozen berries for sauce or use fresh ripe berries; if using frozen, drain excess liquid before puréeing.

Nutritional Analysis (Per Serving)
✦ Calories: 162   ✦ Protein: 2 g   ✦ Cholesterol: 0 mg
✦ Sodium: 35 mg   ✦ Fat: 0.3 g   ✦ Carbohydrates: 39 g

Melon Balls with Warm Ginger Sauce

1	small ripe honeydew melon	1
2	small ripe cantaloupes	2
Sauce		
2 cups	orange juice	500 mL
2 tbsp	minced gingerroot or 1/2 tsp (2 mL) ground ginger	25 mL
1 tbsp	raspberry or red wine vinegar	15 mL
1 tsp	honey	5 mL
1/2 tsp	lemon juice	2 mL
	Fresh mint leaves	

If you don't have a melon baller, use a small spoon to scoop melon flesh, or cut flesh into small cubes.

Serves 6

1. Cut melons in half and discard seeds. With a melon baller, scoop out flesh. Divide melon balls among 6 individual dessert dishes.

2. In a saucepan combine orange juice, ginger, vinegar, honey and lemon juice. Bring to a boil; cook until reduced to 1/2 cup (125 mL). Spoon warm sauce over melon balls and serve garnished with mint leaves.

Make Ahead
✦ Make sauce in advance and store covered in refrigerator up to 2 days; reheat before serving.

Nutritional Analysis (Per Serving)
✦ Calories: 109 ✦ Protein: 2 g ✦ Cholesterol: 0 mg
✦ Sodium: 19 mg ✦ Fat: 1 g ✦ Carbohydrates: 26 g

Poached Pears in Chocolate Sauce

2 tbsp	lemon juice	25 mL
6	small ripe pears	6
1 1/2 cups	pear nectar (or other fruit nectar)	375 mL
1/4 cup	semi-sweet chocolate chips	50 mL
1 tbsp	2% evaporated milk	15 mL

Use a firm pear such as a Bosc.

Serves 6

1. Put lemon juice and 6 cups (1.5 L) water in a bowl. Peel pears, leaving whole with stems intact and dropping each in water mixture as it is peeled. Drain. In a saucepan, combine pears and pear nectar. Bring to a boil, reduce heat to medium-low, cover and cook, turning pears over halfway through, for 20 to 25 minutes or until tender when pierced with a knife. Transfer pears and syrup to a bowl; chill.

2. Before serving, drain pears, reserving syrup. Bring syrup to a boil; cook until reduced to 1/4 cup (50 mL). Stir in chocolate chips until melted. Beat in evaporated milk until smooth.

3. Serve chilled pears on top of a pool of hot chocolate sauce.

Nutritional Analysis (Per Serving)
✦ Calories: 167 ✦ Protein: 1 g ✦ Cholesterol: 0 mg
✦ Sodium: 7 mg ✦ Fat: 3 g ✦ Carbohydrates: 37 g

Lemon Meringue Pie

Filling

1¼ cups	water	300 mL
½ cup	fructose	125 mL
1 tsp	grated lemon zest	5 mL
¼ cup	lemon juice	50 mL
¼ cup	cornstarch	50 mL
¾ cup	water	175 mL
1 tsp	margarine	5 mL

Meringue

2	egg whites	2
1 tbsp	fructose	15 mL

Separate eggs carefully for meringue — egg whites contaminated with yolk will not beat properly. Also, make sure your bowls and beaters are perfectly clean when making meringue.

When using margarine, choose a soft (non-hydrogenated) version.

Serves 6
Preheat oven to 450°F (220°C)
Six ½-cup (125 mL) ovenproof dishes
Baking sheet

1. *Make pie filling:* In a saucepan combine 1¼ cups (300 mL) water, fructose, lemon zest and juice. Bring to a boil. In a bowl, stir together cornstarch and ¾ cup (175 mL) water until dissolved. Stir into boiling lemon mixture. Cook, stirring, until thickened. Remove from heat. Stir in margarine. Divide among dishes. Cool.

2. *Make the meringue:* In a bowl, beat egg whites until soft peaks form. Gradually add fructose, beating until stiff peaks form. Spoon over filling; transfer dishes to baking sheet. Bake 5 minutes or until golden. Cool to room temperature. Chill before serving.

Nutritional Analysis (Per Serving)
- Calories: 110
- Protein: 1 g
- Cholesterol: 0 mg
- Sodium: 26 mg
- Fat: 1 g
- Carbohydrates: 25 g

Pumpkin Flan

¾ cup	canned pumpkin	175 mL
2½ tbsp	fructose	32 mL
2	egg whites	2
1	egg	1
½ tsp	almond extract	2 mL
½ tsp	vanilla extract	2 mL
¼ tsp	cinnamon	1 mL
⅛ tsp	ground cloves	0.5 mL
1 cup	2% milk	250 mL

Cinnamon Cream

1 cup	5% ricotta cheese	250 mL
4 tsp	maple syrup or honey	20 mL
¾ tsp	cinnamon	4 mL

For individual servings, use six ¾-cup (175 mL) custard cups or ramekins and bake for 20 minutes.

Serves 6
Preheat oven to 325°F (160°C)
4-cup (1 L) soufflé or casserole dish

1. In a bowl, beat pumpkin, fructose, egg whites, whole egg, almond extract, vanilla extract, cinnamon and cloves until smooth. In a saucepan, heat milk until almost boiling; remove from heat. Whisk hot milk into pumpkin mixture. Pour into dish.

2. Set dish in larger pan; pour in enough hot water to come halfway up sides. Bake for 40 minutes or until set. Remove from water bath; cool on wire rack. Chill.

3. *Make the cinnamon cream:* In a food processor, purée ricotta, maple syrup and cinnamon until smooth. Serve with flan.

Nutritional Analysis (Per Serving)
- Calories: 111
- Protein: 6 g
- Cholesterol: 60 mg
- Sodium: 75 mg
- Fat: 3 g
- Carbohydrates: 13 g

Fresh Fruit Tart

1	8-inch (20 cm) pastry shell, baked	1

Filling

1 cup	skim milk	250 mL
2 tbsp	granulated sugar	25 mL
1 tsp	grated lemon zest	5 mL
1 tsp	grated orange zest	5 mL
½ tsp	vanilla extract	2 mL
1	egg, beaten	1
1 tbsp	cornstarch	15 mL
	Fresh berries and/or sliced fruit	
2 tbsp	red currant jelly	25 mL

Serves 10

1. *Make the filling:* In a saucepan heat milk over medium heat until hot. Stir in sugar, lemon zest, orange zest and vanilla. In a bowl, beat egg with cornstarch until blended. Whisk a little of the hot milk into egg mixture, then pour back into remaining milk. Whisk constantly until mixture is thick enough to coat a spoon; do not boil. Chill.
2. Spread custard over baked crust. Decorate with fruit and berries. In a saucepan, melt jelly. Brush over fruit.

Tip

✦ To save time, use a store-bought pre-baked pastry shell.

Nutritional Analysis (Per Serving)
- ✦ Calories: 220
- ✦ Protein: 1 g
- ✦ Cholesterol: 11 mg
- ✦ Sodium: 58 mg
- ✦ Fat: 4 g
- ✦ Carbohydrates: 44 g

Maple Flan with Walnuts

2	egg whites	2
1	egg	1
2½ tbsp	maple syrup	32 mL
1 tsp	vanilla extract	5 mL
1 tsp	maple extract	5 mL
1½ cups	2% milk	375 mL
	Toasted chopped nuts (optional)	
	Cinnamon Cream (optional) (see recipe, page 394)	

Serves 6
Preheat oven to 325°F (160°C)
4-cup (1 L) soufflé or casserole dish

1. In a bowl whisk together egg whites, whole egg, maple syrup, vanilla and maple extract until smooth. Gradually add milk, whisking constantly. Pour into soufflé dish.
2. Set dish in larger pan; pour in enough hot water to come halfway up sides. Bake for 60 minutes or until set. Remove from water bath; cool on wire rack. Chill.
3. Serve with toasted chopped nuts and/or cinnamon cream, if desired.

Tip

✦ For extra maple flavor, omit the vanilla and use 2 tsp (10 mL) maple extract.

Nutritional Analysis (Per Serving)
- ✦ Calories: 87
- ✦ Protein: 4 g
- ✦ Cholesterol: 54 mg
- ✦ Sodium: 65 mg
- ✦ Fat: 3 g
- ✦ Carbohydrates: 10 g

Frozen Lemon Roulade

Genoise Cake

5	eggs	5
½ cup	fructose	125 mL
1¼ tsp	nutmeg	6 mL
1 tsp	grated lemon zest	5 mL
1 tsp	vanilla extract	5 mL
¾ cup	all-purpose flour	175 mL
	Icing sugar	

Lemon Ice Milk

4 cups	vanilla ice milk or frozen vanilla yogurt, softened	1 L
2 tbsp	grated lemon zest	25 mL
½ cup	lemon juice	125 mL
1 tsp	lemon extract (optional)	5 mL
½ cup	strawberry purée	125 mL
	Extra grated lemon zest	

Serves 20
Preheat oven to 375°F (190°C)
15- by 10-inch (40 by 25 cm) jelly roll pan, lined with parchment paper and sprayed with baking spray

1. *Make the genoise:* Beat eggs with fructose until thick and creamy. Stir in nutmeg, lemon zest and vanilla. Fold in flour. Pour into prepared jelly roll pan, spreading to edges. Bake for 12 to 15 minutes or until puffy and golden. Let cool 5 minutes. Invert onto a clean tea towel dusted with sifted icing sugar. Dust with more sifted icing sugar. Remove jelly roll pan and carefully peel paper away from cake. Starting at the short end, roll cake and tea towel up together. Cool completely.

2. *Make the lemon ice milk:* In a bowl, beat ice milk, lemon zest, lemon juice and, if desired, lemon extract until well combined. Unroll cake and tea towel. Spread lemon ice milk evenly over genoise. Roll cake up. Wrap in plastic wrap. Freeze until firm.

3. Dust roulade with sifted icing sugar. Cut cake into ½-inch (1 cm) slices. Serve on top of a pool of strawberry purée and garnish with lemon zest.

Tip

✦ Omit strawberry purée and serve with 1 cup (250 mL) of sliced strawberries instead.

Nutritional Analysis (Per Serving)

✦ Calories: 135 ✦ Protein: 3 g ✦ Cholesterol: 87 mg
✦ Sodium: 43 mg ✦ Fat: 4 g ✦ Carbohydrates: 20 g

Honey Vanilla Ice Cream with Hot Spiced Apples

Ice Cream

2 cups	2% milk	500 mL
3 tbsp	honey	45 mL
1/8 tsp	vanilla extract	0.5 mL
6	egg yolks	6

Spiced Apple Mixture

3	apples	3
2 cups	apple juice	500 mL
1/4 tsp	cinnamon	1 mL
1/8 tsp	ground ginger	0.5 mL
1/8 tsp	nutmeg	0.5 mL
2 tbsp	cornstarch	25 mL
1 tbsp	water	15 mL

Don't worry if you don't have an ice cream maker. Pour chilled ice cream mixture into a loaf pan lined with plastic wrap and freeze until solid. Break into small pieces; in a food processor, pulse on and off until smooth. Store in freezer until ready to serve.

Serves 6

1. *Make the ice cream:* In a saucepan bring milk, honey and vanilla to a boil; reduce heat to low. In a bowl, beat egg yolks. Whisk a little of the hot milk into yolk mixture, then pour back into remaining milk. Whisk constantly over low heat until mixture is thick enough to coat a spoon; do not boil. Remove from heat. Chill. In an ice cream maker, freeze according to manufacturer's directions.

2. *Make the spiced apple mixture:* Peel, core and thinly slice the apples. Put in a saucepan along with apple juice, cinnamon, ginger and nutmeg. Bring to a boil, reduce heat and simmer 5 minutes. Dissolve cornstarch in water; stir into simmering apple mixture and cook 1 minute longer or until thickened. Remove from heat. Cool slightly. Serve over ice cream.

Nutritional Analysis (Per Serving)

✦ Calories: 186 ✦ Protein: 6 g ✦ Cholesterol: 276 mg
✦ Sodium: 41 mg ✦ Fat: 6 g ✦ Carbohydrates: 27 g

Frozen Jamoca Mousse

1 cup	5% ricotta cheese	250 mL
2 cups	low-fat yogurt	500 mL
1/2 cup	fructose	125 mL
4 tsp	cocoa	20 mL
2 tsp	instant coffee granules	10 mL
1 tsp	vanilla extract	5 mL

Serves 12

1. In a food processor or blender, purée ricotta, yogurt, fructose, cocoa, coffee granules and vanilla until smooth.

2. In an ice cream maker, freeze according to manufacturer's directions.

Tips

✦ Buy extra-smooth ricotta for the smoothest mousse.

✦ If don't have an ice cream maker, pour into a baking dish and freeze until solid. Break into small pieces; in a food processor, pulse on and off until smooth. Store in freezer until ready to serve.

Nutritional Analysis (Per Serving)

✦ Calories: 77 ✦ Protein: 3 g ✦ Cholesterol: 7 mg
✦ Sodium: 39 mg ✦ Fat: 2 g ✦ Carbohydrates: 11 g

Raspberry Ice with Fresh Strawberries

4½ cups	fresh raspberries	1.125 L
	Honey to taste	
6 tbsp	low-fat yogurt (optional)	90 mL
6	large fresh strawberries	6
	Fresh mint leaves	

Serves 6

1. In a blender or food processor, purée raspberries. Strain to remove seeds. Stir in honey to taste. In an ice cream maker, freeze according to manufacturer's directions.
2. Divide among 6 individual dessert dishes. Spoon 1 tbsp (15 mL) yogurt on top of each serving, if desired. Garnish each serving with a strawberry and mint leaves.

Nutritional Analysis (Per Serving)
- Calories: 60
- Protein: 1 g
- Cholesterol: 1 mg
- Sodium: 10 mg
- Fat: 0.4 g
- Carbohydrates: 14 g

Pineapple Lime Sorbet

1¼ cups	pineapple purée	300 mL
2 tsp	grated lime or lemon zest	10 mL
¾ cup	freshly squeezed lime or lemon juice	175 mL
¼ cup	water	50 mL
	Granulated sugar to taste (optional)	
	Thin slices lime or lemon	

Serves 4

1. In a bowl, stir together pineapple purée, lime zest and juice, water and, if desired, sugar.
2. In an ice cream maker, freeze according to manufacturer's directions.
3. Divide among 4 individual dessert dishes. Serve garnished with thin slices of lime.

Nutritional Analysis (Per Serving)
- Calories: 56
- Protein: 1 g
- Cholesterol: 0 mg
- Sodium: 10 mg
- Fat: 0.2 g
- Carbohydrates: 15 g

Fresh Fruit Sorbet

| 2½ cups | chopped peeled soft fresh fruit (bananas, peaches, strawberries, etc.) | 625 mL |

Serves 4 to 6

1. Spread fruit on baking sheet and freeze. Purée frozen fruit in food processor and serve immediately.

Tip
- Try a combination of fresh fruits.

Make Ahead
- Best if served immediately. If refreezing, purée again before serving.

Nutritional Analysis (Per Serving)
- Calories: 40
- Protein: 0 g
- Cholesterol: 0 mg
- Sodium: 0 mg
- Fat: 0 g
- Carbohydrates: 10 g
- Fiber: 1 g

Strawberry Orange Buttermilk Sorbet

1 cup	buttermilk or soured milk	250 mL
½ cup	puréed strawberries	125 mL
¼ cup	water	50 mL
¼ cup	honey	50 mL
½ tsp	grated orange rind	2 mL
1 tbsp	orange juice	15 mL

To make soured milk, place 2 tsp (10 mL) lemon juice or vinegar in measuring cup; pour in milk to 1 cup (250 mL) level and let stand for 10 minutes, then stir.

Serves 3 or 4

1. In bowl, mix together buttermilk, strawberries, water, honey, orange rind and juice.
2. Freeze in ice cream machine according to manufacturer's directions. (Or pour into cake pan and freeze until nearly solid. Chop into chunks and beat with electric mixer or process in food processor until smooth. Freeze again until solid.)

Make Ahead

+ Although sorbets are best prepared just before eating so they do not crystallize, they can be prepared up to 2 days in advance.

Nutritional Analysis (Per Serving)
+ Calories: 103   + Protein: 2 g   + Cholesterol: 3 mg
+ Sodium: 65 mg   + Fat: 1 g   + Carbohydrates: 22 g
+ Fiber: 0.5 g

Mocha Ice Cream

2 cups	2% milk	500 mL
1	egg	1
½ cup	granulated sugar	125 mL
2 tbsp	sifted unsweetened cocoa powder	25 mL
1 tsp	instant coffee granules	5 mL

Omit coffee if desired.

Serves 4

1. In saucepan, heat 1 cup (250 mL) of the milk just until bubbles form around edge of pan.
2. Meanwhile, in small bowl, beat egg with sugar until combined; stir in half of the warm milk. Pour egg mixture back into saucepan; stir in cocoa and coffee granules. Cook, stirring, on low heat for 4 minutes or until slightly thickened. (Do not let boil or egg will curdle.) Let cool completely.
3. Stir in remaining milk. Pour into ice cream machine and freeze according to manufacturer's instructions. (Or pour into cake pan and freeze until nearly solid. Chop into chunks and beat with electric mixer or process in food processor until smooth. Freeze again until solid.)

Nutritional Analysis (Per Serving)
+ Calories: 183   + Protein: 6 g   + Cholesterol: 62 mg
+ Sodium: 78 mg   + Fat: 4 g   + Carbohydrates: 32 g
+ Fiber: 1 g

Tulip Cookies with Fruit Sorbet

¾ cup	buttermilk	175 mL
1	egg	1
6 tbsp	granulated sugar	90 mL
⅓ cup	whole wheat flour	75 mL
⅓ cup	all-purpose flour	75 mL
⅛ tsp	cinnamon	0.5 mL
⅛ tsp	salt	0.5 mL
	Raspberry or mango sorbet	
	Fresh raspberries or sliced ripe mango	

Serves 20
Preheat oven to 350°F (180°C)
Baking sheet sprayed with baking spray

1. In a bowl stir together buttermilk, egg, sugar, whole wheat flour, flour, cinnamon and salt until smooth. Let batter rest for 20 minutes.
2. Place 1 tbsp (15 mL) batter at one end of prepared baking sheet. With the back of a spoon, spread to form a circle 5 inches (12 cm) in diameter. Repeat with another 1 tbsp (15 mL) batter on other half of baking sheet. Bake for 9 to 11 minutes or until golden. With a spatula, remove hot cookies from baking sheet and place each over bottom of a glass, pressing gently to create fluted effect. Cool completely on glass.
3. Repeat with remaining batter, respraying baking sheet between batches.
4. Serve each tulip cup with a small scoop of sorbet, garnished with fresh fruit.

Tips

✦ Use your favorite flavor of sorbet, or use ice milk.

✦ To save time, make the tulip cups assembly-line fashion. Use 2 baking sheets; while one tray bakes, spread the batter on the next tray, then put it in the oven just as you remove the last batch.

✦ The cookies must be shaped while they are warm, so work quickly. If cookie cools and is too firm to shape, return to oven for 30 seconds or until softened.

Nutritional Analysis (Per Serving)
✦ Calories: 60 ✦ Protein: 2 g ✦ Cholesterol: 12 mg
✦ Sodium: 37 mg ✦ Fat: 0.4 g ✦ Carbohydrates: 13 g

Frozen Orange Cream

1 tbsp	grated orange zest	15 mL
1⅓ cups	orange juice	325 mL
⅔ cup	skim milk	150 mL

Serves 4

1. In a food processor or blender, purée orange zest, orange juice and milk.
2. In an ice cream maker, freeze according to manufacturer's directions.

Tips

✦ This makes an excellent palate cleanser between courses of a meal, as well as a refreshing dessert.

✦ If don't have an ice cream maker, pour into a baking dish and freeze until solid. Break into small pieces; in a food processor, pulse on and off until smooth. Store in freezer until ready to serve.

Nutritional Analysis (Per Serving)
- ✦ Calories: 49
- ✦ Protein: 2 g
- ✦ Cholesterol: 1 mg
- ✦ Sodium: 22 mg
- ✦ Fat: 0.1 g
- ✦ Carbohydrates: 10 g

Chocolate Kahlúa Fudge Sauce

⅓ cup	granulated sugar	75 mL
3 tbsp	2% milk	45 mL
1 tbsp	Kahlúa or other chocolate liqueur	15 mL
2 tbsp	sifted unsweetened cocoa powder	25 mL

Makes ⅓ cup (75 mL)

1. In small saucepan, combine sugar, milk, Kahlúa and cocoa; simmer for 5 minutes, stirring often.

Tip

✦ Serve over frozen yogurt or ice cream, or over cake. Pierce top of cake to make holes and pour sauce over top.

Make Ahead

✦ Prepare up to 3 days ahead. Reheat gently, stirring until smooth and adding a little more milk if too thick.

✦ Sauce will thicken if not used immediately; reheat gently to serve.

Nutritional Analysis (Per Serving)
- ✦ Calories: 52
- ✦ Protein: 1 g
- ✦ Cholesterol: 1 mg
- ✦ Sodium: 7 mg
- ✦ Fat: 1 g
- ✦ Carbohydrates: 15 g
- ✦ Fiber: 1 g

National Library of Canada Cataloguing in Publication

Roblin, Lynn
    500 best healthy recipes / Lynn Roblin.

Includes index.
ISBN 0-7788-0094-6

1. Cookery. 2. Nutrition. I. Title. II. Title: Five hundred best healthy recipes.

TX714.R62 2004   641.5'63   C2003-906486-7

index

Sour cream
  apple pie, 385
  brownies, 362
  orange apple cake, 384
  topping, 345
Sour milk, to make, 399
Southwest barley salad, 113
Soya
  orange dressing, 115
  sauce, tip, 49
Soynuts, healthy snack food, 138
Spaghetti
  chicken Tetrazzini, 270
  salmon and tomato sauce over,
    161
  with sun-dried tomatoes and
    broccoli, 139
Spaghettini
  parsley and basil pesto, 142
  with tomatoes, basil and fish,
    166
Spice cake
  banana, 357
  prune orange, 350
Spiced apples, 397
Spicy meatball and pasta stew,
  306
Spicy Mexican dip, 41
Spicy rice, bean and lentil
  casserole, 218
Spicy rice with feta cheese, 214
Spinach
  cheese
    dressing, 328
    tortellini, 155
    tortellini in vegetable sauce,
      147
  chicken breasts stuffed with, 276
  and mushroom salad, 93
  mushrooms stuffed with ricotta
    and, 38
  orange and mushroom salad, 94
  and oyster mushrooms over rice
    noodles, 151
  pesto, 97, 142
    creamy dip, 42
    with pasta, 143
  quesadillas, filled with cheese
    and, 234
  with rice and pine nuts, 214
  and ricotta dip, 36
  and scallops over linguine, 170
  with sole and cream sauce, 241
  tomatoes stuffed with cheese
    and, 321
  tortellini minestrone with, 76
  turkey scallopini, stuffed with
    cheese and, 294
Split pea(s)
  barley vegetable soup, 82
  mushroom soup, 78
Spreads
  tuna and white bean, 34
  vegetable feta cheese, 44

Squares
  date oatmeal, 365
  lemon poppy seed, 365
Squash
  acorn
    about, 327
    with wild rice and pineapple,
      327
  butternut
    and carrot soup, 58
    curried, risotto, 219
    with maple syrup, 326
    and sweet potato soup, 58
  spaghetti, with vegetables and
    tomato sauce, 322
Squid
  macaroni salad, 110
  with tomato sauce, 252
Stew
  beef, vegetable, 303
  chickpea and pasta, with
    meatballs, 306
  chili bean, 307
  lamb, 192
    vegetable, 303
  mushroom potato, 317
  seafood tomato, 253
  veal, vegetable, 303
Stir-fries
  beef with vegetables, 299
  chicken teriyaki with asparagus
    and red peppers, 274
Stock
  beef, 53
  chicken, 53
  fish, 53
  seafood, 53
  vegetable, 52
Strawberry(ies)
  -banana mousse, 391
  blueberry pear crisp, 388
  chocolate-dipped, 344
  filling, 364
  orange buttermilk sorbet, 399
  sauce, 347
  shortcake, 353
Streusel
  apple cake, 359
  apple muffins, 371
  apricot date cake, 358
Strudel
  apple and pear, 386
  cauliflower, leek and sweet
    potato, 320
  mango blueberry, 387
Stuffing, apple, raisin and rice, 288
Sugar snap peas
  about, 144
  with sesame sauce, 339
Surimi. See Crabmeat
Sweet-and-sour
  chicken meatballs over rice, 289
  sauce, with pork stir-fry, 308
  shrimp over rice fettuccine, 169

Sweet peas. See Green pea(s)
Sweet potato(es)
  and apple casserole, 334
  and brussels sprouts, 336
  carrot and parsnip soup, 57
  and carrot casserole, 318
  cauliflower and leek strudel,
    320
  chicken, with leeks and, 282
  curried
    broccoli soup, 71
    carrot orange soup, 56
    lamb with, 311
    risotto, 219
  with maple syrup, 326
  orange soup with maple syrup,
    59
  red lentil soup, with cheese
    tortellini, 77
  split pea and ham soup, 86
  and squash soup, 58
  white bean and orzo soup, 75
Swiss cheese
  artichoke bake, 33
  artichoke dill sauce, 141
  rigatoni with eggplant, tomatoes
    and, 156
  turkey scallopini, stuffed with
    spinach and, 294
Swordfish
  fettuccine with leeks and, 160
  gratin, 246
  kebabs, in apricot glaze, 250
  with lemon sauce, 247
  with linguine in tomato sauce,
    165
  with mango salsa, 246
  salad, 119
    with tarragon and pecans,
      121
  and salsa over rotini, 164
  Tetrazzini, 270

T

Tabbouleh
  Asian-style, 115
  Greek-style, 116
Tahini
  about, 221, 222
  dressing, 223
  hummus, 35
  tip, 35
Tarragon, chicken salad, 122
Tart
  fruit, 395
  tropical, 386
Tartar sauce, about, 259
Teriyaki
  chicken
    with sesame seeds over rotini,
      178
    stir-fry with asparagus and red
      peppers, 274